Complications of Neuroendovascular Procedures and Bailout Techniques

Complications of Neuroendovascular Procedures and Bailout Techniques

Edited by

Rakesh Khatri
Fort Wayne Neurological Center, Fort Wayne, IN, USA

Gustavo J. Rodriguez
Paul L. Foster School of Medicine, Texas Tech University Health Sciences Center, El Paso, TX, USA

Jean Raymond
Centre Hospitalier de l'Universitéde Montréal, Montreal, Canada

Adnan I. Qureshi
Zeenat Qureshi Stroke Institute, St Cloud, MN, and University of Minnesota, Minneapolis, MN, USA

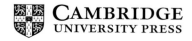

CAMBRIDGE
UNIVERSITY PRESS

CAMBRIDGE
UNIVERSITY PRESS

University Printing House, Cambridge CB2 8BS, United Kingdom

Cambridge University Press is part of the University of Cambridge.

It furthers the University's mission by disseminating knowledge in the pursuit of education, learning and research at the highest international levels of excellence.

www.cambridge.org
Information on this title: www.cambridge.org/9781107030022

© Cambridge University Press 2016

First published 2016

Printed in the United Kingdom by Clays, St Ives plc

A catalog record for this publication is available from the British Library

Library of Congress Cataloging in Publication data
Names: Khatri, Rakesh, editor. | Rodriguez, Gustavo J., editor. | Raymond, Jean (Radiologist), editor. | Qureshi, Adnan I., editor.
Title: Complications of neuroendovascular procedures and bailout techniques / edited by Rakesh Khatri, Gustavo J. Rodriguez, Jean Raymond, Adnan I. Qureshi.
Description: Cambridge ; New York : Cambridge University Press, 2016. | Includes bibliographical references and index.
Identifiers: LCCN 2015049720 | ISBN 9781107030022 (Hardback : alk. paper)
Subjects: | MESH: Neurosurgical Procedures–adverse effects | Cerebrovascular Disorders
Classification: LCC RD594 | NLM WL 368 | DDC 617.4/8101–dc23
LC record available at http://lccn.loc.gov/2015049720

ISBN 978-1-107-03002-2 Hardback

Contents

Contributors

Karanpal Dhaliwal, MBBS
Zeenat Qureshi Stroke Research Center,
Departments of Neurology, Neurosurgery,
and Radiology, University of Minnesota,
Minneapolis, MN, USA

Tenbit Emiru, MD PhD
Chief of Neurology, Hennepin County
Medical Center, Assistant Professor,
Neurology Department, University of
Minnesota, Minneapolis, MN, USA

Ricardo Hanel

Ameer E. Hassan, DO
Associate Professor of Neurology,
Radiology, and Neurosurgery at the
University of Texas Health Science Center,
San Antonio, and Director, Endovascular
Surgical Neuroradiology, Neurocritical
Care, and Clinical Neuroscience research,
Valley Baptist Medical Center, Harlingen,
TX, USA

Nazli Janjua, MD
Asia Pacific Comprehensive Stroke
Institute, Pomona, CA, and Medical
Director, NeuroInterventional Services,
Pomona Valley Hospital Medical Center,
Adjunct Faculty, University of California at
Riverside Medical School, Riverside,
CA, USA

Hunar Kainth, BS
Zeenat Qureshi Stroke Research Center,
Departments of Neurology, Neurosurgery,
and Radiology, University of Minnesota,
Minneapolis, MN, USA

Daraspreet Kainth, MD
Zeenat Qureshi Stroke Research Center,
Departments of Neurology, Neurosurgery,
and Radiology, University of Minnesota,
Minneapolis, MN, USA

Asif Khan, MD
Interventional Neurology Fellow,
Zeenat Qureshi Stroke Institute,
Centracare/St. Cloud Hospital, St. Cloud,
MN, USA

Rakesh Khatri, MD
Director of Stroke Care Now Network and
Director Vascular Neurology, Neurocritical
Care and Neurointervention, Fort Wayne
Neurological Center, Fort Wayne,
IN, USA

Neil Kothari, MD
Department of Medicine, Division of
Nephrology & Hypertension and
General Internal Medicine Rutgers
New Jersey Medical School, Newark,
NJ, USA

Venkata K. Lanka, MD
Radiation/MRI/Laser Safety Officer,
Radiation Safety Office, VA Hospital,
Washington DC, USA

Alberto Maud, MD
Stroke Medical Director, UMC of El Paso,
and Associate Professor, Departments of
Neurology and Radiology, Paul L. Foster
School of Medicine, Texas Tech University
Health Sciences Center of El Paso, El Paso,
TX, USA

Jefferson T. Miley, MD
Vascular and Interventional Neurology,
Seton Brain and Spine Institute, and
Assistant Professor of Neurology at Dell
Medical School, University of Texas at
Austin, Austin, TX, USA

Adnan I. Qureshi, MD
Associate Head and Professor at the
Zeenat Qureshi Stroke Research Center,
Department of Neurology, University of
Minnesota, Minneapolis, MN, USA

Mushtaq H. Qureshi, MD
Departments of Neurology, Paul L. Foster
School of Medicine, Texas Tech University
Health Sciences Center, El Paso, TX, USA

Alluru S. Reddi, MD
Professor of Medicine and Chief,
Department of Medicine, Division of
Nephrology and Hypertension and General
Internal Medicine, Rutgers New Jersey
Medical School, Newark, NJ, USA

Gustavo J. Rodriguez, MD
Associate Professor and Vice Chair,
Department of Neurology and Clinical
Associate Professor, Department of
Radiology, Paul L. Foster School of
Medicine, Texas Tech University Health
Sciences Center of El Paso, El Paso, TX, USA

James J. Roy, PharmD BCPS
Critical Care Clinical Pharmacist at
Parkview Regional Medical Center, Fort
Wayne, IN, USA

Farhan Siddiq, MD
Co-director, Harris Methodist Hospital
Stroke Center, Texas Health Resources,
Fort Worth, TX, USA

John Slaby, MD
Vascular and Interventional Radiologist,
Fort Wayne, IN, USA

Jose I. Suarez, MD
Professor of Neurology at the
Baylor College of Medicine, Houston,
TX, USA

Bryan M. Statz, PharmD
Clinical Pharmacist at Parkview
Regional Medical Center, Fort Wayne,
IN, USA

Megan Straub, PharmD
Clinical Pharmacist at Parkview Regional
Medical Center, Fort Wayne, IN, USA

M. Fareed K. Suri, MD
Director, Stroke Program,
Centracare/St. Cloud Hospital, St. Cloud,
MN, USA

Wondwossen G. Tekle, MD
Adjunct Assistant Professor of
Neurology, University of Texas Health
Science Center of San Antonio,
Endovascular Surgical Neuroradiology,
Vascular and Critical Care Neurology,
Valley Baptist Medical Center, Harlingen,
TX, USA

Ramachandra P. Tummala, MD
Associate Professor at the Departments of
Neurosurgery and Neurology, University of
Minnesota Medical School, Minneapolis,
MN, USA

Haralabos Zacharatos, DO
Neurointerventional Surgery,
Neurocritical Care Director, Vassar
Brothers Medical Center, Poughkeepsie,
NY, USA

Preface

Although it is well known that complications during neurointerventional procedures happen even in the most experienced hands, conversations about these events are scant, as it may be hard to acknowledge them, or the memories may be uncomfortable and quickly buried. We would like to congratulate and thank all the authors for their contribution to this book, the purpose of which is to share the experience of experts in the field, as evidence-based medicine for many of these procedures is lacking. Ultimately the goal is to improve the outcomes of our patients and contribute to a rapidly growing field.

This book is intended for those performing neurointerventional procedures. It is detailed but concise, to be used as a quick reference for tips to help with prevention or early detection of complications and/or to be prepared to face them when they happen. Such knowledge will help in avoiding common mistakes when time is crucial.

It is comprehensive but not complete, as new devices are constantly being developed, and new neurointerventional techniques described. Given the dynamic nature of this subspecialty, it would be impossible for an updated edition of the book to cover the latest technology by the time of its publication. Devices may soon become obsolete and techniques abandoned. We emphasize, however, that basic safety principles will not change, and good planning and preparation will provide the operator with the required confidence to deal with adversity, even if complications are unforeseen. The keen operator will adjust and come up with new bailout techniques.

Our patient population is characterized by severe cerebral and cardiac vascular disease. Patients often present with a prior history of cerebrovascular events predisposing them to adverse events during the neurointerventional procedure. A significant proportion of periprocedural complications related to neurointerventional procedures can be mitigated by appropriate preprocedural planning and preparation. Therefore we have included a chapter that covers perioperative planning and a chapter that covers the neurocritical care aspects of these patients. Although they need only a small incision for access, neurointerventional procedures have become a potential source of exposure to cumulative radiation for both patients and operators. We therefore decided to include a radiation safety chapter. Not only is this a hot topic at present, but it is our commitment to provide safety knowledge for the short and long term, and to keep operators conscious of the potential dangers.

We hope this work helps to provide operators with insight into treatment conditions, so that proper judgment, planning, and preparation of a structured procedure becomes a comfortable journey, and dealing with common and uncommon scenarios will result in the desired clinical outcome for our patients.

Chapter 1

Groin complications during neuroendovascular procedures

John Slaby

Many challenging scenarios can occur before, during, and after percutaneous arterial access has been attempted or obtained for endovascular procedures. Anatomic knowledge of the access region and the patient's past history is important in planning the endovascular approach and treating associated complications. It is always important to review any available prior imaging studies to assess the aortic arch and vascular tree anatomy. Despite careful planning, access complications occur, and some common problems along with treatment options are presented in this chapter.

Risk factors for percutaneous access site complications

Risk factors include the patient's age, peripheral vascular disease, obesity, female gender, periprocedural anticoagulation/antiplatelet medication, thrombolytic therapy, and larger caliber sheaths used during procedures. If heparin was administered during procedure, an activated clotting time (ACT) level could be obtained at the appropriate time to determine when sheath removal will be safer with less bleeding risk. Depending on institution protocols and size of sheath used, the ACT value should be less than 150–200 seconds prior to sheath removal (unless transradial access was used)[1,2].

Accessing "pulseless" femoral region

Large body habitus or atherosclerosis may impair palpation of the femoral pulse. A large soft tissue pannus can be retracted and restrained with assistance from technologist or taped across patient onto table. Ultrasound can be used to identify and access the artery, but if vessels are heavily calcified, consider using a larger gauge needle (instead of a 21 gauge micropuncture needle) to allow passage of a 0.035 guidewire. Otherwise, it may be difficult to advance the smaller micropuncture sheath through the calcified vessel over the smaller 0.018 guidewire. Alternatively, a stiff micropuncture sheath may be used. Using ultrasound in the transverse plane is preferred, and the femoral artery is located lateral to the compressible femoral vein. If calcified plaque is present in the artery, sonographic shadowing can be seen at the location of the artery.

The groin crease is not a reliable site for identifying the location of the common femoral artery (CFA), owing to variation with body soft tissue habitus. Therefore, fluoroscopy can be used as a guide to target bony landmarks or a calcified atherosclerotic vessel. Typically, the CFA overlies the medial third of the femoral head and should be accessed over the

Complications of Neuroendovascular Procedures and Bailout Techniques, ed. Rakesh Khatri,
Gustavo J. Rodriguez, Jean Raymond and Adnan I. Qureshi. Published by Cambridge University Press.
© Cambridge University Press 2016.

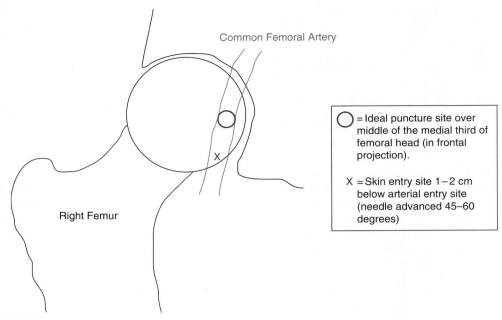

Common Femoral Artery

Right Femur

X

○ = Ideal puncture site over middle of the medial third of femoral head (in frontal projection).

X = Skin entry site 1–2 cm below arterial entry site (needle advanced 45–60 degrees)

Figure 1.1 Landmarks for access to common femoral artery.

femoral head to allow for compression at conclusion of procedure (Figure 1.1). To avoid parallax, the femoral head should be centered on the fluoroscopic image.

An alternative method to localize the femoral artery is to perform a contralateral femoral artery puncture with subsequent angiogram to roadmap the ipsilateral femoral artery, or advancing a guidewire across the bifurcation into the ipsilateral artery. The guidewire can be used as a target for puncture. This method is helpful for iliac interventions but likely unnecessary for neurovascular interventions unless an additional access site is required. Upper extremity access may be necessary if the common femoral or iliac arteries are occluded[3].

Accessing "bypass" graft at site of femoral puncture

See Figure 1.4. Aortobifemoral bypass grafts can be directly accessed with similar rates of complications as native vessels. Typically, aortobifemoral bypass grafts are placed anterior to the native vessels and can be easily palpated. If inadvertent access of the native vessel is performed, a second puncture may be necessary unless the anastomosis is more proximal. In this scenario, the guidewire may need to be negotiated into the bypass graft with the aid of a curved catheter or angled guidewire. Knowledge of anatomy and location of anastomosis may be helpful in determining where to access, particularly if there are imaging studies available for review prior to the start of procedure[4].

Complications subsequent to percutaneous access

Femoral arterial dissection

Dissections related to femoral puncture can occur from subintimal passage of guidewire during initial arterial access or the use of vascular closure devices[5]. Caution must be taken

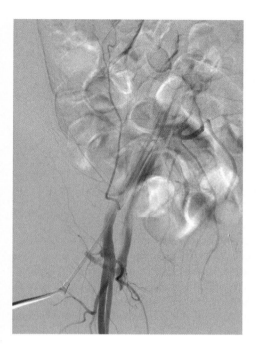

Figure 1.2 Right common femoral artery injection demonstrates early filling of femoral vein, confirming fistulous connection.

when advancing a guidewire if there is poor blood flow from the needle, as the distal end of the needle may be in a subintimal location. Femoral arterial dissections may extend into the external iliac artery or result in local arterial thrombosis and occlusion.

Endovascular repair and surgery are treatment options. Contralateral groin access may be necessary if dissection is located near the ipsilateral access. Prolonged balloon inflation may be sufficient to allow for intimal apposition, although a stent may be necessary. If thrombotic occlusion has occurred, catheter-directed thrombolysis followed by prolonged balloon angioplasty or stent placement may be necessary.

Anatomic considerations need to be factored into the decision to place a stent into the CFA. Care must be taken to avoid occluding the bifurcating vessels. Additionally, self-expanding nitinol stent grafts are preferred in the femoral artery because of their resistance to compression and deformity at the hip joint[6].

Hematoma /retroperitoneal hematoma

See Figure 1.3. Retroperitoneal hemorrhage may be caused by puncture above the inguinal ligament resulting in arterial puncture in the anterior or posterior wall after the artery has entered the retroperitoneal space. Symptoms include back or flank pain with a drop in hemoglobin, hypotension, and tachycardia. Hypotension may be a late sign, although in some cases, hypotension resistant to standard fluid resuscitation may occur early on. There may be compression signs to adjacent structures such as femoral vein compression leading to thrombosis/edema, or femoral nerve compression leading to sensory or motor deficit and skin necrosis.

Diagnosis is confirmed with non-contrast computed tomography (CT) scan of abdomen and pelvis. For groin hematomas, ultrasound may be adequate to evaluate for

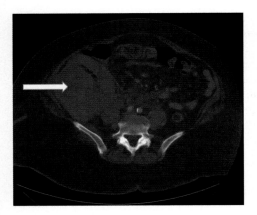

Figure 1.3 CT abdomen and pelvis: large right-sided retroperitoneum hematoma measuring 11.8 × 12.8 cm. Patient was stabilized with fluids, discontinuation of antiplatelet medications, and transfusion of packed red blood cells.

pseudoaneurysm (see below). Bleeding is exacerbated by anticoagulation which should be discontinued or reversed using protamine sulfate. If the hematoma is small, conservative management may be sufficient. Treatment strategies include endovascular stent graft placement from contralateral approach, using caution to prevent occlusion of the deep femoral or superficial femoral arteries during deployment. Surgery for hematoma evaluation and arterial repair may be required if there are anatomic limitations or if the source of bleeding is located at the CFA bifurcation. Balloon occlusion may be necessary as a temporizing measure to allow for surgical procedure if life-threatening hemorrhage is ongoing.

Every neurointerventionalist should have a policy to deal with these situations. Following steps are not in any particular order, but typically our strategy includes:

1. Stat hemoglobin and hematocrit measurements.
2. Mark the hematoma in groin and abdomen with skin marker to have some visual objective idea of hematoma dimensions for early identification of expansion. Such markings may not be a reliable criteria for hematoma expansion or amount of blood loss; however, manual compression should be instituted if visible enlarging swelling is noticed while other steps are being taken.
3. Reverse anticoagulation and antiplatelet medications if possible depending on clinical situation.
4. Ensure good intravenous access in case intravenous vasopressors are needed. May need to place central line or peripherally inserted central catheter (PICC line) if situation warrants. Start intravenous fluids. Intravenous fluid boluses may be required for hypotension.
5. Type and screen blood. If rapid drop in hemoglobin and while vascular surgery team is being contacted, packed red blood cell transfusion may be needed along with fluids.

Arterial pseudoaneurysm at site of percutaneous access

A common complication of percutaneous access is pseudoaneurysm development, which is a cavity within hematoma or dilatation at arteriotomy site. The risk increases if large caliber catheters and sheaths are used, or if poor compression occurs after sheath removal. Symptoms include pain, swelling, and pulsatile mass with or without bruit. Diagnosis is confirmed with color Doppler ultrasonography which reveals an anechoic mass with internal flow and typically bidirectional blood flow, commonly referred to as a 'yin-yang' appearance.

The two most commonly described treatments are compression and percutaneous thrombin injection, whereas stent grafts and surgery are used in complex cases. Assessment of distal pulses is important before and after treatment.

Prolonged compression is performed with ultrasound probe, orthogonal or perpendicular to the neck of the pseudoaneurysm in an effort to compress the neck. The minimum amount of pressure to occlude the pseudoaneurysm is preferred in order to minimize occlusion of the adjacent artery or vein. This is typically performed at 5–30 minute intervals until complete thrombosis is achieved. Other manual compression devices can be used with or without ultrasound, such as the FemoStop device (St. Jude Medical, Minnetonka, MN). Poor candidates for compression would include large complex pseudoaneurysms with a wide neck, or in presence of comorbities such as obesity, pain, or hemodynamically unstable patients.

Thrombin injection is preferred by many interventionalists since the procedure can be performed rapidly without sedation, particularly in a pseudoaneurysm with a small neck. An arteriovenous fistula (AVF) is a contraindication to thrombin injection, while a wide or short neck of the pseudoaneurysm can be difficult to successfully obliterate and increases the risk of distal embolization[7]. Some interventionalists have suggested using simultaneous balloon occlusion during thrombin injection at the site of the pseudoaneurysm to minimize distal embolization if the neck is large or complex, but this procedure has only been evaluated with a small series of patients. This technique may require contralateral femoral artery access, crossing the aortic bifurcation with administration of heparin to prevent distal thrombus formation during balloon inflation.

Lastly, surgery is a viable option, while stent grafts could be placed in poor surgical candidates. Infected pseudoaneurysm may necessitate surgical debridement with arterial repair and autologous venous graft placement. Careful selection of patients is required for stent placement, and anatomical considerations such as location, tortuosity of the vessel, or mobility of the hip joint may be limiting factors.

Complications related to arteriotomy vascular closure devices

Percutaneous closure devices allow for earlier ambulation and discharge post procedure. Typically, patients are required to spend 4–6 hours lying flat after sheath removal to ensure adequate hemostasis, but the use of a closure device decreases this time to 1–2 hours. There are several different devices that achieve hemostasis through methods including suture-mediated closure, collagen plugs, or nitinol clips. It is important to understand the specific indications and contraindications with each device before deployment, and an anatomic overview may be necessary with a femoral angiogram. An important consideration in the decision to use a closure device is whether a repeat procedure will be needed, as some devices require a certain amount of time before repeat puncture is recommended.

Complications from these devices can result in arterial occlusion or distal embolization. Treatment options include surgical extraction or angioplasty. Angioplasty can be used for stenosis or occlusions and has been described as a treatment related to stenosis from suture-mediated closure devices[8]. Steno-occlusive disease related to collagen plug closure may require surgery if angioplasty or stenting is unsuccessful. Surgery would also be necessary if the closure device material embolized distally or if not accessible by endovascular approach.

If the closure device fails or guidewire access is lost, hemostasis may be necessary with manual compression or stent graft placement.

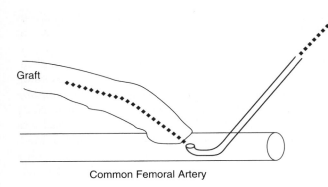

Figure 1.4 Accessing aortofemoral bypass graft. Curved catheter with guidewire (dashed line) to redirect into aortofemoral bypass graft.

Graft

Common Femoral Artery

Arteriovenous fistula formation

Arteriovenous fistulas (AVFs) are generally caused by distal punctures resulting in formation of communicating channels between artery and adjacent vein. AVFs may be suspected with palpation or continuous bruit on auscultation, and diagnosed with duplex ultrasonography. Ultrasound may show monophasic flow within the proximal portion of the artery and arterialized pulsatile flow within the outflow vein (Figure 1.2). The site of communication may or may not be visualized with ultrasound, while anatomic details are better demonstrated with angiography or cross-sectional imaging. AVFs can be asymptomatic or associated with pain, swelling, distal ischemia, deep venous thrombosis, bleeding, or high-output states.

Conservative treatment measures such as ultrasound-guided compression has variable results and is frequently limited by size of the fistula or periprocedural anticoagulation. More definitive treatment options would include surgical closure or exclusion with endovascular stent graft. Evaluation for stent graft placement is typically performed from the contralateral femoral approach, and care must be taken to avoid occluding the deep femoral or superficial femoral arteries during intervention. Shorter length stents may be needed in the CFA to prevent occlusion of the deep and superficial femoral arteries. Mobility of the hip joint may be a problem with deformity or fracture of the stent if placed in the CFA. Nitinol stent grafts are preferred, owing to the mechanical resistance to external distortion and deformation at a mobile joint. Stent placement may limit future percutaneous access of the groin, although shorter length stents can minimize this problem and maintain an uncovered portion of the artery for future puncture.

Acute lower extremity ischemia

Although rare, femoral artery thrombosis and occlusion may result in acute ischemia of the lower extremity. The ischemia may be due to large sheath size in a relatively smaller caliber artery, unrecognized pre-existing atherosclerosis, dissection, closure device complication (as mentioned above), and arterial spasm.

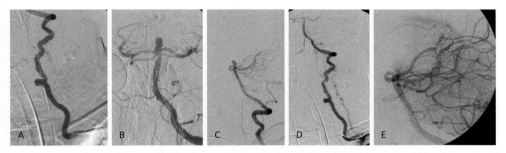

Figure 1.5 Transbrachial approach to basilar tip aneurysm endovascular coiling. This 79-year-old female presented with subarachnoid hemorrhage. She had severe peripheral vascular disease and therefore left-side transbrachial approach was undertaken. A: AP view demonstrating that left vertebral artery was catheterized with 4 French catheter which was exchanged for 6 French Neuron catheter. B, C: AP and lateral view demonstrating basilar tip aneurysm measuring 7.3 mm × 3.5 mm sharing origin of right posterior cerebral artery. D, E: AP and lateral view demonstrating near-complete obliteration achieved with minimal neck residual.

Recognizing occurrence of ischemia as soon as possible is very important. Examining the pulses after procedure is extremely important in every case where femoral artery is punctured for access. Anticoagulation with heparin may be considered if it can be used safely to prevent thrombus propagation. If time allows, CT angiography with aorta run off can be considered; however, if considered emergent then vascular surgeon consult should be made and patient taken to operating room. Emergent revascularization may be performed and, if needed, angiography can be done intra-operatively. Depending on the severity of ischemia, fasciotomy may be considered to prevent morbidity from reperfusion compartment syndrome.

Depending on the suspected etiology, contralateral femoral puncture can be considered to treat thrombotic occlusion with catheter-directed thrombolysis, followed by prolonged balloon angioplasty or stent placement as mentioned above under dissection treatment.

Alternative percutaneous arterial access routes

See Figure 1.5. The radial, axillary and brachial arteries provide an alternative approach to arterial access if the femoral arteries are occluded. These routes are a secondary approach, owing to the additional risks related to brachial plexus injury, distal embolism, hematoma formation, and stroke. The upper extremity arteries have a smaller caliber, increasing the chance of occlusion from the sheaths and resulting in distal upper extremity ischemia. The brachial artery is preferred over the axillary artery since it is easier to compress against the adjacent humerus bone. Obtaining bilateral upper extremity blood pressures is an important consideration to evaluate for a subclavian arterial stenosis. If there is a differential measurement greater than 10–20 mmHg, this finding suggests a stenosis in the side with the lower pressure, and puncture should be made in the opposite arm if clinically feasible. If available, ultrasound guidance with micropuncture needle is preferred.

When evaluating the abdominal aorta or mesenteric arteries, the left upper extremity is preferred to minimize risk of stroke since the carotid arteries are avoided during navigation of the catheter. The right upper extremity may be a better option if imaging the supra-aortic cerebral vessels is desired, especially in the setting of a "bovine" arch (normal anatomic variant with common origin of the brachiocephalic and left common carotid arteries). The left approach would allow easy access to the left vertebral artery if this is a vessel of interest, unless it takes origin directly off the aortic arch (another common anatomic variant).

The radial artery has gained popularity as an alternative to femoral artery access but has certain advantages and disadvantages. The dual blood supply to the wrist limits the potential for limb ischemia, but a normal Allen's test is necessary to confirm patency of the ulnar artery and palmar arch. Others advocate performing pulse oximetry of the thumb before and after compression of ipsilateral radial artery to confirm adequate collateral circulation in the event of radial artery compression.

Some advantages of transradial access include earlier patient ambulation with less frequent vascular complications since the artery is easily compressible. Some disadvantages are related to the smaller size of the vessel requiring smaller sheaths and the potential for vessel spasm. Most 6 French sheaths are well tolerated, and antispasm medications are helpful. Contraindications to transradial access include abnormal Allen's test or known upper extremity vascular disease. If future dialysis access is considered, then the radial artery should be avoided.

The radial artery is typically accessed with a 21 gauge needle approximately 2–3 cm cephalic to the wrist flexion crease (or radial styloid), since it is larger and less tortuous at the crease. A micropuncture set may be used to cannulate the radial artery with a 5 French introducer sheath. A mixture of heparin (5000 IU/ml), verapamil (2.5 mg), lidocaine (2%, 1.0 ml), and nitroglycerin (0.1 mg) is infused through the introducer sheath immediately after insertion to relieve and prevent local vasospasm. Heparin administration to prevent thrombosis or occlusion during the procedure is recommended. Wrist immobilization is also recommended during and briefly after radial artery catheterization to minimize bleeding complications. There are several devices on the market to assist with hemostasis and compression at the wrist, although gauze with pressure dressing or inflatable blood pressure cuff can be used. Sheath removal can be done without reversal of anticoagulation, unlike transfemoral punctures[3,9].

Almost any other artery can be accessed percutaneously, but the small size of distal arteries limits the catheters and sheaths available for use, while potentially increasing risk of complications. If the popliteal artery is chosen, ultrasound guidance is recommended to avoid the adjacent superficial popliteal vein.

Lastly, translumbar access to the abdominal aorta is another infrequently used alternative. This approach requires a prone position with fluoroscopic guidance using bony landmarks. Contraindications include uncontrolled hypertension, coagulopathy, aortic aneurysm, severe atherosclerosis, or severe scoliosis. Self-contained retroperitoneal hematomas are common, but mostly are predominantly asymptomatic.

References

1. Muller DW, Shamir KJ, Ellis SG, Topol EJ. Peripheral vascular complications after conventional and complex percutaneous coronary interventional procedures. *The American Journal of Cardiology* 1992;69:63–8.

2. Nasser TK, Mohler ER 3rd, Wilensky RL, Hathaway DR. Peripheral vascular complications following coronary interventional procedures. *Clinical Cardiology* 1995;18:609–14.

3. Layton KF, Kallmes DF, Cloft HJ. The radial artery access site for interventional

neuroradiology procedures. *American Journal of Neuroradiology* 2006;27: 1151–4.

4. Cowling MG, Belli AM, Buckenham TM. Evaluation and complications of direct graft puncture in thrombolysis and other interventional techniques. *Cardiovascular and Interventional Radiology* 1996;19:82–4.

5. Deitch SG, Gupta R. Radioembolization complicated by dissection of the common femoral artery. *Seminars in Interventional Radiology* 2011;28:133–6.

6. Tsetis D. Endovascular treatment of complications of femoral arterial access. *Cardiovascular and Interventional Radiology* 2010;33:457–68.

7. Loose HW, Haslam PJ. The management of peripheral arterial aneurysms using percutaneous injection of fibrin adhesive. *The British Journal of Radiology* 1998;71:1255–9.

8. Kim YJ, Yoon HK, Ko GY, Shin JH, Sung KB. Percutaneous transluminal angioplasty of suture-mediated closure device-related femoral artery stenosis or occlusive disease. *The British Journal of Radiology* 2009;82:486–90.

9. Nohara AM, Kallmes DF. Transradial cerebral angiography: technique and outcomes. *American Journal of Neuroradiology* 2003;24:1247–50.

Complications in endovascular embolization of intracranial aneurysms: prevention and bailout techniques

Gustavo J. Rodriguez, Alberto Maud, and
Mushtaq H. Qureshi

Introduction

Endovascular coil embolization, in which microcoils are inserted into the aneurysm to promote clotting and sealing, emerged as an alternative therapeutic option to surgical clip placement in the treatment of intracranial aneurysms. At present, there is an increasing trend to undergo endovascular treatment in the United States, irrespective of whether the aneurysm is ruptured or unruptured[1,2]. In addition to coil embolization, newer techniques have emerged in the endovascular embolization of intracranial aneurysms. Endovascular embolization is not, however, exempt from complications including fatality. The two most feared complications are intraprocedural aneurysm rupture and thromboembolism. Overall, the largest series of endovascular coil embolization report less than 5% risk of intraprocedural aneurysm rupture and less than 10% of thromboembolic complications[3,4]. However, these numbers vary according to different types of aneurysms and whether the aneurysm has previously ruptured.

Endovascular embolization of intracranial aneurysms is a complex treatment with multiple variables to take into consideration. A good outcome usually starts with meticulous planning, adequate informed consent, understanding of the aneurysm's characteristics, consideration of treatment options, and appropriate postprocedural care. Complications may happen even in the most experienced hands. In such cases, early recognition and management are key factors for a favorable outcome. Knowledge of possible complications not only increases confidence in the operator, and the confidence conveyed to the patient and/or relatives, but also may reduce the morbidity and mortality associated with complications.

This chapter covers an overview of the practice of endovascular embolization of intracranial aneurysms, complications that may arise depending on the aneurysm characteristics, ways to approach difficult aneurysms, and suggested bailout techniques in case of complications.

Informed consent

Informed consent starts with the establishment of a good patient–physician relationship. It is important to spend the necessary time to ensure that the procedure, the risks and benefits or alternative options, and potential complications are explained and understood. Considerations of whether the aneurysm is or not ruptured, its size and location, the patient's age,

Complications of Neuroendovascular Procedures and Bailout Techniques, ed. Rakesh Khatri, Gustavo J. Rodriguez, Jean Raymond and Adnan I. Qureshi. Published by Cambridge University Press. © Cambridge University Press 2016.

Table 2.1 Size of aneurysms

Categories	By convention[7]	ISUIA (propensity to rupture)[9]
Small	≤5 mm (very small ≤3 mm)	<7 mm
Medium	>5 to ≤15 mm	≥7 to ≤12 mm
Large	>15 to ≤24 mm	≥13 to 24 mm
Giant	≥25 mm	≥24 mm

ISUIA, International Study of Unruptured Intracranial Aneurysms

history of hypertension, and previous history of subarachnoid hemorrhage are among the important elements in determination of the benefit–risk ratio[5]. Not only should we inform the patient about complications reported in the literature at centers of excellence, but each institution should also keep track of its local complication rates[6]. In the absence of an emergency, all questions and concerns should be answered and addressed before the procedure starts. The management of endovascular complications starts with good, informed consent.

Intracranial aneurysm characterization

It is important to standardize the definitions and characteristics of intracranial aneurysms, not only for documentation but also for research purposes[7]. Most aneurysms are true aneurysms (also known as berry or saccular aneurysms) and are located in the circle of Willis. These are usually bifurcation or side wall aneurysms. Fusiform or peripheral (distal) aneurysms are pseudoaneurysms, not true aneurysms.

The size (see Table 2.1), location, and morphology, including the presence of irregularities or daughter sacs, are also important features that need documentation. These aneurysm characteristics are better obtained from cerebral digital subtracted imaging. Although 3D rotational angiography increases the detection of very small aneurysms, measurements are more accurate when obtained from high-resolution planar images as 3D images can easily be artefactual[8]. This is the time to look for the best working projection, the projection that separates the aneurysm from the parent vessel so that the neck is well visualized. The neck characteristics should also be documented. Wide neck aneurysms are those with a neck larger than 4 mm. The dome-to-neck ratio is of great importance and should be reported. A dome-to-neck ratio <2 may be unfavorable for primary coil embolization. Wide neck and unfavorable dome-to-neck aneurysms may require additional treatment methods or assistance, as discussed later in this chapter. It is also important to document the size of the parent vessel, as small parent vessels may not be amenable to accommodating devices for assistance.

General considerations in endovascular aneurysmal embolization

General anesthesia versus conscious sedation

It is a common practice to perform intracranial aneurysm embolization under general anesthesia. Advantages of this approach include better imaging quality due to lack of patient motion, control of the airway, and hemodynamics. There have, however, been several institutional reports on the treatment of ruptured and unruptured aneurysms under conscious sedation with local anesthesia[10–12]. In those retrospective studies, complication rates were similar to those for aneurysm embolization under general anesthesia. Patients with a low-grade subarachnoid hemorrhage and those with unruptured aneurysms formed most of the groups undergoing conscious sedation with local anesthesia. Advantages included avoidance of general anesthesia complications and a rapid and accurate neurological assessment. In addition, authors also claimed a better turnover time between procedures, given the absence of induction and recovery periods, with resultant estimated lower costs[12]. In a few patients, conscious sedation with local anesthesia was either aborted or converted into general anesthesia, mainly because of endovascular complications, anatomical difficulties, or restlessness of the patient. The group of Kan et al.[11] suggested having anesthesia available per protocol, which allowed them to convert a case to general anesthesia in less than 10 minutes. In conclusion, conscious sedation with local anesthesia can be an alternative to general anesthesia in patients with low-grade subarachnoid hemorrhage or unruptured aneurysms.

Antithrombotic use during aneurysm embolization

There are two main circumstances in which one needs to pay close attention to antithrombotic treatment to decrease complications during embolization of intracranial aneurysms. One is during the actual procedure when anticoagulation is used, and the other is in stent-assisted procedures where antiplatelet use is important.

In unruptured aneurysms when full anticoagulation is used, an activated clotting time (ACT) >250 seconds should be pursued, and hourly monitoring should be performed, especially in procedures that are prolonged beyond the expected duration time. In the case of ruptured aneurysms, the decision is more complex. The treatment of ruptured aneurysms increases the risk of thromboembolic events. A prospective study, in which magnetic resonance imaging (MRI) of the brain was performed during coil embolization, demonstrated the presence of lesions detected by diffusion-weighted imaging (DWI) in 71% of patients with ruptured aneurysms and in 24% of those with unruptured aneurysms[13]. Partial anticoagulation may be considered if the risk of hemorrhage is low, with the initial bolus at the microcatheterization time and full anticoagulation once a few coils have been detached. The presence of factors that may predispose to aneurysm rupture (such as very small size, aneurysm irregularities, or difficult microcatheterization for reasons including tortuous anatomy) or active hemorrhage elsewhere may prevent administration of any anticoagulation until the aneurysm is secured and/or the active hemorrhage is under control.

In preparation for treatment of wide neck aneurysms, and when stent placement, liquid embolic agent use, or flow diversion are anticipated, the appropriate antiplatelet regimen consisting of dual antiplatelet agents (usually aspirin at doses in the range 81–325 mg/day and clopidogrel at 75 mg/day) should be started at least 5 days previously. Alternatively, loading doses can be used. Continuation of dual antiplatelet therapy for the short term (one to three months) may also be considered in wide neck aneurysms, large aneurysms, or those that are incompletely embolized, even if primary coil embolization was performed independent of coil protrusion. In a transcranial Doppler study, this high-risk population was found to have a higher rate of distal microemboli and clinical events during aneurysm embolization[14]. In a study of 154 patients undergoing endovascular embolization of unruptured intracranial aneurysms, patients receiving dual antiplatelet agents were less likely to have cerebrovascular ischemic events than those receiving a single antiplatelet agent (4 cases, representing 4.4% of the 90 who received dual agents) vs. 5 cases (7.8% of the 64 patients who received a single agent) or DWI lesions on MRI (31 cases (34%) vs. 27 cases (42%)) with similar hemorrhagic complications. Significant differences in the rate of symptomatic ischemic complications (single, 21.7%; dual, 3.5%; $P = 0.014$) and DWI abnormalities (single, 37.8%; dual, 20.9%; $P = 0.048$) were found when wide neck aneurysms were analyzed independent of the treatment, including whether a stent was placed[15]. Long-term dual antiplatelet use should be considered in cases of flow diversion.

Primary coil embolization

In the 1990s the first coils were introduced in endovascular embolization of intracranial aneurysms. The Guglielmi detachable coil (GDC; Boston Scientific/Target Therapeutics, Fremont, CA) incorporating an electrolysis detachable system was approved by the US Food and Drug Administration (FDA) in 1995. The technology has continued to evolve, and today we have many coil sizes and configurations. By placing platinum coils within the aneurysm, subsequent thrombosis will be promoted. The ultimate purpose is to isolate the aneurysm from the parent vessel, decreasing the chances of further growth and/or rupture. Often, in the presence of a wide neck aneurysm, there is a risk of parent vessel occlusion by herniation of the coils into the parent vessel, and its treatment requires assistance from a balloon or a stent placement. Newer concepts include the use of liquid embolic agents to obliterate the aneurysm or the use of stents with a dense strut design for flow diversion.

Coil structure

A coil has a complex structure. The primary structure is the "stock" wire, which is fabricated in a linear form with a diameter (D1) of a variable range. This then undergoes a series of transformations or looping into a secondary configuration (diameter D2) and further looping into a tertiary configuration (D3). All these factors contribute to the physical properties of the coil, including softness and spatial configuration, in a simple 2D helical or more complex 3D shape[16].

Selection of the first coil

Inappropriate coil selection and placement techniques may be responsible for most intra-procedural ruptures (83% in a meta-analysis of 17 reports)[17], and up to 50% of these ruptures occur during the first coil placement[18]. In one study[19] of the 172 aneurysms treated in 158 patients, failure of the lead coil placement was observed in 24 procedures (14%). The majority of aneurysms (83.7%) were located in the anterior circulation. Coils with 3D configuration were used as the lead coil in 80% of embolization procedures, except in aneurysms with size <3 mm, for which 3D configuration was used in 60% of the procedures and 2D in the rest. There were 24 (14%) lead coil placement failure procedures in 172 aneurysm embolization procedures; in 23 of 24 (96%) patients with failure of lead coil placement, the failure occurred in aneurysms less than 10 mm in size (see Table 2.2). The main technical factors associated with lead coil placement failure were related to the coil (length, diameter, and type) followed by microcatheter support failure. Among these patients, 21 (87.5%) required a change in the coil length, 17 (70.8%) a change in coil diameter, and 10 (41.7%) a change in coil type (brand and/or configuration) for successful placement of the lead coil (see Table 2.3). A total of four (16.7%) patients required a change

Table 2.2 Distribution of successful first coil placement in relationship to length factor for aneurysm <10 mm

Length factor (F)	Aneurysm size (mm)		
	≤3	3.1–6	6.1–10
1	77%	93%	90%
1.5	22%	63%	82%
2	11%	36%	69%
2.5	–	30%	40%

Table 2.3 A summary of rescue strategies to overcome lead (first) coil placement failure in various strata defined by aneurysm diameter

	Aneurysm diameter (mm)				Total N (%)
	≤3	3.1–6	6.1–10	>10	
Lead coil failure (n)	3	11	9	1	24
Coil diameter change n (%)	3 (100%)	5 (45.5%)	8 (88.9%)	1 (100%)	17 (70.8%)
Coil length change n (%)	3 (100%)	8 (72.7%)	9 (100%)	1 (100%)	21 (87.5%)
Decrease in length n (%)	3 (100%)	8 (72.7%)	6 (66.7%)	1 (100%)	18 (75%)
Increase in length n (%)	0	0	3 (33.3%)	0	3 (12.5%)
Coil type change n (%)	0	5 (45.5%)	4 (44.4%)	1 (100%)	10 (41.7%)
Microcatheter change n (%)	0	3 (27.3%)	1 (11.1%)	0	4 (16.7%)
Balloon assistance n (%)	1 (33.30%)	1 (9.1%)	3 (33.3%)	0	5 (20.8%)

in microcatheter, and six (25%) patients had balloon/stent assistance for successful lead coil placement. Two of 24 (8.3%) patients had rupture of their aneurysms during the attempt to reposition the lead coil. The rupture complication rate in the lead coil placement failure group was 8% (2 of 24 patients) compared with 1.3% (2 of 148 patients) in the successful lead coil placement group. The rate of lead coil failure is mainly determined by the coil length, which is probably the most essential factor to be considered, particularly in small aneurysms. The observations can be summarized by using a novel mathematical concept of length factor (F): Optimal lead coil length (L) cm = largest dimension of the aneurysm (D) mm × 10 × F. The F factor, which should be kept close to 1 for aneurysms of <3 mm, should be between 1 and 2 for aneurysms measuring 3 to 6 mm. A higher factor would be acceptable for larger aneurysms. The authors acknowledge the oversimplification of a complex calculation; however, this formula may offer help and a practical approach to the operator in the selection of the first coil[19].

Failure of coil placement

Coil placement may be unsuccessful owing to the inability of the coil to adequately deploy within the aneurysm sac. This may result in protrusion of the coil or complete prolapse of the microcatheter in addition to coil outside the sac.

If the coil is not adequately deployed within the aneurysm sac, repositioning should be attempted by retraction of the coil and relocation of the microcatheter within the aneurysm sac. If the coil cannot be deployed without protrusion, the coil may be retracted and another coil of a different size or configuration may be considered. The operator may have to decide whether additional coils are necessary or if the procedure should be concluded. If the microcatheter has been displaced from the aneurysm sac, an attempt can be made to advance the microcatheter over the coil length back into the sac. Whether such an attempt will be successful depends upon what component of the coil is within the aneurysm and whether enough support can be provided to move the microcatheter back into the aneurysm sac. Not infrequently, the coil may have to be retracted and the microwire reintroduced through the lumen of the microcatheter to re-enter the aneurysm sac. The microcatheter is subsequently advanced into the aneurysm sac and imbedded further into the aneurysm for greater stability.

Coil misplacement or migration

Misplacement of a coil occurs in 2–6% of occasions[20]. Little agreement exists about the terminology used in coil misplacement or migration. These, however, are the definitions that we have selected in this chapter: Detachment of a coil in an unintended location, or movement after the detachment, is considered coil misplacement or migration. Coil protrusion is when the coil or part of the coil protrudes into the parent vessel. Distal migration is when the coil is completely outside the aneurysmal sac.

Coil protrusion and distal migration

An infrequent occurrence during endovascular treatment is protrusion of detachable coils into the parent lumen, causing subsequent thrombosis within the parent vessel and/or embolic events[21,22]. Overall, thromboembolic complications occur in 2.5–28% of cases, with a variable and often uncategorized component related to coil protrusion[3,23]. Coil protrusion may result from size mismatch between the aneurysm or residual aneurysm and the selected coils, inadequate positioning of the microcatheter within the aneurysm, and/or the presence of low dome-to-neck ratio including wide neck aneurysms[21,24]. Several techniques for managing coil protrusions into parent vessels have been described in case reports, including removal and repositioning of the coil before electrolytic detachment[25], removal of an already detached coil by using a retrieval device[26–28], repositioning or redirecting the protruding coil by using balloon inflation and additional coil placement[29,30], or stent reconstruction of the lumen of the parent vessel[21,25,31].

The protrusion severity can be graded using a three-point scheme as previously described[22]. A schematic representation of the various grades of the scheme is shown in Figure 2.1. If a loop or coil protrudes into the parent vessel lumen by less than half the parent artery diameter, it is given a grade I. When either a coil or loop protrudes into the parent vessel lumen by more than half of the parent artery diameter, it is given a grade II or III. Retrieval of the coil has to be carefully executed. Entrapment of the coil within the coil mass or between the microcatheter and coil mass may lead to coil stretching. If the coil cannot be placed without protrusion, the coil may be retracted and another coil of smaller size may be considered.

If the protruding coil is already deployed and detached, the operator must determine whether protrusion is associated with hemodynamic alterations evident from delay in

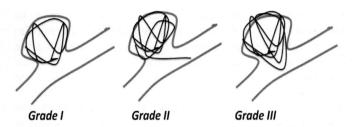

Figure 2.1 Schematic representation of the various grades of coil protrusion severity, using a three-point scheme.

Grade I   *Grade II*   *Grade III*

contrast opacification in the parent vessel adjacent or distal to the segment with protrusion, particularly in grade II and III protrusions. In the event of coil protrusion and active hemodynamic alteration or pulsating coil segment, deployment of a self-expandable intracranial stent may be considered. When the decision is made to place a self-expanding stent, the microcatheter is withdrawn from the aneurysmal sac and advanced past the ostium of the aneurysm into the distal arterial segment by using a micro-guidewire. Then a self-expandable intracranial stent Enterprise (Cordis, (Johnson and Johnson, Raynham, MA) or Neuroform (Stryker Neurovascular, Kalamazoo, MI)) is deployed across the aneurysm neck, either through the microcatheter or through the delivery catheter after this has been exchanged for the initial catheter over an exchange length microwire. The aim of stent placement is to push back the protruded coil or loop into the aneurysm sac, or to trap the protruding mass between the wall of the parent artery and the stent. Intravascular thrombus formation during the embolization procedure, diagnosed by an angiographic filling defect with occlusion of the parent vessel, can occur with coil protrusion. In the event of intravascular thrombus, intra-arterial (IA) infusion of platelet glycoprotein IIB/IIIA inhibitors may be administered through a microcatheter placed next to the thrombus, as discussed in other sections. As an alternative, intravenous administration of IIB/IIIA inhibitor can be considered, leading to a systemic effect. Oral antiplatelet medication, usually a combination of aspirin and clopidogrel, is recommended, especially if a stent has been placed.

In one study[22], of the 10 patients with grade II or III protrusions, five protrusions were associated with hemodynamic changes. A balloon was inflated in front of the aneurysm neck in two patients in an unsuccessful attempt to reposition the protruding coil into the aneurysm. Intravascular thrombus formation occurred in two patients, both of whom were undergoing embolization of an anterior communicating artery aneurysm. In patient 6, a 2 mg bolus of Abciximab (0.2 mg/ml) was administered intra-arterially through a microcatheter placed next to the thrombus for 20 minutes. After the administration of Abciximab, there was complete resolution of the filling defect with good distal flow. In another patient, a bolus of eptifibatide, 10 mg (143 µg/kg), was administered intra-arterially through the microcatheter placed within the thrombus. After 15 minutes, the patient had some flow through the thrombus but no distal flow was observed. The patient was then placed on continuous intravenous infusion of eptifibatide, 41 µg/min, for 24 hours. Six patients underwent stent placement within the same procedure after coil protrusion was detected. No antiplatelet therapy was administered before the stent deployment in any of the six patients. One patient with a grade I coil protrusion pulsating in the parent vessel underwent self-expandable intracranial stent deployment (Neuroform). Five patients with grade II or III protrusions and active hemodynamic alteration underwent self-expandable intracranial stent deployment: four Neuroform stents and one Enterprise stent were used, followed by antiplatelet therapy. The coil embolization procedure was resumed after the stent deployment in only one patient. Eighteen of the 19 patients were given aspirin, 325 mg orally or 300 mg as a suppository, after coil or loop protrusions were detected, in the angiographic suite. Aspirin was continued as a 325-mg daily dose.

In another study[21], nine procedures were complicated by coil protrusion. The causes of coil herniation appeared to be coil instability after detachment ($n = 6$), excessive embolization ($n = 1$), microcatheter-related problems ($n = 1$), or being pushed by embolization of subsequent coils ($n = 1$). Endovascular stent placement to reconstruct the lumen and/or flow of the internal carotid artery (ICA) was technically successful in all nine patients; one needed a second stent because of further coil migration. No significant procedure-related complications were found. The studies demonstrated that delayed thrombosis or progression of coil protrusion appears to be uncommon after antiplatelet treatment alone or in combination with self-expanding stents. Intravascular stent placement appears to be an effective option if treatment is required owing to hemodynamic compromise. On occasions, unraveling or stretching is the cause of coil protrusion (Figure 2.1).

Distal migration of a coil refers to the migration of a complete coil outside the aneurysmal sac. The most common causes are undersized coil, wide neck aneurysms, or unfavorable neck-to-dome ratio[32,33]. Interestingly, on rare occasions coil migration has also been described as a delayed phenomenon. Patients have presented weeks after the initial treatment with coil protrusion or ischemic events despite single antiplatelet use[34,35], or distal migration has been found incidentally even after stent placement[36,37].

Coil stretching, unraveling, and fracture

See Figures 2.2 to 2.5. Loss of coil configuration can make proper placement of a coil impossible, or lead to coil protrusion or distal migration. "Stretched coil" is a term used to

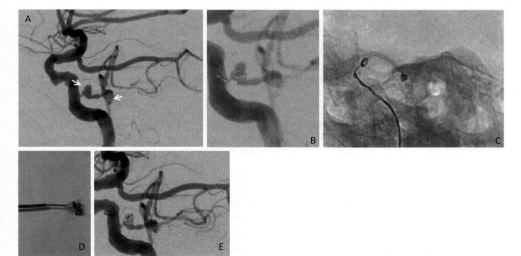

Figure 2.2 A 71-year-old woman who presented with Hut and Hess grade 3 subarachnoid hemorrhage centered in the posterior fossa. Cerebral digital subtracted angiography demonstrated a dysplastic trigeminal artery with two pseudoaneurysmatic areas (A). The patient underwent endovascular coil embolization. During the coil embolization of the more proximal pseudoaneurysm, the microcoil failed to detach initially, and then detached inappropriately, occluding the main feeder of the basilar artery (B). A 4 mm Alligator retrieval device (Covidien, Mansfield, MA) was used to remove the coil (C, D) and this was followed by successful coil embolization (E).

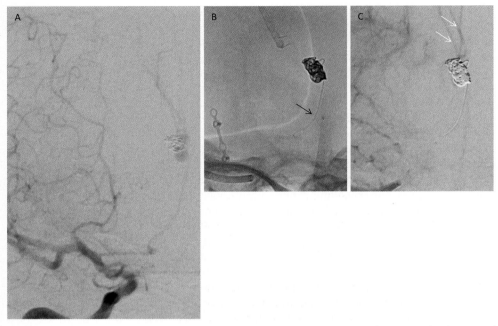

Figure 2.3 A 33-year-old woman with past medical history of bifrontal lobe trauma, who presented with Hunt and Hess grade 3, Fisher grade 3 subarachnoid hemorrhage and a right pericallosal/callosal marginal bifurcation pseudoaneurysm. During manipulation of the last coil, it unraveled with occlusion of the parent vessel (black arrow). Prior to its retrieval, it was decided to assess the collateral flow, and it was noted that both right callosal marginal and pericallosal arteries were filling in a retrograde fashion (white arrows). No further intervention was performed and the case ended. The patient was clinically unchanged and suffered no infarct on computed tomography (CT).

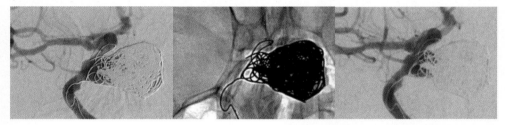

Figure 2.4 A 64-year-old woman with a giant right superior hypophyseal aneurysm causing compression of the right optic nerve, resulting in right eye blindness. The patient had been prepped with aspirin and clopidogrel a week prior. During coil embolization, there was premature detachment of a coil, and the coil herniated into the proximal parent vessel. It was decided to stent-trap the coil. A Neuroform EZ (Stryker Neurovascular, Kalamazoo, MI) was used. The parent vessel remained patent. The patient suffered no clinical consequences.

describe when a portion of the coil loses its configuration. An unraveled coil occurs when a larger portion of the coil loses its tertiary and secondary configuration, usually preventing normal forward push of the coil. Often, if the pull continues, the coil ends up completely unraveling or fracturing. Entrapment of the coil within the coil mass, or between the microcatheter and the coil mass, can lead to stretching or unraveling during manipulation, especially during retrieval. If an attempt to push the coil forward inside the aneurysm fails,

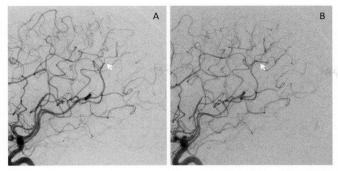

Figure 2.5 A 32-year-old woman with history of previous subarachnoid hemorrhage underwent coil embolization of an unruptured 2.5 mm right M1 segment, origin of the anterior temporal artery aneurysm. The first coil was a HyperSoft 1.5 mm × 2 cm coil (MicroPlex; MicroVention, Aliso Viejo, CA). Upon detachment the coil quickly migrated to the distal middle cerebral artery vasculature and became lodged at a branching point, with occlusion of the inferior branch (A). The flow was restored after initial infusion of Integrilin for 20 hours, and aspirin and clopidogrel load. The patient remained asymptomatic at all times. The aneurysm was later treated with stent-assisted coil embolization (B). Note restoration of the flow in a follow-up angiogram; the patient remained asymptomatic.

different techniques can be attempted to withdraw the coil before its fracture. Before retrieval is attempted, however, the inflation of a non-detachable balloon at the neck of the aneurysm may help in pushing a stretched coil inside the aneurysmal sac[25]. Several techniques have been described to withdraw coils that are already unraveled, such as using a 2 or 4 mm Amplatz Goose neck microsnare (Microvena, White Bear Lake, MN) with the loop around the microcatheter and advancing it until the loop is around the healthy portion of the coil, followed by entrapment within the snare loop and its microcatheter[26]. The introduction of two 0.010 inch microwires inside the microcatheter has also been reported in the retrieval of an unraveled coil, by trapping the healthy portion of the coil and pulling out all devices as a system[29]. The Alligator retrieval device (Covidien, Irving, CA) has also been used to capture distally migrated coils[33]. Other commonly used devices in the retrieval of migrated coils include those intended for mechanical thrombectomy in ischemic stroke[32,38]. Alternatively, some authors have reported good clinical outcomes from conservative management with the use of antithrombotic agents, or the deliberate placement of a proximal unraveled coil into an extracerebral artery[39]. A conservative approach can also be considered when the damaged coil creates no hemodynamic compromise and/or there is presence of good collateral flow (see Figure 2.3).

Thromboembolic complications

See Figures 2.6 and 2.7. Intraprocedural thrombosis can occur through a combination of enhanced intrinsic thrombogenicity seen in patients with subarachnoid hemorrhage, and reaction to foreign bodies such as platinum-based coils or nitinol stents. The process of obliteration of the aneurysm requires thrombus formation within the matrix of coils deployed within the aneurysmal sac. However, if thrombosis extends into the parent artery, partial or complete occlusion of the artery may occur, with or without distal embolism. A non-occlusive thrombus is difficult to identify, and filling defects that are radiotranslucent without a clear configuration may be the only finding. Flow stasis in the vicinity and distal artery may be seen. Intraprocedural thrombosis can occur with or without coil

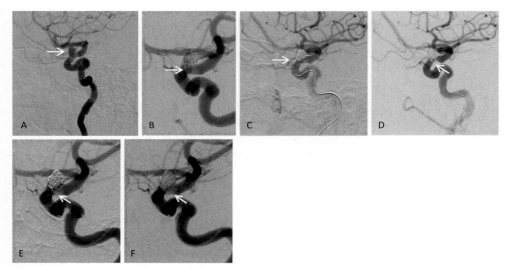

Figure 2.6 Coil prolapse and thrombosis during aneurysm embolization. **A:** Internal carotid artery aneurysm protruding in anterior and superior direction (arrow). **B:** Prolapse of coil loops into the parent artery (arrow). **C:** A self-expanding nitinol stent 4.5 × 22 mm positioned across the aneurysm neck (arrow). **D:** Filling defect (thrombus) in internal carotid artery in proximity to the stent and coil mass (arrow). **E:** Partial resolution of filling defect (thrombus) in internal carotid artery in proximity to the stent and coil mass after administration of intra-arterial glycoprotein IIB/IIIA inhibitor Eptifibatide 5 mg (arrow). **F:** Continued resolution of filling defect (thrombus) in internal carotid artery in proximity to the stent and coil mass after administration of intra-arterial glycoprotein IIB/IIIA inhibitor Eptifibatide 5 mg (arrow).

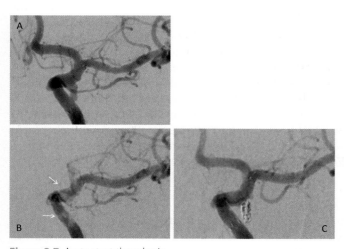

Figure 2.7 Acute stent thrombosis.
A: A 50-year-old female with a 5 mm, "tall" left posterior communicating artery aneurysm (**A**). The patient had been prepped with aspirin and clopidogrel for a week prior to the treatment. After placement of the Enterprise stent (Cordis, Johnson and Johnson, Raynham, MA), hyperacute stent thrombosis was noted. **B:** Areas of filling defect (arrows). Note its thermodynamic effect on the loss of anterior cerebral artery flow. Epifibate 135 micrograms/kg was given as bolus intravenously following an infusion 0.5 mg/kg per min for 20 hours. The thrombus resolved completely, and procedure was continued with successful coil embolization of the aneurysm. The patient was neurologically intact after the procedure. A follow-up angiogram demonstrates stable stent and coil mass, no filling of the aneurysm (**C**).

protrusion into the parent artery. In one systematic review, the overall risk of symptomatic thromboembolic complications was 11% in 109 patients who underwent aneurysm embolization[40].

Because the majority of thromboembolic events associated with GDC treatment occur intraoperatively, the emphasis is on intraoperative anticoagulation therapy. For patients with subarachnoid hemorrhage, heparin should be administered concurrently with microcatheter placement and deployment of the first coil, and the dose should be titrated to maintained ACTs of 200 to 250 seconds. For patients with unruptured aneurysms, heparin should be administered early, before placement of the guide catheter. No clear benefit was observed[40] with the postoperative use of aspirin or heparin, although a slightly lower rate of thromboembolic complications was observed with each postoperative regimen in the cumulative analysis. Given the risk of bleeding, we do not recommend the routine postoperative use of heparin. However, for selected patients, heparin administration may be continued for 24 hours postoperatively, to maintain aPTTs (activated partial thromboplastin times) of 1.5 to 2.5 times the control values. Such patients include those with a coil protrusion in the parent vessel, angiographic evidence of thrombus outside the aneurysmal sac, or ischemic symptoms in the intra- or postoperative period. The aPTT should be measured every 6 hours. A weight-based nomogram ensures safe and effective anticoagulation[41]. After a 24-hour course of heparin, a combination of aspirin (325 mg, daily) with ticlopidine (250 mg, twice daily) or clopidogrel (75 mg, twice daily) may be used for 4 weeks, especially in patients with low risk for rupture, to ensure endothelialization of thrombogenic surfaces. As discussed previously, the risk of thromboembolic events is very low after the first 4 weeks.

Intraprocedural thrombosis without coil prolapse

These events occur when the parent artery is small and there is a relative large interface between the coil mass and the parent artery. Thrombus formation within the aneurysm has relatively easy access into the parent artery, and additional thrombosis occurs owing to turbulence at the junction between the parent artery and coil mass. This occurrence is usually seen after the majority of the aneurysm has been obliterated by the coil mass. Therefore, the chance of rebleeding from the aneurysm is relatively low. Intra-arterial bolus or infusion of platelet glycoprotein IIB/IIIA inhibitors has become the first line of treatment in those scenarios.

Thrombolytics have not often been used, owing to risk of rebleeding from the intracranial aneurysm or at the site of ischemic intraparenchymal injury. The original microcatheter may be withdrawn from the aneurysmal sac into the parent artery if further coil placement is not anticipated, or a new microcatheter may be placed in the parent artery in the vicinity of the aneurysm for intravascular thrombus treatment. Agents such as Abciximab (2–20 mg) or Eptifibatide (1000–9000 μg) are commonly used in various dilutions (low volume is preferred). Intermittent boluses are administered until resolution of intravascular thrombus or occlusion is angiographically documented. An intravenous infusion may be infrequently chosen if resolution of thrombus or occlusion is not adequate. The mechanism by which platelet glycoprotein IIB/IIIA inhibitors lyse intravascular thrombus is unknown but is attributable to potentiation of the intrinsic lytic system and/or platelet deaggregation in the early phase of thrombus formation. Anecdotal use of mechanical thrombectomy devices in the event of complete arterial occlusion has been reported in the literature. Jeong and Jin[42] have reported the safety and recanalization rates of intra-arterial Abciximab and intra-arterial Tirofiban infusions for thromboembolism occurring during coiling. According to their report, thromboembolism was completely ($n = 1$) or partially ($n = 7$) resolved in eight cases (72.7%) at the time of the final angiographic control in the Abciximab group. Complete ($n = 9$) or partial ($n = 2$) resolution was achieved in all cases at the time of follow-up angiography (<3 days after the procedure). In the Tirofiban group, thromboembolism was completely ($n = 4$) or partially ($n = 6$) resolved in 10 cases (90.9%) at the time of the final control angiography. The thrombus resolution in the two groups was not significantly different (final angiography, $P = 0.311$; follow-up angiography, $P = 0.707$). Hemorrhagic complications did not develop in either group. Aggour et al.[43] reported and compared the safety and efficacy of using combined intra-arterial and intravenous Abciximab to treat thrombi complicating endovascular cerebral aneurysm coil embolization. Amelioration, as measured by the Thrombolysis in Myocardial Infarction flow grade score, was observed in 17 of 23 patients (73.9%). Six of 23 patients demonstrated no change (26.1%) whereas complete recanalization was achieved in 13 patients (56.5%). Eleven patients (47.8%) demonstrated ischemic lesions. Hemorrhagic complication did not occur in any patient. Seventeen out of 23 patients demonstrated a modified Rankin Scale (mRS) of ≤ 2 whereas 6 of 23 patients demonstrated a mRS of >2. Ries et al.[44] also reported and estimated the safety and efficacy of Abciximab in combination with prophylactic heparin, acetylsalicylic acid (ASA), and clopidogrel application in cases of thrombus formed as a complication of endovascular coil embolization. In their series, no infarcts on follow-up CT were noted after treatment with Abciximab in 29 out of 42 patients (69.0%, 95% CI: 52.9 to 82.4%). Coagulant rescue therapy was not applied in five patients because of a small non-occlusive thrombus or good collateral blood supply. Of these, consecutive infarction was seen on follow-up CT in three cases. Periprocedural or rebleeding was not observed in any case.

Intraprocedural thrombosis with coil prolapse

Coil prolapse creates a mechanical component to flow alteration and turbulence as discussed previously in other sections.

Intraprocedural aneurysm rupture

See Figure 2.8. Aneurysmal rupture is reported in less than 5% of cases. It may happen during the initial diagnostic angiography owing to microwire, microcatheter, or coil manipulation.

General management of patients with intraprocedural aneurysm rupture

In patients undergoing general anesthesia, if aneurysmal rupture occurs, immediate steps such as control of intracranial hypertension using hyperventilation, Mannitol, hypertonic saline, and judicious use of intravenous antihypertensive agents in the event of acute hypertensive response are appropriate. The neurological assessment is limited, and mainly focused on pupillary reaction. Reversal of large and unreactive pupils should be the goal. If not previously present, the placement of external ventricular drainage may also be required to treat and monitor the intracranial pressure. When intravenous heparin has already been administered, reversal using protamine sulfate may be necessary. At the same time it is

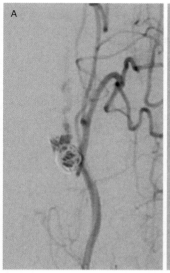
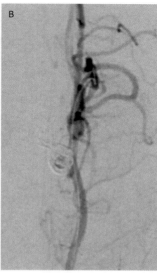

Figure 2.8 A 55-year-old woman presented with a ruptured left pericallosal aneurysm. During the placement of the second coil, contrast extravasation was noted (A). No assistance device could be accommodated, owing to the size of the parent vessel. Additional coils were immediately placed within the aneurysmal sac, and the parent vessel was preserved (B). The neurological status remained unchanged.

important to secure the aneurysm to stop the hemorrhage. The method varies depending on the treatment stage, as discussed later. If a balloon catheter is already in position across the neck of the aneurysm, the balloon can be inflated to stop the hemorrhage. If the balloon is not in the proximity of the aneurysm, preparing and advancing a *de novo* balloon catheter may not be a time-effective strategy; instead, rapid aneurysm obliteration with coils should be attempted.

When the patient is under conscious sedation, rapid intubation is usually required to continue the treatment properly, in order to avoid restless movements. A neurological evaluation at the time of rupture may be possible and necessary to help guide management immediately before patients undergo general anesthesia.

Intraprocedural aneurysm rupture: stages

Intraprocedural aneurysmal rupture can occur at any stage of the procedure, including during the initial diagnostic angiography. Selective injections from diagnostic or guide catheters placed in the internal carotid or vertebral arteries can result in aneurysmal rupture, particularly in those patients with primary aneurysmal rupture within the past 12 hours. Programmed automated contrast injection is common in the evaluation of patients with intracranial aneurysm, to acquire multiple images using rotational angiography. Pressure transmission can be considerable if the diagnostic or guide catheter is placed at high cervical positions within internal carotid or vertebral arteries, or if there is considerable straightening of proximal arteries by guide catheters. Outflow resistance due to distal vasospasm also increases the pressure transmitted to the aneurysmal wall. A decision must be made at that time, based on the clinical and anatomical information, as to whether surgical clip placement or endovascular treatment is required after the general management.

Intraprocedural rupture can also happen during microcatheterization, with the initial placement of the microcatheter and microwire. The microwire is advanced into the aneurysmal sac under direct visualization using a road mapping technique. The micro-catheter is advanced over the microwire to an appropriate position, usually 2/3 into the aneurysmal sac, prior to the microwire withdrawal. Aneurysm rupture during microwire manipulation is infrequent and probably under-recognized. Most wire perforations that are noted lead to no clinical sequel; reversal of anticoagulation and continued coil embolization to secure the aneurysm are the key elements in its management. Sometimes a larger segment of microwire may have to be advanced within the aneurysm sac to provide a more stable platform for the microcatheter to be advanced through an angulated or tortuous entrance point. Careful manipulation of the devices during this step is advised. Forward propulsion of the microwire and microcatheter can be seen owing to straightening of the microwire and further advance of the microcatheter. When the vasculature is straightened, the effective length of the devices increases, leading to forward movement.

In case of aneurysm perforation by the microcatheter, the operator has to be careful with the magnitude of microcatheter withdrawal that will bring the microcatheter within the aneurysmal sac. Too much withdrawal could bring the microcatheter too proximal into the parent artery, delaying hemostasis. An appropriate coil can be deployed within the aneurysmal sac to ensure temporary stability. Some operators recommend not withdrawing the microcatheter if it has protruded outside the wall of the aneurysm in the subarachnoid space until a coil is advanced to the end of the microcatheter ready for deployment. Placement of a coil from the subarachnoid space across the ruptured area into the aneurys-mal sac may also help ensure cessation of the bleeding.

During coil deployment, the risk of aneurysmal rupture is highest at the time of the first or second coil deployment. Usually, in cases of rupture, the coil is pushed outside the wall of the aneurysm into the subarachnoid space. A coil that is larger than necessary, or a microcatheter tip placed close to the aneurysm wall, will increase the probability of such an event. Verification of the position of the distal end of the microcatheter in two different views allows a better assessment of the microcatheter tip in relation to the aneurysm wall. A distance of approximately 1 mm between the aneurysm wall and microcatheter tip ensures safe advance of the coil, so the coil starts to acquire its configuration prior to touching the wall.

The operator must take care to reposition the coil within the sac of the aneurysm to ensure temporary stability. Some operators recommend that if a small portion of the coil is in the subarachnoid space, deployment of the coil can be initiated from there. However, further coil deployment must occur not by advancing the coil but by withdrawing the microcatheter, ensuring that the majority of the deployment is within the aneurysmal sac. The risk of rupture with second or subsequent coil deployment needs to be recognized because the distal end of the microcatheter or aneurysm wall may be obscured. The shell provided by one coil is quite porous, and new coils can easily move outside the shell provided by the first coil and aneurysm wall.

Treatment of aneurysms with wide neck or unfavorable neck-to-dome ratio

The standard definition of a wide neck aneurysm is when the neck is greater than 4 mm. Aneurysms with a dome-to-neck ratio <2 are also not favorable for primary coil embolization. Alternative assistant techniques exist in the treatment of these aneurysms, including balloon remodeling, stent assistance, liquid embolic agents, and flow

Table 2.4 Comparison of ATENA and CLARITY

	ATENA[47]		CLARITY[4]	
	Primary coil embolization	Balloon remodeling	Primary coil embolization	Balloon remodeling
Complete occlusion	59.8%	59.8%	46.9	50%
Neck remnant	24.3%	20.1%	41.6%	44.9%
Aneurysm remnant	16%	20.1%	11.5%	5.1%
Thromboembolic complications	6.2%	5.4%	12.7%	11.3%
Aneurysmal rupture	2.2%	3.2%	4.4%	4.4%
Overall complications	10.8%	11.7%	17.4%	16.9%

ATENA: Analysis of Treatment by Endovascular Approach of Nonruptured Aneurysms study. CLARITY: CLinical and Anatomical Results In the Treatment of ruptured intracranial aneurysms study.

diversion. Except for the balloon remodeling technique, use of dual antiplatelet agent treatment is usually required.

Balloon remodeling technique/balloon-assisted coil embolization

Moret *et al.*[45] described the balloon remodeling technique in 1994 for the treatment of wide neck aneurysms. Although initially this was thought to be a technique with a higher risk of thromboembolic complications[46], more recent studies show complication rates and clinical outcome similar to those for primary coil embolization in ruptured[4] and unruptured aneurysms[47]. One of the main limitations is navigation through a tortuous anatomy. When single-lumen microcatheter balloons were used, complete withdrawal of the balloon micro-catheter was required for reshaping of the wire. An alternative to complete withdrawal is to withdraw only the microwire. A continuous hand-flush of the mix (contrast and saline) used to inflate the balloon is slowly injected through the single-lumen microcatheter while the wire is taken out for reshaping before being reintroduced. This step prevents back flow of blood without the need to reposition the balloon catheter in the distal vasculature. The recent introduction of double-lumen microcatheter balloons not only obviates this step but allows the use of larger microwires with a better torque profile for better navigation.

The usual technique consists of placement of the balloon microcatheter along the neck of the aneurysm. The balloon is inflated, with the aim of prevention of coil protrusion into the parent vessel during coil embolization or cessation of hemorrhage in the case of aneurysmal rupture. There are two types of compliant balloons: the low-compliance balloons such as the Hyperglide (ev3/Covidien, Irvine, CA) that maintain a cylindrical shape during inflation, and the high-compliance balloons such as the Hyperform (ev3/Covidien, Irvine, CA) that acquire a "pear-like" shape when inflated, for more complex aneurysms[48]. Given the high compliance of these balloons, the technique can sometimes be modified by using the front of the balloon to partially introduce it in the aneurysmal sac (toe technique) or the back of the balloon (heel technique), in order to protect not only the neck/parent vessel but also the adjacent branches. In some circumstances, the microcatheter

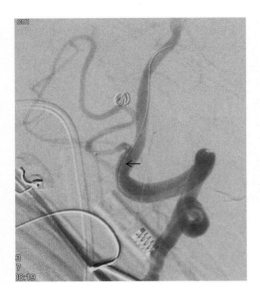

Figure 2.9 A 43-year-old woman who presented with Fisher 3 and Hunt–Hess 1 subarachnoid hemorrhage was found to have a 3.7 × 3.1 × 2.4(neck) mm aneurysm originating from the choroidal point segment of the left posterior-inferior cerebellar artery (PICA). A 6 French 80 cm Shuttle ® (Cook Inc., Bloomington, IN) in the left subclavian and a 6 French Neuron® 070 guide catheter (Penumbra Inc., Alameda, CA) in the left vertebral artery were used for access. The aneurysm was then catheterized with an Excelsior ® SL-10 (Stryker Neurovascular, Kalamazoo, MI), pre-shaped 90 degrees. Repeated attempts to advance the first coil (Cashmere®; Codman Neurovascular, Raynham, MA) in the aneurysm led to repeated microcatheter tip herniation out of the aneurysm or herniation of the microcatheter into the distal left vertebral artery. A HyperForm® 4 × 7 mm balloon microcatheter (Covidien Plc, Dublin, Ireland) was advanced and placed across the origin of the left PICA (black arrow). The balloon was then inflated at the origin of the left PICA for stabilization of the microcatheter. This was sufficient to enable stable coil embolization with preservation of the parent vessel. A total of four coils were deployed with obliteration of the aneurysm. The patient was extubated with no change in her neurological examination.

may be unstable and the balloon cannot be placed near the aneurysm neck. In these cases, the balloon can sometimes be placed proximally to support and stabilize the microcatheter (Figure 2.9). A double microcatheter technique can be used in cases where balloon or stent-assisted coiling cannot be achieved or is not preferred (Figure 2.10).

Stent-assisted coil embolization

Stent-assisted coil embolization has emerged as an alternative to treat wide neck aneurysms. It was first described by Higashida et al.[49] in 1997 using a balloon-expandable stent in the treatment of a basilar aneurysm. Later, self-expandable stents were designed, and these are currently the most commonly used for intracranial coil assistance. The first stent to be approved by the FDA was the Neuroform. The most commonly used stents for coil assistance in the United States are the Neuroform and Enterprise. The stent is positioned with the intention of keeping the coils within the aneurysmal sac by creating a scaffold across the neck. Stent placement requires dual antiplatelet therapy, which is not ideal for ruptured aneurysms.

Based on their cell configuration, stents are classified as open (Neuroform, Stryker Neurovascular, Kalamazoo, MI) and closed cell design (Enterprise, Codman & Shurtleff, Raynham, MA). The different cell configurations provide the stent with different properties. The Enterprise, with its closed cell design, has a larger radial force (the resistance of a stent to being compressed) in straight anatomies; however, in tortuous anatomies, it has more ovalization (narrowing of the lumen) but less "gator backing" (protrusion of the struts into the aneurysmal sac) and kinking (protrusion of the struts within the lumen, making navigation through the stent difficult). The Neuroform in tortuous anatomies has a larger outward radial force and better conformability (less bending stiffness, or better ability to adapt to the vessel as opposed to straightening the vessel) and wall apposition (ability to be in contact with the vessel wall). The Neuroform has larger cells but also needs a larger microcatheter system, 0.027 vs. 0.021 inch[50,51].

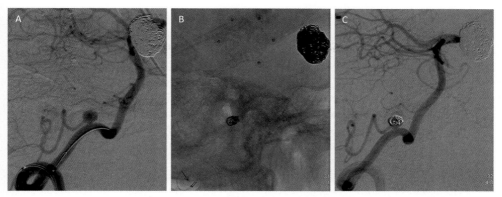

Figure 2.10 A 44-year-old woman with history of ruptured right middle cerebral artery aneurysm and good clinical recovery underwent right PICA aneurysm embolization. The aneurysm was located in the anterior medullary segment and measured 5 × 4 mm (A). A 6 French Neuron® 070 guide catheter (Penumbra Inc, Alameda, CA) was placed in the right vertebral artery. An Excelsior® SL-10 (Boston Scientific, Natick, MA), pre-shaped 45 degrees, was advanced into the aneurysm. Through the microcatheter, a coil (Cashmere 14 4 mm × 4.5 cm; Micrus Endovascular, San Jose, CA) was advanced into the aneurysm. Despite multiple repositioning attempts, an appropriate position away from the PICA lumen could not be obtained. Through the guide catheter, a second Excelsior® SL-10 (pre-shaped 45 degrees; Boston Scientific, Natick, MA) was advanced into the aneurysm, and a coil (HydroSoft 10 Helical 2 mm × 4 cm; Microvention, Tustin, CA) was placed parallel with the previous one. Both coils were advanced simultaneously, remaining in the aneurysmal sac. The combined coil mass was thought to be stable in the aneurysm sac, away from the right PICA lumen, and the coils were detached (B). The larger coil was detached first. Follow-up angiography showed no coil herniation (C).

Two main microcatheterization techniques are commonly used with stent assistance: primary stent placement and the jailing technique[52]. Primary stent placement entails the placement of the stent with no additional devices in the guide catheter, the placement of the stent is then followed by coiling that can be done in the same procedure or in a delayed one. The jailing technique implies the need to have, in addition to the delivery microcatheter, a microcatheter that will be placed in the aneurysmal sac prior to stent deployment. Disadvantages of primary stent placement are the need to cross through the stent and the struts, which may lead to failure, stent movement, and deformity of the stent. We favor the jailing technique if difficulties are anticipated given a tortuous anatomy. The jailing technique can lead to microcatheter herniation at the time of stent placement. This can be overcome with partial stretch-resistant coil placement that can help to guide the microcatheter back into the aneurysmal sac.

The safety of stent-assisted coil embolization practice in ruptured aneurysms has yet to be determined. In a large study in which ruptured aneurysms were treated within 72 hours, the authors found a technique-related complication rate of 21% and a 30-day mortality rate of 20% with most complications being thromboembolic[53]. Another large study, in which 216 patients were treated with stent and 1109 patients without stent, found neurological morbidity and mortality related to the procedure of 7.4 and 4.6% compared with 3.8 and 1.2% in those without stent placement, despite similar angiographic results. Multivariate analysis associated stent placement in ruptured aneurysms with an increased risk of complications (P: 0.027; OR: 0.508; 95% CI: 0.279 to 0.925)[54]. The current guidelines recommend stent avoidance unless no other method can be used in treating ruptured aneurysms[55].

Liquid embolic agents

In 2007, the FDA approved the liquid embolic agent Onyx HD 500 (Covidien, Inc., Irvine, CA) as a Humanitarian Exemption device for side wall aneurysms with a wide neck (>4 mm) or dome-to-neck ratio <2.

The Onyx liquid embolic system is a combination agent of ethylene-vinyl alcohol copolymer (EVOH) and dimethylsulfoxide (DMSO), opacified with micronized tantalum powder, that has been primarily used in the endovascular treatment of arteriovenous malformations (AVMs). Originally, different EVOH concentrations, viscosities 18 (concentration 6%) and 34 (8%), were used in AVM embolization. An EVOH 12% polymer concentration was initially used for aneurysm embolization until Onyx HD (viscosity 500) was finally developed with a 20% EVOH concentration. Its increased viscosity lessens the likelihood of reflux into the parent vessel. When Onyx comes into contact with blood or water, the EVOH precipitates and solidifies because of the rapid diffusion of the DMSO solvent. The technique requires preparation with dual antiplatelet therapy. A compliant balloon is used for remodeling and is inflated to keep the Onyx in the aneurysmal sac for brief periods of time.

The first European trial to report on experience with Onyx HD 500 in 22 aneurysms showed an immediate occlusion rate of 82% and 91% at approximately 1 year. The main clinical complications were transient ischemic events and cranial neuropathies. Technical complications included propagation of the Onyx into the parent vessel in 12 patients, occlusion of the ophthalmic artery in four cases without clinical consequences, one vessel rupture that required vessel occlusion, and one vessel occlusion found incidentally on follow-up. MRI-DWI lesions were found in six patients; five had transient symptoms. Cranial neuropathies were present in two of the six patients with space-occupying aneurysms. No mortality was reported[56]. The largest Onyx HD 500 trial to date, with 84 wide neck aneurysms, reported total aneurysm occlusion of 85% at 6 months, and 90% at 18 months. Retreatment was required in 3%, permanent morbidity present in 7%, and procedure-related mortality of 2.9%. One patient was not treated with antiplatelet agents owing to the rupture of the aneurysm and further thrombosis of the ipsilateral ICA; the other patient suffered a wire perforation and a large hemorrhage 5 hours after the procedure[57].

It is not uncommon to see the Onyx cast protrude into the parent vessel; the Onyx protrusion may or may not be unstable. Instability of the Onyx cast can be due to pulsatility of a tail or to protrusion of the cast, as when aneurysms have a base broader than the dome. In cases of unstable protrusion of the Onyx cast, stent placement has been suggested, to push the cast back into place. Other recommendations include slower injections towards the end, when the Onyx cast is approaching the neck, and the use of a straight microcatheter tip, so its withdrawal at the end of the procedure is more predictable[58].

Flow diversion

A new generation of flexible stent-like devices has emerged. These are self-expanding, microcatheter-delivered, and offer high metal surface area with small cells, thus acting as flow diverters. The idea of reconstructing the endothelial wall at the neck of the aneurysm is behind this new generation of devices, called flow diverters. In 2011 the FDA approved the Pipeline (Covidien, Fremont, CA).

A triaxial system is used for deployment of flow diverters. The Navien catheter (ev3 Endovascular, Plymouth, MN) (5 Fr, 0.070 inch outer diameter, 0.058 inch inner diameter,

115 cm) is used and tracked into position over a Marksman microcatheter (ev3 Endovascular, Plymouth, MN). In one study of 78 procedures[59], a Navien catheter tip was placed in the cervical ICA (1/78 procedures, 1%), petrous ICA (23/78, 30%), proximal cavernous ICA (48/78, 62%), distal cavernous/clinoidal ICA (3/78, 4%), supraclinoid ICA (2/78, 2%) and the M1 segment (1/78, 2%).

Difficulty in release of distal end of flow-diverting stent

The distal end of a flow-diverting stent is held tightly closed by a coil that is incorporated into the wire 15 mm from the distal end of the microwire. Initially, the stent is pushed forward through a Marksman microcatheter (ev3 Endovascular, Plymouth, MN) which releases the distal portion of the stent except the part contained within the retention coil. Two clockwise rotations of the microwire are required to release the distal end of the stent and allow it to expand. Occasionally, the most distal portion of the stent is not released despite advancement of the stent and rotations of the microwire. This difficulty is more likely to be encountered if the junction between retention coil and stent is angled. Therefore, reattempting disengagement in a relatively straight segment (such as a horizontal section of the proximal middle cerebral artery) by advancing or retracting the delivery system should be considered. More exposure of the distal portion of the stent in front of the microcatheter increases the radial force at the stent/retention coil junction and may result in expansion. Once the distal end is expanded, the whole delivery system can be repositioned as needed.

Deployment in collapsed form

During deployment, the stent may remain elongated and collapsed rather than expanding properly with the withdrawal of the catheter, because the radial force of the stent structure is not as high as for other self-expanding stents. In some instances, additional retraction of the microcatheter by advancing the microwire may be adequate. However, if expansion is not seen after a quarter of the stent has been exposed, forward movement of the system (deployed stent and microcatheter) as one unit is required to force the struts to push out, resulting in subsequent expansion of the stent. Several such forward movements may be required to achieve the desired result. If forward pushing of the system does not result in the desired expansion, repositioning the stent to allow a different trajectory of the propulsion may be helpful. The operator must be aware that the stent length is reduced in its expanded state compared with that in the partly collapsed state. Therefore, appropriate adjustments may be necessary to avoid malpositioning of the stent. If the stent is deployed completely and appears to be partly collapsed in certain segments, a compliant angioplasty balloon may be required to perform angioplasty within the lumen of the stent to achieve adequate expansion. If the operator is considering this option, the microwire should preferably be left in position for advancing the balloon catheter through the lumen of the stent. The operator may be required to re-enter the space within the lumen using a microwire. It is recommended that such entry be done using a J configuration on the distal end to avoid entanglement of wire within the struts of the stent.

Misalignment of the deployed stent

The segment of the stent deployed within the fusiform aneurysmal segment or in front of the ostium of the aneurysm may prolapse into the aneurysmal sac. Such prolapse is seen during forward movement of the system (deployed stent and microcatheter) as one unit, because the segment of the system without any encircling wall can bow out in the path of least resistance. The system has to be retracted and realigned to ensure that deployment occurs within the desired segment of the stent. Such events can be prevented by ensuring that an adequate segment of the stent is deployed distal to the aneurysm to ensure alignment. Nevertheless, frequent realignment may be necessary during deployment.

Loss of distal access

If the microwire is removed unintentionally or intentionally (as when inability to pass the microcatheter over the retention coil mandates withdrawal of the microwire and micro-catheter), the lumen of the stent requires accessing again and crossing by the microwire to establish connection with distal segment of the artery. This step is required if post-stent deployment angioplasty is required. A more complex scenario is if the proximal end of the stent is deployed within the fusiform aneurysmal segment or in front of the ostium of the aneurysm. If the stent is not anchored by a microwire traversing the lumen, the proximal end may lose its alignment and deviate into the aneurysmal sac. The central lumen of deployed stent may no longer be accessible by a microwire or microcatheter, preventing the placement of an overlapping stent to create an artificial lumen. The deviation of the proximal end of the stent and contact with the aneurysm wall may result in undue stress on the wall, which can manifest as worsening of mass effect or rupture. Accessing again and crossing the lumen of the stent by microwire may not be possible without realignment of the proximal end of the stent. Such realignment may require placing and inflating the balloon within the aneurysmal sac[60] or capturing the proximal end using a snare and retracting it enough to change the alignment[61]. However, if distal access cannot be regained and thus overlapping stent placement is no longer an option, the operator may have to decide whether obliteration of the aneurysm using coil placement is possible. Aneurysmal obliteration in these circumstances may result in parent arterial occlusion. An assessment of tolerance to such an occlusion and status of collateral circulation may be required prior to permanent occlusion. Temporary balloon occlusion testing may be required in these settings to confirm tolerance to parent artery occlusion. Open surgical access with retrieval of the delivered stent may be infrequently required. A surgical bypass, connecting the superficial temporal artery to a middle cerebral artery branch, may be required prior to permanent occlusion of the parent artery.

Complications

According to data for the Silk flow diversion stent, intra- and postprocedural ischemic stroke was observed in 22 cases (7.7%) in which a flow diverter was used[62]. In the Italian multicenter experience, ischemic events were observed in 13 (4.8%) patients, with 8 (3%) and 5 (2%) attributed to the Silk stent and to PED (Pipeline embolization device) respectively[63]. Four cases were considered procedure-related while the remainder were attributed to the device. The report from the early postmarket result from the United States multicentric study with PED demonstrated a total of six (1.6%) periprocedural ischemic events[64], but there are no data about postprocedural ischemic events. In the results from the "Pipeline for uncoilable or failed aneurysms" trial, which is a multicenter trial[65], we observe that intraprocedural ischemic stroke was present in three (2.8%) patients, whereas no such cases were noted to be postprocedural.

According to Silk data, postprocedural or delayed (occurring past 7 days) rupture of aneurysm was observed in 10 cases in which flow diverters were used (3.5%)[62]. In the Italian multicenter experience, the occurrence of hemorrhagic events when using the Silk stent was a total of 15 (5.4%)[63], whereas in the patients treated with PED it was 10 (2.7%). Seven (2.6%) cases of aneurysm rupture were considered intraprocedural, while the remaining cases were attributed to the device. The report from the early postmarket result from the United States multicenter study with PED[64] demonstrated a total of four (6.9%) post-operative hemorrhages, but there is no intraprocedural hemorrhage noted. According to the "Pipeline for uncoilable or failed aneurysms"[65] trial, intraprocedural hemorrhage rupture was observed in two (1.9%) patients, whereas no such cases were noted to be postprocedural.

Carotid-cavernous fistula occurred in 2 of 44 patients treated with the Pipeline device in the "Pipeline for uncoilable or failed aneurysms" trial[65]. The aneurysmal segment of the ICA is vulnerable to perforation by flow diversion, mechanical distension, or device manipulation. If the source of the fistula can be identified in the aneurysmal wall, it may be necessary to obliterate the segment of origin by using coil placement. If the source is identified within the parent artery, the operator may consider placing a covered stent across the arterial segment. If neither step is possible, parent arterial occlusion may be required after assessment of tolerance to such an occlusion and status of collateral circulation. Temporary balloon occlusion testing may be required in the same settings to confirm tolerance to parent artery occlusion. A transvenous approach may be possible by obliter-ation of the cavernous sinus, but this is difficult in settings of arterial procedure and perforation of parent artery or aneurysmal segment. Carotid-cavernous fistula has been reported with intracranial angioplasty in a patient with high grade stenosis of the left cavernous ICA due to perforation[65]. A coronary stent was used to treat the fistula.

In one study of treated aneurysms[66], a SILK flow diverter (Balt Extrusion, Montmor-ency, France) was used in 16 patients (47%, single device in 15) and the Pipeline emboliza-tion device (ev3/Covidien, Fremont, CA) was used in 18 (53%, single device in 16). In-stent stenosis was observed in 38% of SILK devices and 39% of Pipeline devices on follow-up angiography and was asymptomatic in 12 of 13 patients. One woman presented with transient ischemic attacks and required stent angioplasty due to end tapering and mild, diffuse in-stent stenosis.

Table 2.5 Complications associated with the SILK flow diverter[62]

Stroke	22 (7.7%)
TIA	7 (2.5%)
ICH	4 (1.4%)
Parent artery occlusion	29 (10.2)
In-stent thrombosis	17 (4.9%)
Aneurysm	10 (3.5%)
Mortality	14 (4.9%)
Periprocedural complications	36 (12.5%)
Delayed complications	28 (9.9%)

ICH: intracerebral hemorrhage; TIA: transient ischemic attack

Table 2.6 Clinical complications with the SILK device in Italian multicenter experience[63]

Clinical complications	Class of complications		Clinical outcome		
	Procedure-related	Device-related	Silent	Clinical sign	Death
Ischemic events	4	4	1	5	2
Hemorrhagic events	3	2	-	1	4
Hydrocephalus	1	-	-	-	1
Total	8	6	1	6	7

Table 2.7 Clinical complications with the Pipeline embolization device in Italian multicenter experience[63]

Clinical complications	Class of complications		Clinical outcome		
	Procedure-related	Device-related	Silent	Clinical sign	Death
Ischemic events	-	5	-	2	3
Hemorrhagic events	4	6	2	2	6
Hydrocephalus	-	-	-	-	-
Total	4	11	2	4	9

Table 2.8 Clinical complications with the Pipeline embolization device in a US multicenter experience[64]

Total PED procedures	62
Aneurysms treated	58
Total number of PED deployed	123
Major complication rate (permanent disability or death resulting from perioperative or delayed complication)	8.5%
Periprocedural TEEs (transient ischemic attack or stroke)	6 (1.6%)
Fatal postoperative hemorrhages	4 (6.9%)
Flow-limiting distal in-stent stenosis identified on follow-up angiograms	2 (0.3%)

PED, Pipeline embolization device

Aneurysms with special circumstances

Very small intracranial aneurysms

See Figure 2.11. Very small aneurysms are those that are 3 mm or less in their largest diameter and are more commonly seen in the anterior communicating artery[67]. They were not studied in the International Subarachnoid Aneurysm Trial (ISAT); however, they have been associated with an increased risk of intraprocedural rupture based on several reports.

Table 2.9 Serious adverse events in the "Pipeline for uncoilable or failed aneurysms" trial: results from multicenter trial[65]

Amaurosis fugax	5 (4.7)
Headache	5 (4.7)
Intracranial hemorrhage	5 (4.7)
Non-neurologic bleeding	5 (4.7)
Ischemic stroke	4 (3.7)
Cardiac arrhythmia	3 (2.8)
Dizziness or tinnitus	2 (1.9)
Carotid cavernous fistula	2 (1.9)
Carotid occlusion; patient also counted as ischemic stroke	1 (0.9)
Cilioretinal artery embolism	1 (0.9)
Diplopia	1 (0.9)
Possible intracranial hemorrhage	1 (0.9)
Colitis	1 (0.9)
Deep venous thrombosis	1 (0.9)
Lightheadedness or palpitations	1 (0.9)
Lung cancer	1 (0.9)
Pulmonary embolism	1 (0.9)
Rectovaginal fistula	1 (0.9)
Recurrent breast cancer	1 (0.9)
Pneumonia or urinary tract infection	1 (0.9)
Visual field worsened	1 (0.9)
Total number of patients (out of 107)	44

In a meta-analysis, intraprocedural rupture was noted, ranging from 5% in previously unruptured to around 10% in previously ruptured aneurysms, with an associated mortality of 1.2% and 3.1% respectively[68]. Interestingly, it appears that balloon assistance, with a balloon catheter placed at the neck level that can quickly be inflated once perforation is suspected, offers a favorable outcome, likely by prevention of blood extravasation[69]. On the other hand, the rate of recanalization in successfully treated very small aneurysms is very low, with only 5.4% needing retreatment[68].

An important technical consideration in the treatment of these very small aneurysms is that the distal tips of different microcatheters extend by different distances beyond their radiopaque markers. It is crucial to be familiar with the devices to be used when planning endovascular treatment[70].

Patients with very small aneurysms are a population at risk for intraprocedural rupture. Risk and benefits should be well balanced prior to treatment, especially in unruptured aneurysms given the reported natural history[71].

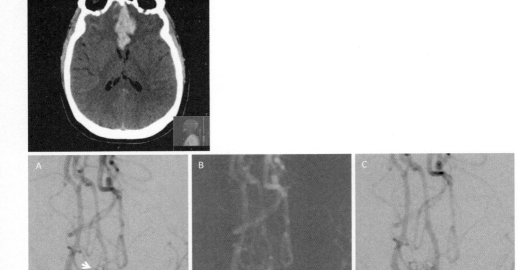

Figure 2.11 A 49-year-old woman who presented with Hunt and Hess grade 1 subarachnoid hemorrhage and a flame-like intraparenchymal hemorrhage (top left image). **A:** Cerebral angiography demonstrated 1.5 mm anterior communicating artery aneurysm. **B:** The patient underwent endovascular coil embolization: note the Excelsior SL-10 (Boston Scientific, Natick, MA) microcatheter within the aneurysm, the radiopaque marker and distal end of the aneurysm. **C:** Final image after a single Helical HyperSoft 1.5 mm × 1 cm coil (MicroPlex; MicroVention, Aliso Viejo, CA).

Peripheral aneurysms

See Figure 2.12. Distal or peripheral aneurysms are infrequent. Morphologically they can be fusiform or saccular; however, when saccular, the neck is usually wide and not necessarily arising from a branching point. In pathological studies, the most common findings are vessel wall injury with dissection and pseudoaneurysm formation[72]. Etiologies associated include infection, cancer, trauma, radiation, and connective tissue and autoimmune disorders. Surgical and endovascular approaches have been reported. Inability to catheterize the aneurysm adequately may lead to technical complications including aneurysm rupture[73,74]. Retention of the coil mass within the aneurysm may be difficult owing to the width of the neck. At present, other supportive coiling techniques, with balloon remodeling technique or stent placement, are not able to treat peripheral aneurysms, owing to the small caliber of the vessel lumen. Non-selective embolization includes parent vessel occlusion, detachable coils, glue, autologous blood clot, and detachable balloons; all have been used successfully without resultant ischemic consequences owing to the presence of

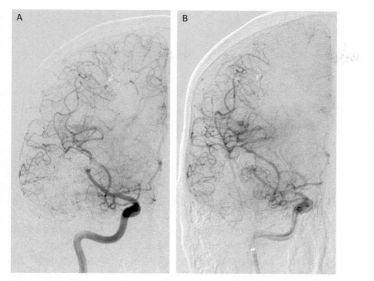

Figure 2.12 A 50-year-old man who presented 3 days after stent-assisted coil embolization of a right middle cerebral artery (MCA) aneurysm with elevated blood pressure and complaints of left arm weakness. Cerebral angiogram demonstrated a 1.3 mm dilation in a right frontal M4 branch of the MCA (A). This was suggestive of a distal dissecting aneurysm that was not seen on previous angiography or brain MRI. Follow-up cerebral angiogram next day showed aneurysm interval enlargement to 2.6 mm × 2.9 mm. A Marathon (ev3, Irvine, CA) microcatheter was advanced over a Synchro 10 (Boston Scientific) microwire into the right MCA frontal M4 branch and embolization was performed using Onyx-18 (ev3, Irvine, CA). The Onyx cast covered the aneurysm and distal and proximal segments of the parent artery to ensure complete parent vessel occlusion (B). The microcatheter was removed, and a follow-up guide run demonstrated no filling of the aneurysm. Patient had good clinical recovery.

leptomeningeal collaterals[75]. Onyx embolization of distal intracranial aneurysms of both the anterior and posterior circulation (M2, M3, and P3 branches) has also been reported[76].

Wide neck bifurcation aneurysms

The classic locations for bifurcation aneurysms sharing the neck with two other vessels are the tip of the basilar/middle cerebral artery bifurcation and some anterior communicating aneurysms. The presence of a wide neck in these locations adds difficulty to the embolization technique. Coil protrusion may occur not only into the parent vessel but also into the bifurcating arteries. A single high-compliance balloon may be sufficient to protect the entire neck and adjacent arteries in a single position[39] or in sequential mode[29]. Different techniques using two balloons or stents, such as the "kissing balloon" technique, "Y" stent reconstruction, "X" configuration stents, and balloon and stent reconstruction have been reported[77–80]. All these endovascular techniques require larger guide support and/or contralateral vessel catheterization.

There have been several cases reporting on closed-cell stent migration in the posterior circulation. The stents were used for coil assistance or flow diversion. The closed-cell design may lead to transmission of forces from the constricted distal end. A discrepancy in luminal diameter between the distal and proximal vessel may result in a constant retrograde force that ultimately moves the stent to a more stable position. The closed-cell design, in conjunction with the angulation of the junction between the P1 vessels and basilar artery, and bending stiffness of the stent, increase forces in a "watermelon seed" fashion, favoring proximal migration of the stent[81,82].

Need for aneurysm re-treatment

Recurrence following endovascular treatment of intracranial aneurysm can be seen in more than one in four treated aneurysms in some case series[83–85]. Most aneurysm recurrences are detected within 6 months of endovascular treatment[83,85,86]. Recurrence is identified from new contrast opacification of neck and/or fundus of a previously treated aneurysm. The mechanism that leads to recurrence is unclear but both coil compaction or aneurysm regrowth have been proposed as potential mechanisms. Coil compaction results from a decrease of interspaces between the loops of the coils. It leads to a smaller coil mesh or coil mass volume, whereas aneurysm regrowth is due to overall increase in aneurysm volume without coil compaction[87].

In one study[88], the pre-, intra-, and postprocedural angiograms were reviewed to confirm and categorize the angiographic severity of aneurysm recurrence. Aneurysm recurrences were stratified according to the Raymond classification[89]. Analyze 9.0 Software (Mayo Clinic, MN) was used to differentiate aneurysm regrowth versus coil compaction in all patients with aneurysm recurrence. The pixel size of the coil mass and aneurysm sac, and the adjacent parent artery, were measured using the Analyze Software. To avoid errors associated with absolute measurements on different images, the pixel sizes of the areas of the coil mass and aneurysmal sac were expressed as a ratio to the pixel sizes of the parent vessel diameter on immediate postprocedural and follow-up angiograms. Increase of aneurysm area or decrease in coil mass of 30% or greater on follow-up angiogram was used to define "aneurysm growth" and "coil compaction," respectively.

A total of 120 ruptured and 92 unruptured intracranial aneurysms in 201 patients were treated using endovascular embolization at our institutions during the selected period. Of these 201 patients, 29 patients had aneurysm recurrence at mean follow-up of 9.1 (±6.3) months; 24 of the 29 patients had subarachnoid hemorrhage as the presenting symptom, 3 had diplopia, and in 1 patient the aneurysm was incidentally found on MRI acquired for investigation of ischemic stroke. After initial treatment, complete aneurysm occlusion was achieved in 12 of the 29 patients, 9 had neck remnants, and 8 had subtotal occlusion detected in the immediate postprocedural angiogram. Of the 29 patients with aneurysm recurrence, 11 (38%) had coil compaction and 18 (62%) had aneurysm growth based on our criteria. Four patients had stent-assisted and one had balloon-assisted coil embolization. There were no patients with both aneurysm growth and coil compaction. Retreatment was performed in 15 of the 18 patients with aneurysm growth, and 8 of the 11 patients with coil compaction. There were no events of new aneurysmal rupture in the 11 patients who had coil compaction or the 18 patients who had aneurysm growth over a mean follow-up period of 22 months (range of 9–42 months).

It is known that aneurysm recurrence rates are higher than aneurysm rebleeding rates[90,91]. Therefore, the clinical significance of aneurysm recurrence is not well understood. Rebleeding after aneurysm recurrence has been reported to be 0.2–7.9%[83,84,90–92]. Byrne et al. reported rebleeding rates of 0.4% and 7.9% for stable and unstable aneurysmal remnants after endovascular treatment[91]. Late rebleeding for aneurysms adequately occluded at 6 month follow-up was found to be 2.5%[93]. We propose that rebleeding events in different series could be explained by the different contributions of coil compaction and aneurysm regrowth in those series. Coil compaction would theoretically pose little or no risk of rebleeding while aneurysm regrowth would indicate instability within the aneurysm wall and thus greater vulnerability to rupture.

Selection of patients with aneurysm recurrence who require retreatment is based on anecdotal evidence. In patients who have a new aneurysm rupture associated with aneurysm recurrence, retreatment is strongly suggested. A lower threshold for treatment is maintained in those with recurrence after treatment for a ruptured intracranial aneurysm. Retreatment options vary between placement of additional coils, stent placement and additional coil deployment, and placement of flow diverters. Additional coil deployment without placement of stent or flow diverter is probably a suboptimal option in most instances of aneurysm recurrence. The option selected depends upon the aneurysm morphology, ability to achieve high density of coil mass without a stent, and stability of additional coils within the aneurysm sac. Because the aneurysm recurrence provides a small and irregular cavity, stable microcatheter placement and subsequent coil insertion can be challenging. Therefore, stent placement should be considered to provide an adequate platform for microcatheter and coil insertion. Dual antiplatelet medication (aspirin and clopidogrel), at least 5 days prior to planned retreatment, should be strongly considered.

Postprocedure care after endovascular aneurysm embolization

Last but not least is the postprocedure management. Depending on how the procedure has gone, one can predict and foresee further complications. Most patients will spend an overnight stay in the critical care unit, for frequent neurological assessment and hemodynamic monitoring. It is crucial to detect neurological changes so they can quickly be addressed. The onset of a new neurological deficit should prompt neuroimaging to rule out hemorrhage. Blood pressure management is also of importance, especially in those patients with coil migration or vessel occlusion that may depend on perfusion pressure and/or collateral circulation.

References

1. Brinjikji W, Rabinstein AA, Nasr DM, *et al.* Better outcomes with treatment by coiling relative to clipping of unruptured intracranial aneurysms in the United States, 2001–2008. *AJNR American Journal of Neuroradiology* 2011;32:1071–5.

2. Andaluz N, Zuccarello M. Recent trends in the treatment of cerebral aneurysms: analysis of a nationwide inpatient database. *Journal of Neurosurgery* 2008;108:1163–9.

3. Vinuela F, Duckwiler G, Mawad M. Guglielmi detachable coil embolization of acute intracranial aneurysm: perioperative anatomical and clinical outcome in 403 patients. *Journal of Neurosurgery* 1997;86:475–82.

4. Brilstra EH, Rinkel GJE, van der Graaf Y, van Rooij WJJ, Algra A. Treatment of intracranial aneurysms by embolization with coils: a systematic review. *Stroke; A Journal of Cerebral Circulation* 1999;30:470–6.

5. Pierot L, Cognard C, Anxionnat R, Ricolfi F, Investigators C. Ruptured intracranial aneurysms: factors affecting the rate and outcome of endovascular treatment complications in a series of 782 patients (CLARITY study). *Radiology* 2010;256:916–23.

6. Murphy K. ISAT and ISUIA: the impact on informed consent. *Techniques in Vascular And Interventional Radiology* 2005;8:106–7.

7. Meyers PM, Schumacher HC, Higashida RT, *et al.* Reporting standards for

endovascular repair of saccular intracranial cerebral aneurysms. *Stroke; A Journal of Cerebral Circulation* 2009;40:e366–79.

8. van Rooij WJ, Sprengers ME, de Gast AN, Peluso JP, Sluzewski M. 3D rotational angiography: the new gold standard in the detection of additional intracranial aneurysms. *AJNR American Journal of Neuroradiology* 2008;29:976–9.

9. Wiebers DO, Whisnant JP, Huston J 3rd, *et al.* Unruptured intracranial aneurysms: natural history, clinical outcome, and risks of surgical and endovascular treatment. *Lancet* 2003;362:103–10.

10. Ogilvy CS, Yang X, Jamil OA, *et al.* Neurointerventional procedures for unruptured intracranial aneurysms under procedural sedation and local anesthesia: a large-volume, single-center experience. *Journal of Neurosurgery* 2011;114:120–8.

11. Kan P, Jahshan S, Yashar P, *et al.* Feasibility, safety, and periprocedural complications associated with endovascular treatment of selected ruptured aneurysms under conscious sedation and local anesthesia. *Neurosurgery* 2013;72:216–20; discussion 20.

12. Qureshi AI, Suri MF, Khan J, *et al.* Endovascular treatment of intracranial aneurysms by using Guglielmi detachable coils in awake patients: safety and feasibility. *Journal of Neurosurgery* 2001;94:880–5.

13. Cronqvist M, Wirestam R, Ramgren B, *et al.* Diffusion and perfusion MRI in patients with ruptured and unruptured intracranial aneurysms treated by endovascular coiling: complications, procedural results, MR findings and clinical outcome. *Neuroradiology* 2005;47:855–73.

14. Klotzsch C, Nahser HC, Henkes H, Kuhne D, Berlit P. Detection of microemboli distal to cerebral aneurysms before and after therapeutic embolization. *AJNR American Journal of Neuroradiology* 1998;19:1315–8.

15. Nishikawa Y, Satow T, Takagi T, *et al.* Efficacy and safety of single versus dual antiplatelet therapy for coiling of unruptured aneurysms. *Journal of Stroke and Cerebrovascular Diseases: The Official Journal of National Stroke Association* 2013;22:650–5.

16. White JB, Ken CG, Cloft HJ, Kallmes DF. Coils in a nutshell: a review of coil physical properties. *AJNR American Journal of Neuroradiology* 2008;29:1242–6.

17. Cloft HJ, Kallmes DF. Cerebral aneurysm perforations complicating therapy with Guglielmi detachable coils: a meta-analysis. *AJNR American Journal of Neuroradiology* 2002;23:1706–9.

18. Tummala RP, Chu RM, Madison MT, *et al.* Outcomes after aneurysm rupture during endovascular coil embolization. *Neurosurgery* 2001;49:1059–66; discussion 66–7.

19. Khatri R, Chaudhry SA, Rodriguez GJ, *et al.* Frequency and factors associated with unsuccessful lead (first) coil placement in patients undergoing coil embolization of intracranial aneurysms. *Neurosurgery* 2013;72:452–8; discussion 8.

20. Ding D, Liu KC. Management strategies for intraprocedural coil migration during endovascular treatment of intracranial aneurysms. *Journal of Neurointerventional Surgery*, doi:10.1136/neurintsurg-2013-010872 2013.

21. Luo CB, Chang FC, Teng MM, Guo WY, Chang CY. Stent management of coil herniation in embolization of internal carotid aneurysms. *AJNR American Journal of Neuroradiology* 2008;29:1951–5.

22. Abdihalim M, Kim SH, Maud A *et al.* Short- and intermediate-term angiographic and clinical outcomes of patients with various grades of coil protrusions following embolization of intracranial aneurysms. *AJNR American Journal of Neuroradiology* 2011;32:1392–8.

23. Pelz DM, Lownie SP, Fox AJ. Thromboembolic events associated with the treatment of cerebral aneurysms with Guglielmi detachable coils. *AJNR American Journal of Neuroradiology* 1998;19:1541–7.

24. Lanzino G, Wakhloo AK, Fessler RD, *et al.* Efficacy and current limitations of intravascular stents for intracranial internal carotid, vertebral, and basilar artery

aneurysms. *Journal of Neurosurgery* 1999;91:538–46.

25. Fessler RD, Ringer AJ, Qureshi AI, Guterman LR, Hopkins LN. Intracranial stent placement to trap an extruded coil during endovascular aneurysm treatment: technical note. *Neurosurgery* 2000;46:248–51; discussion 51–3.

26. Dinc H, Kuzeyli K, Kosucu P, Sari A, Cekirge S. Retrieval of prolapsed coils during endovascular treatment of cerebral aneurysms. *Neuroradiology* 2006;48:269–72.

27. Kwon OK, Kim SH, Kwon BJ, et al. Endovascular treatment of wide-necked aneurysms by using two microcatheters: techniques and outcomes in 25 patients. *AJNR American Journal of Neuroradiology* 2005;26:894–900.

28. Fourie P, Duncan IC. Microsnare-assisted mechanical removal of intraprocedural distal middle cerebral arterial thromboembolism. *AJNR American Journal of Neuroradiology* 2003;24:630–2.

29. Khatri R, Cordina SM, Hassan AE, Grigoryan M, Rodriguez GJ. Sequential sidelong balloon remodeling technique in coil embolization of a wide-necked basilar tip aneurysm. *Journal of Vascular and Interventional Neurology* 2013;6:7–9.

30. Sugiu K, Martin JB, Jean B, Rufenacht DA. Rescue balloon procedure for an emergency situation during coil embolization for cerebral aneurysms. Technical note. *Journal of Neurosurgery* 2002;96:373–6.

31. Tong FC, Cloft HJ, Dion JE. Endovascular treatment of intracranial aneurysms with Guglielmi Detachable Coils: emphasis on new techniques. *Journal of Clinical Neuroscience: Official Journal of the Neurosurgical Society of Australasia* 2000;7:244–53.

32. Liu KC, Ding D, Starke RM, Geraghty SR, Jensen ME. Intraprocedural retrieval of migrated coils during endovascular aneurysm treatment with the Trevo Stentriever device. *Journal of Clinical Neuroscience: Official Journal of the Neurosurgical Society of Australasia* 2014;21:503–6.

33. Henkes H, Lowens S, Preiss H, et al. A new device for endovascular coil retrieval from intracranial vessels: alligator retrieval device. *AJNR American Journal of Neuroradiology* 2006;27:327–9.

34. Fiorella D, Kelly ME, Moskowitz S, Masaryk TJ. Delayed symptomatic coil migration after initially successful balloon-assisted aneurysm coiling: technical case report. *Neurosurgery* 2009;64:E391–2; discussion E2.

35. Haraguchi K, Houkin K, Nonaka T, Baba T. Delayed thromboembolic infarction associated with reconfiguration of Guglielmi detachable coils–case report. *Neurologia Medico-chirurgica (Tokyo)* 2007;47:79–82.

36. Banerjee AD, Guimaraens L, Cuellar H. Asymptomatic delayed coil migration from an intracranial aneurysm: a case report. *Case Reports in Vascular Medicine* 2011;2011:901925.

37. Gao BL, Li MH, Wang YL, Fang C. Delayed coil migration from a small wide-necked aneurysm after stent-assisted embolization: case report and literature review. *Neuroradiology* 2006;48:333–7.

38. Hopf-Jensen S, Hensler HM, Preiss M, Muller-Hulsbeck S. Solitaire(R) stent for endovascular coil retrieval. *Journal of Clinical Neuroscience: Official Journal of the Neurosurgical Society of Australasia* 2013;20:884–6.

39. Wang C, Xie X. Treatment of an unraveled intracerebral coil. *Catheterization and Cardiovascular Interventions: Official Journal of the Society for Cardiac Angiography & Interventions* 2010;76:746–50.

40. Qureshi AI, Luft AR, Sharma M, Guterman LR, Hopkins LN. Prevention and treatment of thromboembolic and ischemic complications associated with endovascular procedures: Part II–Clinical aspects and recommendations. *Neurosurgery* 2000;46:1360–75; discussion 75–6.

41. Raschke RA, Reilly BM, Guidry JR, Fontana JR, Srinivas S. The weight-based heparin dosing nomogram compared with a "standard care" nomogram.

A randomized controlled trial. *Annals of Internal Medicine* 1993;119:874–81.

42. Jeong HW, Jin SC. Intra-arterial infusion of a glycoprotein IIb/IIIa antagonist for the treatment of thromboembolism during coil embolization of intracranial aneurysm: a comparison of Abciximab and tirofiban. *AJNR American Journal of Neuroradiology* 2013;34:1621–5.

43. Aggour M, Pierot L, Kadziolka K, Gomis P, Graftieaux JP. Abciximab treatment modalities for thromboembolic events related to aneurysm coiling. *Neurosurgery* 2010;67:503–8.

44. Ries T, Siemonsen S, Grzyska U, Zeumer H, Fiehler J. Abciximab is a safe rescue therapy in thromboembolic events complicating cerebral aneurysm coil embolization: single center experience in 42 cases and review of the literature. *Stroke; A Journal of Cerebral Circulation* 2009;40:1750–7.

45. Moret J, Cognard C, Weill A, Castaings L, Rey A. The "Remodelling Technique" in the treatment of wide neck intracranial aneurysms. angiographic results and clinical follow-up in 56 cases. *Interventional Neuroradiology: Journal of Peritherapeutic Neuroradiology, Surgical Procedures and Related Neurosciences* 1997;3:21–35.

46. Sluzewski M, van Rooij WJ, Beute GN, Nijssen PC. Balloon-assisted coil embolization of intracranial aneurysms: incidence, complications, and angiography results. *Journal of Neurosurgery* 2006;105:396–9.

47. Pierot L, Spelle L, Vitry F, Investigators A. Immediate clinical outcome of patients harboring unruptured intracranial aneurysms treated by endovascular approach: results of the ATENA study. *Stroke; A Journal of Cerebral Circulation* 2008;39:2497–504.

48. Baldi S, Mounayer C, Piotin M, Spelle L, Moret J. Balloon-assisted coil placement in wide-neck bifurcation aneurysms by use of a new, compliant balloon microcatheter. *AJNR American Journal of Neuroradiology* 2003;24:1222–5.

49. Higashida RT, Smith W, Gress D, *et al.* Intravascular stent and endovascular coil placement for a ruptured fusiform aneurysm of the basilar artery. Case report and review of the literature. *Journal of Neurosurgery* 1997;87:944–9.

50. Kim BM, Kim DJ, Kim DI. Stent application for the treatment of cerebral aneurysms. *Neurointervention* 2011;6:53–70.

51. Krischek O, Miloslavski E, Fischer S, Shrivastava S, Henkes H. A comparison of functional and physical properties of self-expanding intracranial stents [Neuroform3, Wingspan, Solitaire, Leo+, Enterprise]. *Minimally Invasive Neurosurgery: MIN* 2011;54:21–8.

52. Biondi A, Janardhan V, Katz JM, *et al.* Neuroform stent-assisted coil embolization of wide-neck intracranial aneurysms: strategies in stent deployment and midterm follow-up. *Neurosurgery* 2007;61:460–8; discussion 8–9.

53. Tahtinen OI, Vanninen RL, Manninen HI, *et al.* Wide-necked intracranial aneurysms: treatment with stent-assisted coil embolization during acute (<72 hours) subarachnoid hemorrhage–experience in 61 consecutive patients. *Radiology* 2009;253:199–208.

54. Piotin M, Blanc R, Spelle L, *et al.* Stent-assisted coiling of intracranial aneurysms: clinical and angiographic results in 216 consecutive aneurysms. *Stroke; A Journal of Cerebral Circulation* 2010;41:110–5.

55. Connolly ES, Jr., Rabinstein AA, Carhuapoma JR, *et al.* Guidelines for the management of aneurysmal subarachnoid hemorrhage: a guideline for healthcare professionals from the American Heart Association/American Stroke Association. *Stroke; A Journal of Cerebral Circulation* 2012;43:1711–37.

56. Weber W, Siekmann R, Kis B, Kuehne D. Treatment and follow-up of 22 unruptured wide-necked intracranial aneurysms of the internal carotid artery with Onyx HD 500. *AJNR American Journal of Neuroradiology* 2005;26:1909–15.

57. Piske RL, Kanashiro LH, Paschoal E, *et al.* Evaluation of Onyx HD-500 embolic system in the treatment of 84 wide-neck intracranial aneurysms. *Neurosurgery* 2009;64:E865–75; discussion E75.

58. Simon SD, Lopes DK, Mericle RA. Use of intracranial stenting to secure unstable liquid embolic casts in wide-neck sidewall intracranial aneurysms. *Neurosurgery* 2010;66:92–7; discussion 7–8.

59. Colby GP, Lin LM, Huang J, Tamargo RJ, Coon AL. Utilization of the Navien distal intracranial catheter in 78 cases of anterior circulation aneurysm treatment with the Pipeline embolization device. *Journal of Neurointerventional Surgery* 2013;5 Suppl 3:iii16–21.

60. Crowley RW, Abla AA, Ducruet AF, McDougall CG, Albuquerque FC. Novel application of a balloon-anchoring technique for the realignment of a prolapsed Pipeline Embolization Device: a technical report. *Journal of Neurointerventional Surgery* 2014;6:439–44.

61. Hauck EF, Natarajan SK, Langer DJ, *et al.* Retrograde trans-posterior communicating artery snare-assisted rescue of lost access to a foreshortened pipeline embolization device: complication management. *Neurosurgery* 2010;67:495–502.

62. Murthy SB, Shah S, Shastri A, *et al.* The SILK flow diverter in the treatment of intracranial aneurysms. *Journal of Clinical Neuroscience: Official Journal of the Neurosurgical Society of Australasia* 2014;21:203–6.

63. Briganti F, Napoli M, Tortora F, *et al.* Italian multicenter experience with flow-diverter devices for intracranial unruptured aneurysm treatment with periprocedural complications–a retrospective data analysis. *Neuroradiology* 2012;54:1145–52.

64. Kan P, Siddiqui AH, Veznedaroglu E, *et al.* Early postmarket results after treatment of intracranial aneurysms with the pipeline embolization device: a U.S. multicenter experience. *Neurosurgery* 2012;71:1080–7; discussion 7–8.

65. Becske T, Kallmes DF, Saatci I, *et al.* Pipeline for uncoilable or failed aneurysms:

results from a multicenter clinical trial. *Radiology* 2013;267:858–68.

66. Cohen JE, Gomori JM, Moscovici S, Leker RR, Itshayek E. Delayed complications after flow-diverter stenting: Reactive in-stent stenosis and creeping stents. *Journal of Clinical Neuroscience: Official Journal of the Neurosurgical Society of Australasia* 2014;21:1116–22.

67. Ioannidis I, Lalloo S, Corkill R, Kuker W, Byrne JV. Endovascular treatment of very small intracranial aneurysms. *Journal of Neurosurgery* 2010;112:551–6.

68. Brinjikji W, Lanzino G, Cloft HJ, Rabinstein A, Kallmes DF. Endovascular treatment of very small (3 mm or smaller) intracranial aneurysms: report of a consecutive series and a meta-analysis. *Stroke; A Journal of Cerebral Circulation* 2010;41:116–21.

69. Nguyen TN, Raymond J, Guilbert F, *et al.* Association of endovascular therapy of very small ruptured aneurysms with higher rates of procedure-related rupture. *Journal of Neurosurgery* 2008;108:1088–92.

70. Lim YC, Kim BM, Shin YS, Kim SY, Chung J. Structural limitations of currently available microcatheters and coils for endovascular coiling of very small aneurysms. *Neuroradiology* 2008;50:423–7.

71. Greving JP, Wermer MJH, Brown RD, et al. Development of the PHASES score for prediction of risk of rupture of intracranial aneurysms: a pooled analysis of six prospective cohort studies. *The Lancet Neurology* 2014;13:59–66.

72. Saito A, Fujimura M, Inoue T, Shimizu H, Tominaga T. Lectin-like oxidized low-density lipoprotein receptor 1 and matrix metalloproteinase expression in ruptured and unruptured multiple dissections of distal middle cerebral artery: case report. *Acta Neurochirurgica* 2010;152:1235–40.

73. Bradac GB, Bergui M. Endovascular treatment of the posterior inferior cerebellar artery aneurysms. *Neuroradiology* 2004;46:1006–11.

74. Isokangas JM, Siniluoto T, Tikkakoski T, Kumpulainen T. Endovascular treatment of peripheral aneurysms of the posterior

inferior cerebellar artery. *AJNR American Journal of Neuroradiology* 2008;29:1783–8.

75. Baltacioglu F, Cekirge S, Saatci I, *et al.* Distal middle cerebral artery aneurysms. Endovascular treatment results with literature review. *Interventional Neuroradiology: Journal of Peritherapeutic Neuroradiology, Surgical Procedures and Related Neurosciences* 2002;8:399–407.

76. Zhao PC, Li J, He M, You C. Infectious intracranial aneurysm: endovascular treatment with onyx case report and review of the literature. *Neurology India* 2010;58:131–4.

77. Albuquerque FC, Gonzalez LF, Hu YC, Newman CB, McDougall CG. Transcirculation endovascular treatment of complex cerebral aneurysms: technical considerations and preliminary results. *Neurosurgery* 2011;68:820–9; discussion 9–30.

78. Arat A, Cil B. Double-balloon remodeling of wide-necked aneurysms distal to the circle of Willis. *AJNR American Journal of Neuroradiology* 2005;26:1768–71.

79. Kim BM, Kim DI, Park SI, *et al.* Coil embolization of unruptured middle cerebral artery aneurysms. *Neurosurgery* 2011;68:346–53; discussion 53–4.

80. Saatci I, Geyik S, Yavuz K, Cekirge S. X-configured stent-assisted coiling in the endovascular treatment of complex anterior communicating artery aneurysms: a novel reconstructive technique. *AJNR American Journal of Neuroradiology* 2011;32:E113–7.

81. Khatri R, Rodriguez GJ, Siddiq F, Tummala RP. Early migration of a self-expanding intracranial stent after the treatment of a basilar trunk aneurysm: report of a second case. *Neurosurgery* 2011;69:E513–5; author reply E5–7.

82. Rodriguez GJ, Maud A, Taylor RA. Another delayed migration of an enterprise stent. *AJNR American Journal of Neuroradiology* 2009;30:E57.

83. Raymond J, Guilbert F, Weill A, *et al.* Long-term angiographic recurrences after selective endovascular treatment of aneurysms with detachable coils. *Stroke; A Journal of Cerebral Circulation* 2003;34:1398–403.

84. Naggara ON, White PM, Guilbert F, *et al.* Endovascular treatment of intracranial unruptured aneurysms: systematic review and meta-analysis of the literature on safety and efficacy. *Radiology* 2010;256:887–97.

85. Li MH, Gao BL, Fang C, et al. Angiographic follow-up of cerebral aneurysms treated with Guglielmi detachable coils: an analysis of 162 cases with 173 aneurysms. *AJNR American Journal of Neuroradiology* 2006;27:1107–12.

86. Sluzewski M, van Rooij WJ, Rinkel GJ, Wijnalda D. Endovascular treatment of ruptured intracranial aneurysms with detachable coils: long-term clinical and serial angiographic results. *Radiology* 2003;227:720–4.

87. Sluzewski M, van Rooij WJ, Slob MJ, *et al.* Relation between aneurysm volume, packing, and compaction in 145 cerebral aneurysms treated with coils. *Radiology* 2004;231:653–8.

88. Abdihalim M, Watanabe M, Chaudhry SA, *et al.* Are coil compaction and aneurysmal growth two distinct etiologies leading to recurrence following endovascular treatment of intracranial aneurysm? *Journal of Neuroimaging: Official Journal of the American Society of Neuroimaging* 2013;24:171–5.

89. Wakhloo AK, Gounis MJ, Sandhu JS, *et al.* Complex-shaped platinum coils for brain aneurysms: higher packing density, improved biomechanical stability, and midterm angiographic outcome. *American Journal of Neuroradiology* 2007;28:1395–400.

90. Plowman RS, Clarke A, Clarke M, Byrne JV. Sixteen-year single-surgeon experience with coil embolization for ruptured intracranial aneurysms: recurrence rates and incidence of late rebleeding. Clinical article. *Journal of Neurosurgery* 2011;114:863–74.

91. Byrne JV, Sohn MJ, Molyneux AJ, Chir B. Five-year experience in using coil embolization for ruptured intracranial aneurysms: outcomes and incidence of late rebleeding. *Journal of Neurosurgery* 1999;90:656–63.

92. Sluzewski M, van Rooij WJ. Early rebleeding after coiling of ruptured cerebral aneurysms: incidence, morbidity, and risk factors. *American Journal of Neuroradiology* 2005;26:1739–43.

93. Ferns SP, Sprengers ME, van Rooij WJ, *et al.* Late reopening of adequately coiled intracranial aneurysms: frequency and risk factors in 400 patients with 440 aneurysms. *Stroke; A Journal of Cerebral Circulation* 2011;42:1331–7.

Chapter 3

Complications associated with embolization of arteriovenous malformations and fistulas

Hunar Kainth, Daraspreet Kainth, Karanpal Dhaliwal, Alberto Maud, and Adnan I. Qureshi

Basic principles of treatment of intracranial arteriovenous malformations

The basic principle of endovascular embolization procedures involves percutaneous entry into the femoral, radial, or brachial artery by use of a modification of Seldinger's technique[1,2]. Guide catheters or sheaths are introduced through the aorta into the supra-aortic vessel of interest. Microcatheters and balloon catheter devices are introduced through the guide catheter and guided to the target lesion with flexible microwires. Advanced designs of microcatheters including flow directed microcatheters have allowed highly selective delivery of coils and embolic materials into regions of interest.

In 1930, Brooks reported closure of a carotid-cavernous fistula with surgical introduction of muscle embolus in the carotid artery[3]. Luessenhop and colleagues subsequently reported embolization with silastic spheres and silk sutures introduced into the internal carotid artery to treat cerebral arteriovenous malformations (AVMs)[4]. Technical advances, such as flow directed and other specialized microcatheters and new embolic agents, have increased the therapeutic potential of embolization for cerebral AVMs. However, embolization of cerebral AVMs on its own is curative in less than a quarter of the lesions and is one aspect of a multimodality approach to these lesions.

Endovascular embolization has been utilized in treating AVMs for presurgical embolization to reduce blood loss, morbidity, and mortality. In addition, embolization can be utilized to reduce nidus size prior to radiosurgery, for palliation for symptomatic large non-surgical AVMs, and for embolization of aneurysms associated with AVMs. Palliative embolization to halt progression of symptoms for large non-surgical or non-radiosurgical AVMs has been utilized in patients presenting with progressive neurological deficit secondary to high flow or venous hypertension.

It should be noted that the role of embolization in treatment of AVMs is based mainly on results from observational studies[5]. Embolization is done by placing a microcatheter in the distal portion of an arterial feeder that exclusively supplies the AVM. Any normal branches are excluded on the basis of assessment of vessel architecture and sometimes physiological testing by injection of short-acting amobarbital sodium and lidocaine through the microcatheter.

Embolization is usually done through several arterial feeders. The goals of presurgical embolization are to decrease the nidus size and to occlude deep, surgically inaccessible or deep

Complications of Neuroendovascular Procedures and Bailout Techniques, ed. Rakesh Khatri, Gustavo J. Rodriguez, Jean Raymond and Adnan I. Qureshi. Published by Cambridge University Press.

arterial feeding vessels in large AVMs to facilitate surgical excision. With surgical embolization before excision, the malformation can be removed completely through surgery in up to 96% of patients. Two indirect comparisons have suggested that embolization before surgery can shorten the operative times, reduce intraoperative blood loss, and improve neurological outcomes in patients with complex AVMs such that they are comparable to those with less complex AVMs (i.e., not requiring embolization). The goals of pre-radiosurgical embolization are to decrease target size to <3 cm in diameter, as smaller lesions have a higher cure rate, and to eradicate angiographic predictors of hemorrhage, such as intranidal aneurysms.

In a study of 125 patients who were poor surgical candidates or who had refused surgery, embolization produced total occlusion in 11% of AVMs and reduced the volume in 76% of AVMs, to make radiosurgery possible. Radiosurgery produced total occlusion in 65% of the partly embolized AVMs[6].

Dural arteriovenous fistulas are derived from meningeal arteries and drain into dural sinuses or meningeal veins; they can have retrograde drainage into subarachnoid veins. Treatment includes transarterial, transvenous, or combined endovascular obliteration of the fistula by direct puncture of the affected sinus.

For successful transarterial embolization, the embolic agent must be delivered to obliterate the shunt between the arterial and venous drainage. However, this technique is not always feasible if there are multiple small feeding vessels that cannot be embolized. The risks of transarterial embolization include stroke from embolic agents entering normal blood vessels.

Transvenous embolization of dural arteriovenous fistulas (AVFs) can be achieved by embolization of the affected sinus. However, this can be challenging if the sinus involved also has normal venous drainage. Coil packing can be used to effectively occlude the involved sinus. In cases in which it is difficult to access the involved sinus, direct puncture techniques can be employed to treat dural AVFs. For example, direct puncture of the involved sinus can be achieved through a craniotomy. The risks include blood loss, infection, and air embolism. In other complex dural AVFs, a combination of the above techniques, such as combining transarterial and transvenous approaches, is required in order to obliterate the AVF.

In other instances, a stent can be placed to treat an AVF. This technique is performed to treat fistulas where placing a stent across the arterial vessel involved will obliterate the fistula. For example, in the case of a traumatic AVF involving the internal carotid artery and jugular vein, a stent can be placed across the carotid artery which will preserve flow and help obliterate the fistula.

The treatment of AVMs and fistulas requires evaluation on a case by case basis. However, basic principles guide the management of AVMs and fistulas. A patient's age, medical comorbidities, neurological status, angio-architecture, and prior treatments must be considered when making treatment decisions. The current treatment modalities include surgery, radiosurgery, and endovascular embolization.

Case 1

A 55-year-old man (Figure 3.1) who was admitted with a spontaneous intraventricular and subarachnoid hemorrhage. Computed tomography (CT) angiography and diagnostic cerebral angiography demonstrated the presence of a Borden type III right tentorial arteriovenous fistula with feeders from right occipital and right meningohypophyseal artery. He had successful embolization of right occipital feeders with good penetration into and reduction of the lateral aspect of the fistula. The fistula continued to fill from the right meningohypophyseal feeders, and he then underwent successful surgical disconnection of the fistula.

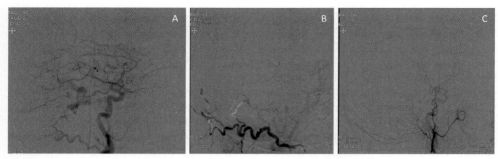

Figure 3.1 A: Pre embolization, B: post NBCA embolization of right occipital feeder, C: post surgical disconnection of the draining vein. No residual fistula present.

Spinal arteriovenous malformations: tips for proper embolization

Arteriovenous lesions of the spinal cord are intricate lesions. The complexity relates to the understanding of the vascular supply of the spinal of the cord and the spatial disposition. To avoid possible complications, it is important to understand the type of lesion to be treated.

Advances in the quality of catheter spinal angiography and microcatheterization of the spinal arteries allow physicians to better understand the angioarchitecture of these vascular lesions. The most common vascular malformation of the spinal cord is AVF followed by AVM. Although genetic hereditary (hereditary hemorrhagic telangiectasia) and non-hereditary diseases (Cobb's syndrome, Klippel–Trenaunay–Weber syndrome, and Parkes–Weber syndrome) can be associated with spinal cord vascular malformation, most of the AVFs affecting the spinal cord are believed to be acquired conditions[7,8].

Spinal cord arteriovenous fistula

Spinal cord arteriovenous fistulas (SCAVFs) can be classified into extradural and intradural according to the location of the fistula point.

Extradural (epidural) SCAVFs are rare, and the fistula point is located in the epidural venous plexus. Extension of SCAVF can go beyond the spine. In the cervical level the deep and ascending cervical arteries are common arterial feeders. In the thoracolumbar segment, arterial feeders arise from the segmental (intercostal and lumbar arteries). The dilated arterialized vein can sometimes compress the dura mater and cause compressive symptoms (myelopathy or radiculopathy). Because of the normal connections between the epidural and intradural venous plexus, the arterialized vein can extend into the coronal venous plexus of the spinal cord and simulate an intradural SCAVF. Extracranial SCAVF are almost exclusively amenable to endovascular treatment.

Intradural SCAVF comprises dural and pial AVF. They differ in the location of the fistula point and the draining vein as well as the arterial feeder.

Dural SCAVF is the most common type of spinal cord vascular malformation found in practice. They typically affect advanced age patients and are more common in men. The fistula point is located at or near the spinal nerve root and the arterial feeder arises from the posterior radicular branch of the segmental artery. The most common location is the thoracic segment. The fistula point contains one or multiple feeders but they are usually microscopic, and the spinal angiogram depicts an early engorged coronal draining vein arising from the fistula point. In general, dural SCAVF are slow flow fistulas, and the arterialization of the coronal venous plexus produces congestion in the dorsal aspect of the spinal cord. Dural SCAVF are successfully treated with surgical ligation of the fistula point. Presurgical embolization is a viable option.

Pial SCAVF involve an arterial feeder arising from the anterior spinal artery and occasionally from the posterior spinal artery. The fistula point is most often located in the ventral aspect of the spinal cord. These high flow fistulas can spontaneously bleed and cause a spinal cord hematoma or subarachnoid hemorrhage. The draining coronal and radicular veins are usually severely arterialized, and it is not uncommon to find aneurysmatic arterial and venous dilatations. The fistula point can occasionally contain dilated veins with glomerular appearance resembling a nidus (pseudonidus). During endovascular and surgical treatment of the pial SCAVF, the preservation of the anterior and posterior spinal arteries is crucial.

Conus medullaris SCAVF is one of the most complex forms of spinal vascular malformation. Fistulas in this particular point of the spinal cord can cause radicular symptoms due to compression of lumbar and sacral spinal roots. They can also bleed in the subarachnoid space of the spinal canal. Owing to the location of the fistula point at the conus medullaris arcade, multiple arterial feeders can contribute to the fistula point. Pial arteries, including the anterior and posterior spinal arteries, participate in the vascular supply of SCAVF in this location. The fistula point can have a nidus or pseudonidus appearance, and because of the reduced parenchymal surface it is sometime difficult to define an intra- or extra-axial location of the nidus. The venous drain is shared by coronal and radicular veins.

Spinal cord arteriovenous malformation

Spinal cord arteriovenous malformations (SCAVM) are relative rare congenital vascular conditions. The nidus of the AVM can be confined to the spinal cord tissue or can extend beyond its limits and involve extradural structures including bone and paravertebral muscles.

Intramedullary SCAVMs are similar to the intracranial AVMs. They are located entirely in the spinal cord parenchyma. The nidus of the lesion can be compact (glomus type) or can be diffuse, extending up and down through more than three metameres. Intramedullary SCAVMs tend to have high flow, and the anterior and posterior spinal arteries are the main arterial feeders. They have propensity to bleed and cause an acute spinal cord hematoma. Chronic symptoms are related to local compression or spinal cord ischemia related to arterial blood-flow steal phenomena. Presurgical embolization helps to reduce hemorrhagic complication during surgical removal. The compact forms are more amenable to complete surgical resection. Correct exposure of the lesion is crucial to obtain a complete surgical excision of the entire vascular lesion and minimize damage of the surrounding normal spinal cord.

Extradural–intradural SCAVMs are congenital genetic non-hereditary vascular lesions that affect the entire somite level. This particular SCAVM is also referred as Cobb's syndrome. They extend away from the spinal canal and involve bone, muscle, nerve roots, and skin. The treatment of these lesions requires a multidisciplinary approach that includes endovascular embolization and palliative surgery.

Physical and chemical properties and mechanism of action of embolic agents

A variety of embolic agents have been used for embolization[9]. Embolic materials are divided into solid or liquid agents. Solid agents consist of polyvinyl alcohol particles, fibers, microcoils, and microballoons. Liquid agents consist of cyanoacrylate monomers such as I-butyl cyanoacrylate and N-butyl cyanoacrylate, and polymer solutions such as ethylene vinyl alcohol. Solid embolic agents such as polyvinyl alcohol (PVA) particles can also be employed to embolize AVMs. To form PVA particles, polyvinyl acetate is hydroxylated to synthesize a highly soluble polymer. The PVA is crosslinked to provide structural stability. Its solubility is indirectly proportional to the amount of hydroxylation and polymerization. In the presence of fluids such as blood or water, the PVA forms a hydrogel. The amount of crosslinking present affects the physical, chemical, and diffusion properties of the polymer. PVA is a non-toxic substance that is heat stable and biocompatible. It works by adhering to vessel walls, thus occluding an AVM. Similar to N-butyl-2-cyanoacrylate (NBCA), PVA elicits an inflammatory response to the vessel wall as well.

Coils are another embolic agent used in embolizing AVMs. Stainless steel coils were originally developed for peripheral embolization and were then utilized to treat cerebrovascular lesions because of their thrombogenic properties. Stainless steel coils were then replaced by more pliable platinum microcoils. Guglielmi et al.[10] first described their experience with the use of detachable platinum coils in 1991. The softer platinum coils allowed better filling of small irregular spaces. Early coil designs were helical and two-dimensional, but this technology was advanced upon with the creation of three-dimensional coils that were spherical when deployed. A platinum coil is deployed through the catheter in a straight state; upon exiting, it returns to a coiled state. The exact mechanism of vessel occlusion induced by coils is not fully understood. Platinum coils are thrombogenic, and histology studies show early thrombus formation with the deployment of coils. Histopathological studies have demonstrated that over time, the intraluminal clot is replaced by fibrous tissue, followed by collagen-rich vascularized tissue surrounding the coils.

Cyanoacrylate monomers are another liquid agent that polymerize on contact with blood. NBCA and isobutyl-2-cyanoacrylate (IBCA) have hemostatic properties providing exceptionally adhesive strength, although this may lead to complications such as causing the catheter to become stuck during the procedure. Cyanoacrylates polymerize on contact with hydroxyl ions in blood. NBCA is mixed with lipiodal in various concentrations to alter the rate at which it will polymerize. In addition, tantalum powder can be added to increase radiopacity. The effects of these polymers are permanent, and thus they have a strong occlusive effect. The chronic inflammatory response induced in the embolized vessel is thought to play a role in the long-term vessel occlusion achieved by NBCA. In order to prevent NBCA from polymerizing in the catheter, the catheter is flushed with 5% dextrose solution before injection of the NBCA.

One agent commonly utilized is ethylene–vinyl alcohol copolymer (EVOH), known as Onyx (Micro Therapeutics, Irvine, CA), which is a non-adhesive non-absorbable liquid agent that is dissolved in dimethyl sulfoxide (DMSO) and tantalum. Tantalum powder is added for radiopacity[11–13]. It was described in 1990 by Taki et al. for use as an embolic agent for treatment of AVMs[14]. It was approved by the Food and Drug Administration (FDA) for presurgical embolization of brain AVMs in 2005. Onyx is available in various viscosities including Onyx 18 (6% EVOH) and Onyx 34 (8% EVOH). Onyx should be shaken for at least 20 minutes before injection to achieve homogenous radiopacity of the mixture. The density and viscosity of the mixtures are proportional to the concentration of EVOH. Precipitation times vary inversely to the concentration of EVOH. Contact with ionic agents such as saline and blood lead to the copolymerization of the Onyx. In order to use Onyx as an embolic agent, first the DMSO solvent is slowly injected into the micro-catheter, filling the dead space to prevent the Onyx from directly contacting blood. Once the Onyx is injected via the catheter, it comes in contact with blood, triggering the solidification process, starting from the exterior of the cast and moving inwards.

Technical complications

There are complications that are related to inadequate placement of microcatheter within the cervical segment. Such complications occur at the point of exit of the microcatheter from a guide catheter placed within the internal carotid artery or vertebral artery. Fre-quently, the operator is focusing on the distal aspect of microcatheter manipulation and navigation. The flow directed microcatheters, in particular because they are advanced without a microwire, tend to collapse at the point of exit from the guide catheter during forward motion of the microcatheter. Lack of responsiveness of the microcatheter to forward pushing, or limited availability of the proximal end of the microcatheter at point of entry into the guide catheter, may be the first indication of such an occurrence. It is imperative that the operator avoids such an occurrence prior to injection of the liquid embolic agent. Loops and tortuosity in the microcatheter lead to increase in resistance to injection of embolic agents, increasing the risk of catheter rupture. The microcatheter also lacks stability and is prone to retropulsion or forward propulsion during injection of embolic material. Therefore, such alterations in axis of the microcatheter should be detected early by intermittent visualization of the exit point from the guide catheter.

Arteriovenous malformations have three major components: arterial feeders; nidus; and venous drainage. The complications related to each of the components and their manage-ment will be described in the following sections.

Arterial feeders

There are six main complications that can occur during embolization that are located within the arterial component of the AVMs as described below:

Reflux into the feeding pedicle and parent artery

During embolization, care must be taken to monitor for reflux into the feeding pedicle or parent artery. Reflux carries the risk of occlusion of the parent vessel, as described in the case below, and increase the chance of adhesion of the microcatheter within the embolic material. Reflux should be minimized by controlled injections and pausing the injection when reflux is seen. Control over potential reflux can also be enhanced with the use of balloon catheter assistance.

(A) Plug and push technique with Onyx, using double or single catheter:

For the first catheter, a Marathon catheter (eV3, Irvine, CA) is placed into the feeding pedicle and the second catheter, usually an Echelon 10 (eV3) is placed in the feeding pedicle, alongside but proximal to the first. Always remember that both catheters must be Onyx compatible, and always plan the device compatibility prior to the procedure. This technique is usually used for a large arterial pedicle with a relatively straight course to avoid the entrapment of the distal microcatheter. Onyx 34 is used through the proximal microcatheter and a plug is formed, usually not more than 1 to 2 cm, or up to operator judgment. Onyx 18 is then injected through the distal microcatheter at a relatively faster rate to penetrate the nidus and then the rate is slowed to complete the obliteration of the nidus.

Some operators may form a plug with Onyx 34 and then push Onyx 18 distally through the same catheter. Care must be taken not to occlude the catheter tip while forming the plug.

(B) Double catheter technique with Onyx 18: For a small sized AVM without fistula and few afferent pedicles. Case series are available using the technique of double simultaneous arterial catheterization as an approach to achieve the complete exclusion of the nidus before reaching the venous drainage, through a more controlled hemodynamic filling. After the intranidal placement of both microcatheters, the first one is washed with 0.3 ml of DMSO, followed by the slow injection of Onyx for 40 seconds to fill the microcatheter lumen. Thereafter, under subtracted fluoroscopy, gradual injection of Onyx occurs, stopping when the first reflux of the material takes place. At this point the second microcatheter is used, with the same steps. As soon as the embolic agent is observed coming out of the second microcatheter, the injection through the first microcatheter is restarted (usually 2 minutes after the first break). The injection of Onyx is then performed simultaneously with a syringe in each hand. At every arterial reflux, the injection is interrupted for 1–2 minutes and then resumed. After the end of the injections, each microcatheter is gently stretched every 1–2 minutes. When the microcatheter acquires a tense and semirectified position, it is withdrawn with gentle short movements.

Case 2

A 31-year-old man with a 1.4 cm × 1.5 cm right temporal AVM with superficial venous drainage (Spetzler and Martin grade 1) was embolized with 30% NBCA following right temporal intracerebral hemorrhage evacuation and partial clipping (Figure 3.2). During embolization of the nidus through the right anterior temporal artery, the NBCA penetrated and obliterated the nidus, but reflux into the M1 trunk was noted. The microcatheter was removed and a glue fragment was found to be present in the M1 trunk. The patient underwent attempted MERCI thrombectomy and then entrapment of the glue fragment with an Enterprise stent, followed by angioplasty with restoration of flow along the length of the M1 segment. There was residual spasm distal to the stent in the anterior M2 segment as well as a paucity of distal MCA branches.

Arterial obliteration with little or no nidus obliteration

The ideal place for microcatheter placement is at the junction of medium-size arterial feeders and branching arterioles. Such positioning ensures that liquid embolic material is deposited in arteriolar and nidus component of the AVMs.

(A) If the microcatheter cannot be placed at the junction, the liquid embolic material may precipitate or polymerize predominantly within the arterial component of the AVMs. The other reason is premature precipitation or polymerization of N-butyl acrylate or Onyx liquid embolic material. Such premature precipitation or

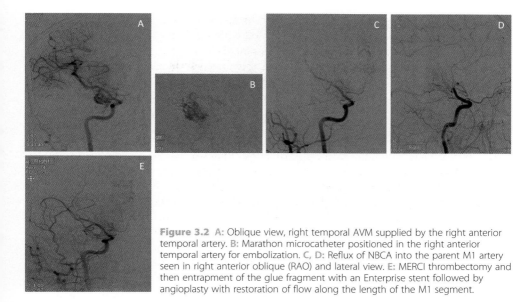

Figure 3.2 **A:** Oblique view, right temporal AVM supplied by the right anterior temporal artery. **B:** Marathon microcatheter positioned in the right anterior temporal artery for embolization. **C, D:** Reflux of NBCA into the parent M1 artery seen in right anterior oblique (RAO) and lateral view. **E:** MERCI thrombectomy and then entrapment of the glue fragment with an Enterprise stent followed by angioplasty with restoration of flow along the length of the M1 segment.

polymerization can occur if the injection is too slow or the concentration of the liquid embolic material is too high. Some operators add minor concentrations of glacial acetic acid to reduce the immediate alkaline pH allowing greater penetration of N-butyl acrylate.

(B) The consequence of arterial obliteration with little to no nidus obliteration is the patency of the nidus maintained through other arterial feeders and prevention of further embolization attempts if other feeders are not accessible to microcatheter placement. In such circumstances, the interventionalist may opt to attempt to access other feeders and if these attempts are not successful, abort the procedures. A second procedure may be attempted after a month: this has a higher likelihood of success following resolution of any arterial spasm and increase in diameter of the alternate feeders due to increased flow that may make them more amenable to catheterization.

In some unique situations, direct access of the feeder artery may be required if only the proximal access is compromised.

Appearance of the invisible artery

A major change occurs in the resistance of the outflow from the arterial side with obliteration of the nidus. Because of pressure increase, small arterial channels that were collapsed previously may become apparent during embolization. Sometimes these arterial channels are alternate feeders into the nidus or fistulas that bypass the nidus. Infrequently, the arterial channels may connect into other arteries that supply viable brain tissue. A high frame rate injection allows distinction of structures such as the high flow AVM, which has rapid contrast clearance, versus the normal flow and opacification of non-AVM arteries which are still visualized after contrast has cleared from the AVM nidus. The best option is to be aware of this occurrence and discontinue embolization at the first appearance of the

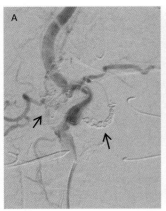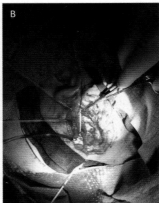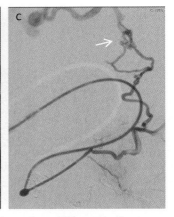

Figure 3.3 A 70-year-old female with past medical history of intracerebral hemorrhage (ICH) requiring hematoma evaluation and second episode 4 years later, diagnosed with dural arteriovenous fistula. She underwent coil embolization in external carotid artery origin and its branches, which were contributing to fistula. Three years later, patient presented to our clinic with increased frequency of headaches and tinnitus. The patient was found to have patency of the left external carotid artery and occipital artery; however, it was not possible to advance a microcatheter through the coil mass (A; note the coils (black arrows)). The occipital artery was then exposed and a small sheath was placed at its origin (B). Angiography through the sheath shows the fistula point (C, white arrow); the microcatheter was advanced through the sheath and the fistula point embolized.

previously occult arterial channels. If inadvertent embolization does occur, the operator must evaluate whether embolic material has penetrated into the normal arterial circulation. If such penetration has occurred, then the operator must assess the ischemic injury either through a neurological examination or angiographic filling of the affected distribution through other arteries. The options are limited except for prevention of any further embolization into the normal arterial circulation.

Adhesion of the microcatheter within the embolic material

The liquid embolic material may precipitate or polymerize predominantly within the arterial component in and around the microcatheter. Such adhesions result in the inability to safely retract the microcatheter from its position in proximity to the AVM.

(A) The operator may attempt to pass a microwire to the end of the microcatheter to reduce the redundancy within the distal end, which may allow disassociation between the catheter and the embolic material.

(B) The operator should pull on the microcatheter very slightly, tighten the RHV (rotating hemostatic valve) to maintain the steady and slow pull on the microcatheter, and then repeat this step every few seconds to minutes depending on the scenario. Sometimes this strategy may take up to an hour but may finally dislodge the microcatheter. Never get impatient and pull on it suddenly as it may avulse the artery. Care should also be taken to avoid catheter fracture, especially at the transition zone.

(C) If a second intermediate catheter such as a Distal access catheter (Stryker, Mountain View, CA) 0.038 inch can be introduced over the original microcatheter after inserting a 0.014 inch microwire through the microcatheter, advance the intermediate catheter until it abuts the Onyx plug if possible, and pull out the microcatheter followed by the intermediate catheter[15]. One should be careful not to inject contrast through the intermediate catheter as it may contain onyx. The last option that the operator has is to infuse vasodilators through the guide catheter or microcatheter (if possible) to reduce arterial spasm around the distal end of the microcatheter. Such vasodilators include nicardipine or verapamil.

(D) If a combination of the above strategies is unable to dislodge the microcatheter, the operator has no choice but to leave the microcatheter in position. The microcatheter is cut and sutured at the point of entry in the femoral artery, either subcutaneously or percutaneously. If surgical resection of the AVM is planned, then the microcatheter may be retracted from the craniotomy site during resection. It may be possible to perform a small arteriotomy in the proximal cervical artery and divide the microcatheter into two parts or trap it with a stent[16]. The distal part can be retracted as part of the excision of the AVM nidus and feeders. The proximal part can be retracted through the femoral end. However, with the exception of the distal portion of the flow directed microcatheter, most microcatheters are reinforced by circumferential coils (braiding), and therefore dividing the microcatheter may only be possible at certain junctions.

A detachable-tip microcatheter has recently been developed, allowing better control and lower risks associated with its retrieval[17,18].

Rupture of microcatheter

The flow directed microcatheters are vulnerable to rupture at the junction where the flow directed distal end is connected to the proximal stiffer braided portion. As more pressure builds up within the microcatheter due to increasing resistance, such rupture becomes a possibility. Therefore, injection of embolic material is inadvisable if excessive resistance is noted. Rupture of the microcatheter during embolization manifests itself as appearance of radiopaque material in the proximal arteries and absence of any further release at the distal end. Further injection should be discontinued immediately. The operator must decide on the safest course to remove the microcatheter without depositing any further liquid material in proximal arteries during microcatheter retraction. If the release occurred in a proximal medium-sized artery, the liquid embolic material may not be completely occlusive to the artery. Sometimes the high flow rate results in fragmentation and distal propagation of the embolic material. The operator may attempt to traverse the in-situ mass of embolic material with a microwire and microcatheter. If the operator is able to traverse the mass successfully, a consideration to primary angioplasty or self-expanding stent placement may be given to maintain the patency of the parent artery. Intra-arterial or intravenous platelet glycoprotein IIB/IIIA inhibitors may be helpful in preventing or treating secondary thrombosis due to foreign body reaction and stasis of blood.

Inadequate obliteration of pre-nidal aneurysm

Obliteration of pre-nidal aneurysms is an important goal of embolization of AVMs. Pre-nidal aneurysms are formed due to hemodynamic stress within the feeding arteries and are a source of rupture. These aneurysms are usually fusiform and without a clear junction between aneurysm and parent artery. If the pre-nidal aneurysm is close to the nidus or in the arteriolar component of the feeder arteries, embolization of the aneurysm with liquid embolic material concurrent with obliteration of nidus may be possible. If the aneurysm is located in the medium-size arterial feeder, simultaneous obliteration of nidus and aneurysm may not be possible. However, obliteration of the aneurysm with detachable or liquid coils inevitably requires obliteration of adjacent arterial feeder. If the nidus can be accessed through other arterial feeders, then coil embolization of the aneurysm may be undertaken first. Subsequently, the nidus may be obliterated by liquid embolization through microcatheter placement in another arterial feeder. If the pre-nidal aneurysm is located in the only accessible arterial feeder, then the operator will have to traverse the aneurysm and place the microcatheter in a distal position that allows adequate penetration of liquid embolic material within the nidus. Once the initial nidus obliteration is performed, the microcatheter is removed. Another microcatheter is placed within or adjacent to the aneurysm and coils are deployed until complete obliteration of aneurysm is achieved. The operator must be aware that the hemodynamic stress on the aneurysm may increase if outflow in the distal arterioles and nidus is reduced or eliminated. Therefore, pre-nidal aneurysm must occur simultaneous to the liquid embolization of AVM nidus and feeders arterioles.

There is one major adverse event that may or may not have any clinical significance which can be seen at the level of the AVM nidus, as described below.

Inadequate obliteration of AVM nidus

Lack of precipitation or polymerization of N-butyl acrylate or Onyx liquid embolic material within the nidus can occur, leading to liquid embolic material fragmenting and dispersing in the venous circulation. Such lack of precipitation or polymerization can occur if the injection is too fast or the concentration of the liquid embolic material is too low. Another reason is the presence of fistulas which are intermingled with the nidus but allow shunting of embolic material preferentially into the fistula, owing to relatively low resistance. The operator frequently uses judgment based on transit time for contrast to clear from the nidus following quick bolus injection, to determine whether rapid flow within AVM requires a complex approach. Ethiodol injections are also used prior to actual embolization to determine the flow pattern within the AVMs. Such information is helpful in planning the dilution of embolic material and rate of injection through the microcatheter. Alternatively, injection of liquid coils or large-size particles prior to liquid embolization may be an option.

When an operator notices that liquid embolic material is not precipitating or polymerizing within the nidus, the first step is to slow the rate of injection or inject in pulsatile fashion. Care must be taken to avoid reducing the rate to the point that precipitation or polymerization occurs around the distal end of the microcatheter, leading to adhesion of the catheter in the intravascular system. Another option is to induce temporary bradycardia or asystole at the time of the injection by systemic administration of intravenous adenosine. Recently, microcatheters with detachable balloons at the distal end have allowed inflation and proximal occlusion at the time of injection of embolic agent, followed by retraction of microcatheter and detachment of the balloon at the arterial feeders of AVMs.

It is quite possible that neither of the above-mentioned strategies is applicable or beneficial in such a scenario. The operator must retract the microcatheter and re-approach the arterial feeders using a new microcatheter which allows injection of liquid coils. Injection and deposition of liquid coils obliterates or delays the flow in the fistulas and large segments of nidus allowing subsequent liquid embolic agent to be delivered without dispersion and fragmentation due to high flow. Compatibility of microcatheter with both liquid coils and embolic material requires a careful review of the manufacturer's instructions prior to introducing the microcatheter. Another technique, which is less commonly used, is injection of high concentrations of ethyl alcohol to introduce thrombosis and spasm within the nidus and fistulas, followed by subsequent injection of liquid embolic material. However, very few microcatheters are compatible with ethyl alcohol and liquid embolic material, limiting such a combined embolization to selected procedures.

There are two major adverse events – obliteration of venous drainage channels, and distant embolization – that may or may not have any clinical significance that can be seen at the level of venous drainage, as described below.

Obliteration of venous drainage channels with or without nidus obliteration

The outflow resistance is an important determinant of pressure within the nidus, and high outflow resistance increases the chance of rupture within the nidus. Deposition of embolic material within the venous channels contributes to increase in outflow resistance, with the magnitude of this increase depending on the residual outflow following embolization. If precipitation or polymerization of liquid embolic material within venous channels is seen, the operator must evaluate the magnitude of nidus obliteration. If the nidus is largely obliterated or if alternate venous channels permit drainage, strict control on blood pressure for a 24–48 hour period maybe adequate. If the nidus is largely patent, the operator must weigh the risks and benefits of a second attempt at obliteration through another arterial feeder to obliterate the nidus, versus aborting the procedure. If catheterization is only possible in the same arterial feeders that were accessed initially, then particulate embolization to obliterate the small nidus channels preceding the occluded venous channels may be an option. If the embolization was part of the pre-surgical approach, then early or emergent surgical excision of the AVM may be another option. The occlusion of venous outflow channels do not have any significant consequences on normal venous drainage because chronic high pressure in these venous channels have rendered them unsuitable for venous drainage of normal brain.

Distant venous embolization

Lack of precipitation or polymerization of N-butyl acrylate or Onyx liquid embolic material within the nidus can occur, leading to liquid embolic material fragmenting and generation of condensed solid material of various sizes. The venous drainage leads the condensed solid material of various sizes into the pulmonary circulation. Temporary hypo-oxygenation may be seen during injection of liquid embolic material. Either further fragmentation leads to clearance of these solid materials and/or vasodilation and shunting allows oxygenation to improve. If prolonged hypo-oxygenation is observed, the image intensifier can be positioned to image the pulmonary section, and frequently radiopaque particles may be seen within the pulmonary circulation. The immediate step is to ensure adequate oxygenation of the patient by intubation and mechanical ventilation, and increasing the fraction of inspired oxygen (FiO_2) and positive end-expiratory pressure titrating to appropriate oxygenation. In the presence of patent foramen ovale, the venous emboli can be transferred into the arterial system leading to arterial occlusion. Treatment is directed towards symptomatic treatment of organ or brain ischemia.

Post-embolization complications: summary

Post-embolization intracerebral hemorrhage (ICH)

Post-embolization ICHs are secondary to increase in outflow resistance leading to high pressure within the nidus or normalization of regional cerebral blood flow to the adjacent normal brain. A state of chronic hypoperfusion exists at the margins of the AVM owing to preferential shunting of blood flow into the high flow AVM. Compensatory vasodilation is frequently seen in the arterioles with gradual loss of vasomotor functions. Post-embolization, there is normalization of regional cerebral blood flow in the chronically dilated arterioles[19]. Such flow is relatively unchecked by loss of vasomotor function within the arterioles, leading to high flow within the capillaries and subsequent rupture. Preventive efforts are focused on stepwise obliteration of AVM, usually limiting embolization to two to three arterial feeders. Such an approach reduces the diversion/normalization of flow into the surrounding tissue and excessive obliteration of venous channels[20]. Reduction in dose of systemic heparin administered during AVM embolization is another approach with reduction in postprocedure ICH rates. Standard treatment including strict control of systemic blood pressure, reversal of any residual anticoagulation, and administration of hyperosmolar treatment must be initiated at the time of initial recognition. If hydrocephalus is seen or anticipated because of large intraventricular hemorrhage, external ventricular drainage may be indicated. If the hematoma is large and surgical evacuation is considered, then evacuation must include surgical excision of any residual AVM to avoid post-surgical rebleeding. An intra- or postoperative angiogram may be necessary to ensure that surgical excision of the residual AVM is complete. Infrequently, postoperative embolization may be necessary to ensure adequate obliteration of residual AVM.

Recurrence of AVMs or AVFs

Recurrence of AVM even after complete angiographic obliteration has been observed in 5–10% of patients[21]. Whether such recurrence is attributed to increased flow into angiographically occult nidus, or represents new proliferation, remains unknown. Continued surveillance using serial angiography at 6–12 month intervals may be of value in early detection of any recurrence. Whether additional embolization, surgical excision, or radiotherapy is required must be decided on a case by case basis. Emergence of new arterial feeders into fistulas is frequent, particularly dural AVFs. If the venous sinus is not obliterated, new arterial feeders can develop within 1–3 months. Therefore, early surveillance may be necessary in patients in whom only arterial embolization was performed. Transvenous embolization with obliteration of major outflow channel may be necessary at the time of repeat embolization. Please note the difference in approach in regard to venous channel obliteration between AVMs and AV fistulas.

References

1. Seldinger SI. Catheter replacement of the needle in percutaneous arteriography; a new technique. *Acta Radiologica* 1953;39:368–76.

2. Kiemeneij F, Laarman GJ, Odekerken D, Slagboom T, van der Wieken R. A randomized comparison of percutaneous transluminal coronary angioplasty by the radial, brachial and femoral approaches: the access study. *Journal of the American College of Cardiology* 1997;29:1269–75.

3. Brooks, B. Discussion of paper by Noland L, Taylor AS. *Transations of the Southern Surgical Association* 1931;43:176–177.

4. Deveikis JP, Manz HJ, Luessenhop AJ, *et al.* A clinical and neuropathologic study of silk suture as an embolic agent for brain arteriovenous malformations. *AJNR American Journal of Neuroradiology* 1994;15:263–71.

5. Ogilvy CS, Stieg PE, Awad I, *et al.* AHA Scientific Statement: Recommendations for the management of intracranial arteriovenous malformations: a statement

for healthcare professionals from a special writing group of the Stroke Council, American Stroke Association. *Stroke; A Journal of Cerebral Circulation* 2001;32:1458–71.

6. Gobin YP, Laurent A, Merienne L, *et al.* Treatment of brain arteriovenous malformations by embolization and radiosurgery. *Journal of Neurosurgery* 1996;85:19–28.

7. Kim LJ, Spetzler RF. Classification and surgical management of spinal arteriovenous lesions: arteriovenous fistulae and arteriovenous malformations. *Neurosurgery* 2006;59:S195–201; discussion S3–13.

8. Patsalides A, Knopman J, Santillan A, *et al.* Endovascular treatment of spinal arteriovenous lesions: beyond the dural fistula. *AJNR American Journal of Neuroradiology* 2011;32:798–808.

9. Purdy PD, Batjer HH, Risser RC, Samson D. Arteriovenous malformations of the brain: choosing embolic materials to enhance safety and ease of excision. *Journal of Neurosurgery* 1992;77:217–22.

10. Guglielmi G, Vinuela F, Sepetka I, Macellari V. Electrothrombosis of saccular aneurysms via endovascular approach. Part 1: Electrochemical basis, technique, and experimental results. *Journal of Neurosurgery* 1991;75:1–7.

11. Song D, Leng B, Gu Y, *et al.* Clinical analysis of 50 cases of BAVM embolization with Onyx, a novel liquid embolic agent. *Interventional Neuroradiology: Journal of Peritherapeutic Neuroradiology, Surgical Procedures and Related Neurosciences* 2005;11:179–84.

12. Abud DG, Riva R, Nakiri GS, *et al.* Treatment of brain arteriovenous malformations by double arterial catheterization with simultaneous injection of Onyx: retrospective series of 17 patients. *AJNR American Journal of Neuroradiology* 2011;32:152–8.

13. Consoli A, Renieri L, Nappini S, Limbucci N, Mangiafico S. Endovascular treatment of deep hemorrhagic brain arteriovenous malformations with transvenous onyx embolization. *AJNR American Journal of Neuroradiology* 2013;34:1805–11.

14. Taki W, Yonekawa Y, Iwata H, *et al.* A new liquid material for embolization of arteriovenous malformations. *AJNR American Journal of Neuroradiology* 1990;11:163–8.

15. Newman CB, Park MS, Kerber CW, *et al.* Over-the-catheter retrieval of a retained microcatheter following Onyx embolization: a technical report. *Journal of Neurointerventional Surgery* 2012;4:e13.

16. Mortimer AM, Nelson RJ, Clifton A, Renowden SA. Retained and fractured microcatheter: a cause of transient ischaemic attacks: endovascular management using carotid stents. *Interventional Neuroradiology: Journal of Peritherapeutic Neuroradiology, Surgical Procedures and Related Neurosciences* 2012;18:381–5.

17. Herial NA, Khan AA, Suri MF, Sherr GT, Qureshi AI. Liquid embolization of brain arteriovenous malformation using novel detachable tip micro catheter: a technical report. *Journal of Vascular and Interventional Neurology* 2014;7:64–8.

18. Paramasivam S, Altschul D, Ortega-Gutiarrez S, Fifi J, Berenstein A. N-butyl cyanoacrylate embolization using a detachable tip microcatheter: initial experience. *Journal of Neurointerventional Surgery* 2014;7:458–61.

19. Kato Y, Sano H, Nagahisa S, *et al.* Control of hemorrhage during AVM surgery–with special reference to treatment of dilated capillaries and arteries around the nidus. *Minimally Invasive Neurosurgery: MIN* 1998;41:62–5.

20. Andrews BT, Wilson CB. Staged treatment of arteriovenous malformations of the brain. *Neurosurgery* 1987;21:314–23.

21. Reig AS, Rajaram R, Simon S, Mericle RA. Complete angiographic obliteration of intracranial AVMs with endovascular embolization: incomplete embolic nidal opacification is associated with AVM recurrence. *Journal of Neurointerventional Surgery* 2010;2:202–7.

Complications during intracranial angioplasty and stent placement

Farhan Siddiq and M. Fareed K. Suri

Introduction

Several studies have evaluated intracranial angioplasty, and deployment of balloon-expandable and self-expanding stents, for treatment of intracranial atherosclerotic stenosis. Initially, angioplasty catheters and balloon-expandable bare metal and drug-eluting stents approved for use in coronary circulation were used "off label" to treat intracranial stenosis. Subsequently, the self-expanding nitinol Wingspan[TM] stent system (Stryker)[1] and three balloon-expandable 316L stainless steel stents used specifically for intracranial stenosis were approved in some countries: these were the Neurolink (Guidant, Advanced Cardiovascular Inc.), Pharos Vitesse[TM] intracranial stent (Micrus Endovascular, San Jose, CA), and the Apollo stent system (MicroPort Medical, Shanghai, China)

The Wingspan stent (Stryker) system is currently the most studied self-expanding stent system. An overview is presented in Figure 4.1.

This stent system is being very closely scrutinized by the US Food and Drug Administration (FDA). Wingspan is now approved only for patients who are between 22 and 80 years old and who meet all of the following criteria:

- who have had two or more strokes despite aggressive medical management;

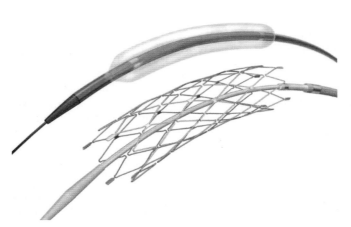

Figure 4.1 Wingspan stent system overview (with permission from Stryker). Configuration 3.5 French/1.17 mm unified over-the-wire (OTW) self-expanding stent system. Nominal stent diameters (mm) 2.5, 3.0, 3.5, 4.0, 4.5. Stent lengths (mm) 9, 15, 20. Recommended guidewire 0.014 in/0.36 mm exchange length (300 cm). Recommended guide catheter 6 French/2 mm (minimum 0.064 in/1.63 mm ID), 90 cm length.

Complications of Neuroendovascular Procedures and Bailout Techniques, ed. Rakesh Khatri, Gustavo J. Rodriguez, Jean Raymond and Adnan I. Qureshi. Published by Cambridge University Press. © Cambridge University Press 2016.

- whose most recent stroke occurred more than 7 days prior to planned treatment with Wingspan;
- who have 70–99% stenosis due to atherosclerosis of the intracranial artery related to the recurrent strokes; and
- who have made good recovery from previous stroke and have a modified Rankin score of 3 or less prior to Wingspan treatment. The Rankin scale is used to measure the degree of disability in stroke patients. Lower scores indicate less disability.

The Wingspan stent system should not be used for:

- the treatment of stroke with an onset of symptoms within 7 days of treatment; or
- for the treatment of transient ischemic attacks (TIAs).

Reported complications in literature

The main complications associated with angioplasty and stent placement are a relatively high rate of perioperative stroke and/or death and angiographic restenosis. The rate of perioperative stroke or death was 10% and 8.4% in systematic reviews of 79 studies (1999 cases)[2] and of 69 studies[3] (2318 cases) respectively. About 6% of strokes or death occurred 1–12 months after the angioplasty and/or stent procedure. The pooled restenosis rate was 14% in the angioplasty-treated group compared with 11% in the stent-treated group[3]. The SSYLVIA[4], Wingspan[1], and ASSIST[5] studies were single-arm studies that reported 1 month rates of periprocedural stroke and death of 6.6%, 4.5%, and 6.5%, respectively. Several post-marketing registries, the US Wingspan registry[6], European INTRASTENT registry[7], and National Institute of Health (NIH) Multi-center Wingspan IAS Registry[8], reported technical success rates of 97% or greater using the new generation of angioplasty catheters and self-expanding stents with acceptable periprocedural stroke or death rates. However, these registries identified a restenosis rate of 25–30% within the first year after the procedure.

In 2007, the SAMMPRIS study[9] compared intensive medical therapy alone with intracranial angioplasty and stent placement combined with intensive medical therapy. The primary endpoint in patients with 70–99% intracranial stenosis who had a TIA or stroke within 30 days prior to enrollment was any stroke or death within 30 days or ipsilateral stroke beyond 30 days within 2 years. Enrollment was discontinued after 451 (59%) of the planned 764 patients had been enrolled, owing to a 14% rate of stroke or death within the first 30 days after enrollment of patients treated with angioplasty and stent placement compared with a 5.8% rate in patients treated with medical therapy alone. There were 5 stroke-related deaths and 10 symptomatic intracranial hemorrhages within 30 days after enrollment in the stent placement arm. The 1 month rate of stroke or death had to be less than 4% in the angioplasty and stent-treated patients to show the superiority stipulated in the primary hypothesis[10]. Numerous explanations have been proposed for the higher than expected rate of stroke or death within 1 month of the procedure, including variations in operator experience, lack of standardization of intensity of anticoagulation measurements, and mandatory policy of stent placement[11]. In the SAMMPRIS trial, intraprocedural heparinization was instituted to a targeted activated coagulation time (ACT) of 250 to 300 seconds without adjustment for variations in the methods of measurement[12], an important consideration given the high rate of intracerebral hemorrhages seen after stent placement.

In an analysis of data derived from three academic centers, the overall 30 day post-procedure stroke and death rate was 7.2% in the SAMMPRIS eligible patients when a mandatory policy of stent placement was not used[13]. The 30 day postprocedure stroke and death rate was 3.3% and 10.2% in the SAMMPRIS eligible patients treated with primary angioplasty or stent placement, respectively. Reacting to these data, interventionalists posit that primary angioplasty as the sole modality or as an alternate to stent placement in selected patients, particularly those with long lesions, tortuous proximal vessels, or limited vessel length available distal to the lesion to allow stable placement of microwire, might achieve the required low 30 day postprocedure stroke and death rates[11].

More recently, the VISSIT trial results were published. The trial was terminated early, after negative results from the SAMMPRIS; an early analysis of outcomes suggested futility after 112 patients of a planned sample size of 250 were enrolled. The 30 day primary safety endpoint occurred in more patients in the stent group (14/58; 24.1%) than in the medical group (5/53; 9.4%) ($P = 0.05$). Intracranial hemorrhage within 30 days occurred in more patients in the stent group (5/58; 8.6%) vs. none in the medical group ($P = 0.06$)[14].

Some precautions are advised in general for these procedures:

1. The recommended guide catheter should be at least 90 cm in length and 1.63 mm (0.064 inches) inner diameter.
2. The length of the balloon should be slightly greater than the lesion to prevent the "watermelon seed" phenomenon; however, it should not be too long either, as it may then be difficult to advance.
3. Do not perform angioplasty in a diseased segment greater than 80% diameter of the normal arterial segment of the same artery.
4. Do not measure a post-stenotic dilated segment.
5. The length of the stent should extend at least 2 mm on either side of the stenotic segment.
6. The diameter of the stent should match the normal diameter of the treated arterial segment.
7. Cross the lesion with microwire and exchange the microcatheter over an exchange length microwire for the balloon microcatheter. Ensure that you keep the exchange length microwire distal to the lesion, allowing some movement during the exchange. Use a soft-tip microwire whenever possible.

Specific complications
Arterial dissection

One of the first recognized complications of intracranial angioplasty was stroke from either abrupt vessel occlusion or arterial dissection[15,16]. Marks *et al.* reported two complications in a series of 23 patients who underwent intracranial angioplasty. One patient had vessel rupture and died from this. A second patient had local thrombosis at the site of the angioplasty which was treated with intra-arterial alteplase without any neurological compromise[16]. Connors and Wojak reported similar complications in a series of 50 patients who underwent intracranial angioplasty[17]. Nahser *et al.*[18] reported two asymptomatic dissections and two strokes during angioplasty of symptomatic vertebrobasilar atherosclerosis in a series of 20 patients. Takis *et al.*[19], in their early experience, reported a significant number of patients having vasospasm during the angioplasty treatment ($n = 5/10$). They also reported two strokes: one related to perforator artery occlusion and the second related to arterial dissection.

Whenever arterial dissection is observed, stent placement to treat intimal dissection may be necessary. If dissection is observed, the operator must decide whether it is flow limiting, owing to protrusion of the intimal flap within the parent lumen or irregularities created by a cleft in the intima or media. Prior to the delivery of stent, the operator must ensure that delivery catheter is in the true lumen. If the microwire is already across the lesion in the parent artery, then immediate stent delivery can occur. If the microwire that served as the base for the original procedure is no longer in position, a microcatheter and microwire in a J configuration may be necessary to traverse the lesion and dissection. The first step must be followed by confirmation by contrast injection through microcatheter to ensure that the distal end of the microcatheter is in the true lumen. Dissections that occur after stent deployment are usually found on either the proximal or distal end of the stent, and second stent placement should provide coverage to the dissected segment. Flow limiting dissections can be treated by placing a second stent. If the intimal flap is not flow limiting but is associated with thrombosis, short-term use of intravenous anticoagulation or platelet glycoprotein IIB/IIIA inhibitors and follow-up angiography may be required. Dissections with small flaps (intimal irregularities) which are asymptomatic may only require observation.

In-stent thrombosis

Stent thrombosis and occlusion have been observed secondary to mechanical plaque disruption, intimal injury, and thrombogenicity of the stent[20–24]. The highest risk of stent thrombosis is within the first 24 hours after placement and the risk decreases substantially after the first 72 hours. The thrombotic process is predominantly platelet-based, initiated after exposure of subintima and platelet adhesion and aggregation at the site of intimal injury. Platelet glycoprotein IIb/IIIa inhibitors may be used to treat in-stent thrombosis. If the thrombosis occurs during the procedure, a microcatheter may be placed in the proximity of the thrombus, and intra-arterial platelet glycoprotein IIb/IIIa inhibitor bolus may be administered. Intra-arterial thrombolysis may also be used to treat parent vessel occlusion. The operator must attempt to identify whether underlying arterial dissection is the causative mechanism, and treatment of dissection as mentioned above may be necessary. Infrequently, flow turbulence due to partially deployed stent or stent distortion may be responsible, and post-stent angioplasty may be necessary for ensuring adequate opposition. If treatment is initiated early, cerebral ischemia can be prevented. Patients must be pretreated with dual antiplatelets (aspirin and clopidogrel), prior to attempting stent placement to prevent in-stent thrombosis. The use of distal protection devices in the treatment of intracranial stenosis has not yet been developed to prevent distal emboli.

Vessel perforation

Vessel perforation is usually caused by use of a balloon or stent that is larger than the size of the parent artery. Such perforation may cause subarachnoid hemorrhage with intraparenchymal extension. These events can be fatal because of the anticoagulation and antiplatelet treatments that are being used. The first sign may be severe pain if the patient is awake during the procedure, followed by contrast extravasation outside the treated artery. Rapid reversal of intravenous heparin using protamine, and platelet transfusion for reversing platelet inhibition by antiplatelet agents, may be considered. Emergent steps to treat intracranial pressure elevation or local mass effect leading to herniation are necessary. The patient should be intubated and intravenous 23.4% sodium chloride or mannitol may be used. If perforation is suspected, the microwire and angioplasty balloon should not be removed without careful understanding of the situation. If the angioplasty balloon is still in the parent lumen, temporary gentle inflation may provide occlusion and stop the hemorrhage. The extravasation may be self-limiting and arterial sacrifice may not be necessary. Since most perforations are secondary to arterial injury and dissection, stent placement may provide support to the dissected segment by opposition of flap and arterial wall, leading to cessation of bleeding. Self-expanding stents and low-porosity stents are recommended, while balloon-expandable stents should be avoided as they may exacerbate the arterial injury. If perforation is confirmed by angiography, the microcatheter should be advanced over the wire just beyond the perforation, and the segment of the vessel should be obliterated by deployment of coils. The patient subsequently may suffer either a fatal intracerebral hemorrhage or an ischemic stroke in the territory of the treated vessel. Infrequently, rupture of cavernous segment internal carotid artery may lead to carotid cavernous fistula. Deployment of a covered stent across the lesion may result in resolution of the fistula and maintain patency of the artery.

Reperfusion hemorrhage

A patient with a recent large ischemic stroke or severe hypoperfusion is particularly at risk of intracranial hemorrhage after intracranial angioplasty and stent placement. The hemorrhage is secondary to restoration of cerebral blood flow (rCBF) in maximally dilated blood vessels (pre-existing owing to long standing hypoperfusion) supplemented by anticoagulation and antiplatelet treatment. In patients with recent ischemic stroke, there is disruption of the blood–brain barrier which is prone to further damage with restoration of perfusion and antithrombitic treatment. The manifestations can range from unilateral cerebral edema to intraparenchymal hemorrhage. Preferably, patients with large ischemic stroke should be treated in a delayed manner. The current approval for Wingspan self-expanding stent by FDA cautions against performance of procedure within 7 days of the index ischemic event. Strict blood pressure control may help to avoid this potentially devastating result. Although the threshold of strict blood pressure control varies among institutions, EMGREG guidelines recommend maintaining systolic blood pressure to less than 120 mmHg after procedure. If the patient has untreated high grade stenosis in other cerebral arteries, maintaining systolic blood pressure to less than 140 mmHg may be acceptable. High-dose anticoagulation and intravenous platelet glycoprotein inhibitors should be avoided in patients at risk. In severe cases, surgical evacuation may be necessary for intraparenchymal hemorrhage.

Vasospasm

Catheter manipulation, microwire placement, or advancement of angioplasty balloon catheter or stent delivery catheter through torturous arteries may lead to vasospasm in the intracranial vessels. Almost all vasospasm is transient and resolves as soon as the devices are withdrawn. If distinction between vasospasm and dissection is required (both can appear as focal and irregular narrowing) without losing access to the distal vessel, a microcatheter can be placed over the microwire with subsequent removal of the microwire. This maneuver relieves some of the distortional stress and relieves the straightening on the vessel wall while preserving distal access. Follow-up angiography after 5–10 minutes may be performed after the procedure to confirm resolution of vasospasm. If vasospasm persists, an intra-arterial vasodilator like calcium channel blocker or

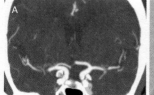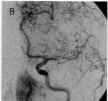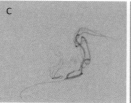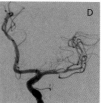

Figure 4.2 Intracranial angioplasty alone: unable to track Wingspan stent. Images are of an 81-year-old female with symptomatic 95% left middle cerebral artery stenosis (A and B), despite medical treatment. A Wingspan stent could not be advanced, and therefore angioplasty with Gateway balloon 1.5 mm × 9 mm was performed alone, with improvement in the lumen (residual 45%). **A:** Computed tomography (CT) head showing left M1 stenosis. **B:** AP angiography showing left distal M1 95% stenosis. **C:** Microcatheter placed distal to stenosis, and run performed to ensure it was placed in true lumen. **D:** Post angioplasty (Gateway balloon 1.5 mm × 9 mm) guide run showing improved lumen.

magnesium may be utilized with varying success. A common site for vasospasm is the distal end of the guide catheter, in particular when the distal end is in the high cervical region of the internal carotid or vertebral artery. Delay in contrast clearance after contrast injection through the guide catheter may be the first manifestation. Retracting the catheter may be adequate to resolve the local vasospasm.

Difficulty in stent delivery

Using an intermediate catheter (at least 5–7 French) for support, and ensuring the stent is well flushed, good proximal support can be obtained by including a 0.014–0.018 inch microwire through the guide catheter into the external or internal carotid artery. The delivery is facilitated by advancement of the guide catheter into the high cervical segment of the internal carotid or vertebral artery, and coaxial introduction of a stiff 0.018 inch microwire through the guide catheter to prevent retropulsion is recommended. If difficulty is still encountered, then performing angioplasty alone may be reasonable (Figure 4.2).

In-stent restenosis

In-stent restenosis typically reaches its maximal severity between 3 and 6 months after the procedure intervention and is reported in as much as 25–30% of cases. The acute component of restenosis may be due to recoil, and delayed component is attributed to proliferation of myocytes and subintimal collagen. Restenosis is mostly asymptomatic and predominantly affects the anterior circulation vessels. The restenosis may be persistent or in-stent depending upon the location in relation to the previously deployed stent. If restenosis is severe or associated with clinical symptoms, repeat angioplasty may be required. Almost 50% of these treated patients may again develop restenosis requiring further procedures.

We typically extend the duration of dual antiplatelet therapy if in-stent restenosis is observed, irrespective of clinical status. In our practice we also encountered a patient with asymptomatic occlusion of the previously placed Neuroform stent (Stryker, USA) that was likely due to progressive in-stent stenosis (Figure 4.3).

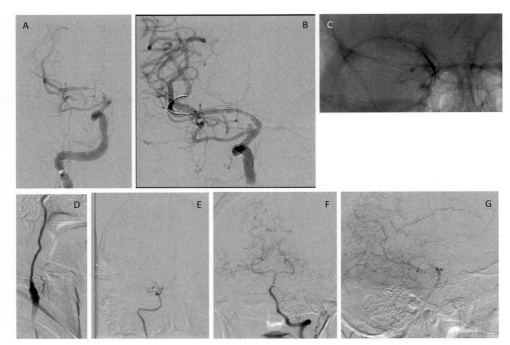

Figure 4.3 A 45-year-old female presented with right hemispheric repeated strokes despite maximum medical management and was noted to have severe stenosis of right middle cerebral artery (MCA) with moderate supraclinoid stenosis (A). Stenosis in MCA was treated with angioplasty with angiographic improvement, but was complicated by a small focal dissection. It was treated by placement of a Neuroform 3.5 mm × 20 mm stent (B, C) with no significant residual stenosis in MCA. The Wingspan stent system was not considered owing to recent stroke, and balloon-mounted coronary stent did not track. Patient has chronic right external carotid artery occlusion (D). She continued with symptoms in right hemisphere TIA requiring indirect bypass surgery with improvement and remained symptom-free for about 1 year. Follow-up after a year demonstrated occluded stent but with collateral flow noted from vertebral artery injection (E, F, G).

References

1. Bose A, Hartmann M, Henkes H, *et al.* A novel, self-expanding, nitinol stent in medically refractory intracranial atherosclerotic stenoses: the Wingspan study. *Stroke; A Journal of Cerebral Circulation* 2007;38:1531–7.

2. Cruz-Flores S, Diamond AL. Angioplasty for intracranial artery stenosis. *The Cochrane Database of Systematic Reviews* 2006:CD004133.

3. Siddiq F, Memon MZ, Vazquez G, Safdar A, Qureshi AI. Comparison between primary angioplasty and stent placement for intracranial atherosclerotic disease: Meta-analysis of case series. *Neurosurgery* 2009; 65:1024–33; discussion 1033–4.

4. Investigators SS. Stenting of Symptomatic Atherosclerotic Lesions in the Vertebral or Intracranial Arteries (SSYLVIA): study results. *Stroke; A Journal of Cerebral Circulation* 2004;35:1388–92.

5. Jiang WJ, Xu XT, Jin M, *et al.* Apollo stent for symptomatic atherosclerotic intracranial stenosis: study results. *AJNR American Journal of Neuroradiology* 2007;28:830–4.

6. Fiorella D, Levy EI, Turk AS, *et al.* US multicenter experience with the wingspan stent system for the treatment of intracranial atheromatous disease: periprocedural results. *Stroke; A Journal of Cerebral Circulation* 2007;38:881–7.

7. Kurre W, Berkefeld J, Brassel F, *et al.* In-hospital complication rates after stent treatment of 388 symptomatic intracranial stenoses: results from the INTRASTENT multicentric registry. *Stroke; A Journal of Cerebral Circulation* 2010;41:494–8.

8. Zaidat OO, Klucznik R, Alexander MJ, *et al.* The NIH registry on use of the Wingspan stent for symptomatic 70–99% intracranial arterial stenosis. *Neurology* 2008;70:1518–24.

9. Derdeyn CP, Chimowitz MI. Angioplasty and stenting for atherosclerotic intracranial stenosis: rationale for a randomized clinical trial. *Neuroimaging Clinics of North America* 2007;17:355–63, viii–ix.

10. Chaudhry SA, Watanabe M, Qureshi AI. The new standard for performance of intracranial angioplasty and stent placement after Stenting versus Aggressive Medical Therapy for Intracranial Arterial Stenosis (SAMMPRIS) Trial. *AJNR American Journal of Neuroradiology* 2011;32:E214.

11. Qureshi AI, Al-Senani FM, Husain S, *et al.* Intracranial angioplasty and stent placement after stenting and aggressive medical management for preventing recurrent stroke in intracranial stenosis (SAMMPRIS) trial: present state and future considerations. *Journal of Neuroimaging: Official Journal of the American Society of Neuroimaging* 2012;22:1–13.

12. Hussein HM, Georgiadis AL, Qureshi AI. Point-of-care testing for anticoagulation monitoring in neuroendovascular procedures. *AJNR American Journal of Neuroradiology* 2012;33:1211–20.

13. Siddiq F, Chaudhry SA, Khatri R, *et al.* Rate of postprocedural stroke and death in SAMMPRIS trial-eligible patients treated with intracranial angioplasty and/or stent placement in practice. *Neurosurgery* 2012;71:68–73.

14. Zaidat OO, Fitzsimmons BF, Woodward BK, *et al.* Effect of a balloon-expandable intracranial stent vs medical therapy on risk of stroke in patients with symptomatic intracranial stenosis: the VISSIT randomized clinical trial. *JAMA* 2015;313:1240–8.

15. Mori T, Kazita K, Chokyu K, Mima T, Mori K. Short-term arteriographic and clinical outcome after cerebral angioplasty and stenting for intracranial vertebrobasilar and carotid atherosclerotic occlusive disease. *AJNR American Journal of Neuroradiology* 2000;21:249–54.

16. Marks MP, Marcellus M, Norbash AM, Steinberg GK, Tong D, Albers GW. Outcome of angioplasty for atherosclerotic intracranial stenosis. *Stroke* 1999;30:1065–1069

17. Connors JJ 3rd, Wojak JC. Percutaneous transluminal angioplasty for intracranial atherosclerotic lesions: evolution of technique and short-term results. *Journal of Neurosurgery* 1999;91:415–23.

18. Nahser HC, Henkes H, Weber W, *et al.* Intracranial vertebrobasilar stenosis: angioplasty and follow-up. *AJNR American Journal of Neuroradiology* 2000;21:1293–301.

19. Takis C, Kwan ES, Pessin MS, Jacobs DH, Caplan LR. Intracranial angioplasty: experience and complications. *AJNR American Journal of Neuroradiology* 1997;18:1661–8.

20. Wholey MH, Wholey MH, Eles G, *et al.* Evaluation of glycoprotein IIb/IIIa inhibitors in carotid angioplasty and stenting. *Journal of Endovascular Therapy: An Official Journal of the International Society of Endovascular Specialists* 2003;10:33–41.

21. Kim JK, Ahn JY, Lee BH, *et al.* Elective stenting for symptomatic middle cerebral artery stenosis presenting as transient ischaemic deficits or stroke attacks: short term arteriographical and clinical outcome. *Journal of Neurology, Neurosurgery, and Psychiatry* 2004;75:847–51.

22. Kim DJ, Lee BH, Kim DI, *et al.* Stent-assisted angioplasty of symptomatic intracranial vertebrobasilar artery stenosis: feasibility and follow-up results. *AJNR American Journal of Neuroradiology* 2005;26:1381–8.

23. Chaturvedi S, Yadav JS. The role of antiplatelet therapy in carotid stenting for ischemic stroke prevention. *Stroke; A Journal of Cerebral Circulation* 2006;37:1572–7.

24. Levy EI, Turk AS, Albuquerque FC, *et al.* Wingspan in-stent restenosis and thrombosis: incidence, clinical presentation, and management. *Neurosurgery* 2007;61:644–50; discussion 50–1.

Chapter 5

Complications during the intra-arterial treatment of ischemic stroke

Nazli Janjua and Rakesh Khatri

Neuro-interventional procedures require impeccable execution to avoid complication. In intra-arterial (IA) stroke cases this must occur under the duress of time for the most critically ill patients, potentially increasing the chance of error. The most feared complication, reperfusion hemorrhage, can occur even with perceived flawless procedures. In various registries and trials[1–3], rates of symptomatic intracranial hemorrhage (sICH) ranged from 8 to 10%. Blind navigation in occluded vessels makes the risk of catheter-related dissection and thromboembolism even greater, and stroke devices come with their own risks. Technical failure, caused by unsuccessful catheterization or treatment, is also more common in these cases with difficult vascular anatomy.

Recent trials studying mechanical thrombectomy for acute ischemic stroke[4–7] have demonstrated the clinical benefit of this approach. These data augment patient triage for such therapies, rendering IA stroke treatment a more widespread procedure, in some cases performed by interventional radiologists or cardiologists, with experiential rather than formalized neuro-interventional treatment. This makes a systemized approach to the potential pitfalls and work-around for these procedures even more essential.

Early endovascular stroke treatment involved local IA thrombolysis, whereby the major risk involved reperfusion. Rates of reperfusion hemorrhage in these trials directly concord with dosage of concomitant intravenous (IV) heparin[8]. This experience has generated knowledge about the use of adjuvant anticoagulant and anti-aggregant agents for patients undergoing stroke treatment. While some studies of IV Abciximab showed overwhelming harm[9], other trials of full-dose systemic thrombolytic followed by additional IA thrombo-lytic have not shown this[10]. In most modern neuro-interventional labs, a practical application of this observation involves admixture of heparin into saline flushes and/or preprocedural bolus dosing of heparin. While no standard guidelines exist, doses of unfractionated heparin 2000–4000 IU/liter of normal saline flush bag with or without pre-intervention bolus of 2000–5000 IU may help balance prevention of further intraprocedural thrombosis against exacerbation of hemorrhage risk.

The first-generation thrombectomy device, the Merci concentric retriever, introduced the use of a removable, navigable metal construct designed to engage the clot. This device has largely fallen out of use in clinical practice, with the more recent trials showing the superiority of current-generation devices (TREVO and SWIFT) over the concentric retriever, and further discussion regarding this device is abbreviated. In brief, experience with the Merci

Complications of Neuroendovascular Procedures and Bailout Techniques, ed. Rakesh Khatri, Gustavo J. Rodriguez, Jean Raymond and Adnan I. Qureshi. Published by Cambridge University Press. © Cambridge University Press 2016.

did have an impact on further iterations of stroke devices. The major worry of any thrombectomy device, brought to light by this first-generation device, is arterial dissection during the retraction process. Techniques to avoid or minimize this risk involve reduction of traction forces directly exhibited against the vessel wall by using soft-tipped guide catheters with good proximal support. These guide catheters can be advanced over inner catheters, or exchanged with other shaped catheters in the parent vasculature, and are atraumatic enough to be advanced well into the petrous carotid or intraforaminal vertebral artery. By doing so, the vector of force of retraction of the device falls into a straight segment within the catheter rather than against turns of the intracranial vessels. This affords more successful retrieval and also prevents backwards pressure against right angled turns in the more vessel segment. Device fracture was noted with the earliest Merci retrievers. This potential complication may be related to the device engineering rather than technician error, a problem remedied in later-generation devices by strengthening the solder point between the device and the delivery wire.

Early-generation Penumbra separators also had initial engineering weaknesses in the proximal aspect of the delivery wire, again, an engineering pitfall, improved upon in the later generation. Several recent mechanical trials now favor performing thrombectomy with stent-retrievers.

Imaging criteria utilized in these trials may be applied in clinical practice to improve patient selection, the first step in avoidance of complications. Triaging patients based on higher ASPECTS scores or small core infarcts based on perfusion imaging[6] identifies the patients most likely to benefit and theoretically least likely to suffer reperfusion hemorrhage. At the same time, many of these trials studied rapid work flow between image acquisition as a primary investigation point, and summarily concluded that obtaining advanced imaging (e.g. computed tomography (CT) angiography or CT perfusion) should not delay the ultimate therapeutic procedure, as delayed time itself may increase the risk of reperfusion hemorrhage. Given the preponderance of data regarding stent-retrievers, these represent the devices in vogue for most thrombectomy treatments, and deserve greater discussion of potential complications and rescue techniques.

As a basic overview, the two most widely available stent-retriever devices include the Trevo device (Stryker) and the Solitaire FR (Covidien/Medtronic, Irvine, CA). Sizes are indicated by two dimensions: the diameter of a fully deployed retriever as well the length. Sizes range from 4 to 6 mm in diameter and 15 to 40 mm in length. Choice in general depends on the vessel occluded (larger diameter device for more proximal occlusion) and length of the clot (longer lengths for large thrombi extending from internal carotid terminus to M1 stem). However, specific geomorphical consideration of each device further affects this choice, although this is beyond the scope of this chapter. Device manufacturers may promote proprietary catheters as "best-fitting" for certain devices, but in general 0.021–0.023" inner diameter catheters may accommodate these stent-retrievers. The microcatheter delivering the device can be navigated directly through the guide catheter or coaxially through an intermediate catheter. The latter technique, as with modern guide catheters designed for more distal delivery, improves the vector of force away from vulnerable aspects of the vessel wall during retraction, thereby improving chances of technical success and minimizing vessel injury.

Complications that happen when things go right

Reperfusion hemorrhage

See Figure 5.1. Here the best strategy is prevention and appropriately selecting patients to minimize risk. Delayed treatment after symptom onset and extensive infarction have been

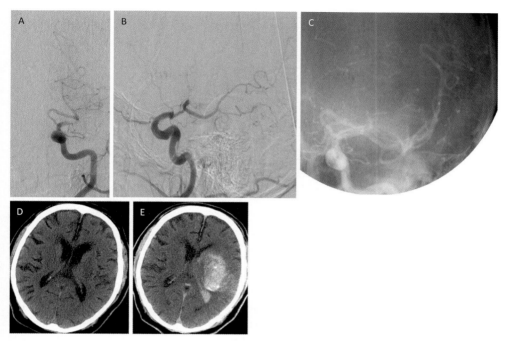

Figure 5.1 An 88-year-old male, with history of diabetes mellitus, received IV alteplase for National Institute of Health Stroke Scale (NIHSS) 22 and was taken for mechanical thrombectomy since no improvement was noted. A: AP view showing left supraclinoid internal carotid artery (ICA) occlusion with left fetal posterior cerebral artery. B: Lateral angiogram showing as above. C: After mechanical thrombectomy with Penumbra Aspiration system, left supraclinoid ICA. Recanalized with partial TICI 2 recanalization of left middle cerebral artery. D: Head CT immediately postprocedure does not show any acute changes. E: 24 hours: head CT shows basal ganglia hemorrhage with intraventricular hemorrhage.

associated with higher risk of hemorrhage[11,12]. Patients with large radiographic evidence of stroke – over 1/3rd middle cerebral artery (MCA) territory or "matched" defects with complete infarction of the target vascular territory – are cutoffs used in clinical practice. Mismatch between penumbra and core as seen on perfusion imaging, as well as between the clinical severity and infarct core on diffusion-weighted magnetic resonance imaging (DWI MRI), or using non-enhanced head CT with the Alberta Stroke Program Early CT Score (ASPECTS) score, may help better select patients[13].

Angiographic signs of bleeding must be recognized. Figure 5.2 shows abnormal pattern of contrast blush or "staining" at each terminal lenticulostriate in a patient undergoing angiography for IA stroke therapy.

In the event of hemorrhage, anticoagulants and fibrinolytics may require reversal. Unfractionated heparin, commonly used in flush systems, is unlikely to affect coagulation parameters. A recently started infusion without bolus can be terminated without specific reversal, as it requires 4–6 hours to achieve a steady state[14]. Bolus doses or any dose resulting in therapeutic anticoagulation is reversed by 1 mg protamine sulfate for every 100 U of heparin given in the last 1 hour[14]. However, this may exacerbate thrombotic conditions and cause severe allergic reaction, which should be considered before its administration.

If recombinant tissue plasminogen activator (tPA) has been administered intravenously or in high IA doses (>20 mg), cryoprecipitate transfusion will replete fibrinogen to help

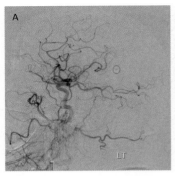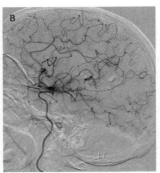

Figure 5.2 (Parenchymal blush). **A:** ICA angiogram, lateral view, in a 74-year-old woman with an acute stroke. Initial contrast injection has already been performed in order to catheterize the ICA. Subsequent angiogram shows a subtle area of subtraction artifact (circled area), which represents contrast retention from the prior injection. This appears in the parietal area, otherwise void of vascularity. On this image it is difficult to appreciate whether this is retained contrast from an occluded distal vessel versus parenchymal staining. **B:** The subsequent angiogram after interval intra-arterial thrombolysis shows much more significant capillary blush on live fluoroscopy (not shown) and contrast retention seen as subtraction artifact on formal angiography (larger circle), making it very clear that this represents parenchymal hemorrhage.

restore homeostasis[15]. For patients previously on warfarin with international normalized ratio (INR) > 1.7, consider reversal with fresh frozen plasma, prothrombin complex concentrate (PCC), vitamin K, or activated factor VIIa[14].

Many patients have longstanding use of aspirin or clopidogrel prior to their acute stroke. Reversal of antiplatelet agents is difficult and requires direct platelet transfusion[14] which has a limited half-life and may be difficult to obtain in a short time frame. Nonetheless, transfusion may be essential, particularly if patients require further surgical intervention of bleeding complications.

Benign contrast staining: risk versus benefit of cessation of anticoagulants post IA stroke therapy

Postprocedural CT often show areas of hyperdensity in the infarcted core of the arterial territory treated (Figures 5.3, 5.4). This contrast staining may be difficult to distinguish from true ICH[16]. Terminology is loose, and includes contrast enhancement, contrast "intravasation", and contrast extravasation, which has been ascribed to either benign or malignant patterns fated for hemorrhage. Predicting the course may be difficult. This pattern of hyperdensity typically dissipates over the next 24 hours, showing it to be more likely to be contrast rather than hemorrhage (Figure 5.3). These findings therefore do not always necessitate discontinuing or reversing antiplatelet and other medications.

The appearance of subarachnoid hemorrhage (SAH) may also be seen on post-treatment CTs, although it is more likely to be attributable to true hemorrhage from vessel injury rather than capillary blood–brain barrier breakdown. It is therefore deemed more worrisome, although the risk of altering antiplatelet regimen should still be weighed carefully. Figure 5.4 demonstrates 24 hour follow-up head CT in a patient presenting with acute stroke left MCA occlusion with pre-existing stenosis. Mechanical thrombectomy and acute stenting was required to maintain patency of the vessel after IA tPA. The patient made significant clinical recovery over the next 24 hours, although follow-up head CT showed

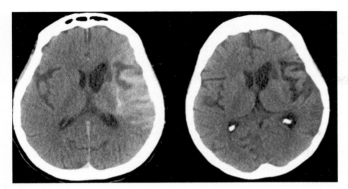

Figure 5.3 (Retained contrast). Axial head CT of a 53-year-old woman who underwent thrombectomy for a left M2 occlusion. She subsequently suffered another stroke in the same location a few days later and underwent a second thrombectomy. This head CT done the day after the second procedure shows a significant hyperdensity in the left MCA territory. It is difficult to differentiate between reperfusion hemorrhage and retained contrast from the angiogram due to breakdown of the blood–brain barrier. Subsequent imaging done 2 days later shows resolution of hyperdensity, supporting the diagnosis of contrast staining rather than hemorrhage.

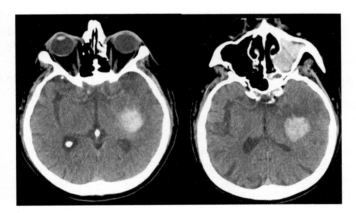

Figure 5.4 Reperfusion hemorrhage. Head CT in a 74-year-old man who underwent thrombectomy for left M1 occlusion. A consolidated area of hyperdensity raises concern for reperfusion hemorrhage. A subsequent head CT done the following day shows largely unchanged appearance, making the diagnosis of hemorrhage more likely than retained contrast in this case.

hyperdensity in left lateral ventricle and adjacent region. This prompted discontinuation of antiplatelets. Two days later the patient suffered in-stent thrombosis.

Antiplatelet regimens in acute stenting

Acute stenting in stroke is a rare occurrence after introduction of stent-retrievers. Converse to the above issue is the scenario of an urgent stent placement during stroke therapy in a patient not pre-treated with antiplatelet agents. Typical "loading" doses for medication-naïve patients are 325 mg of aspirin and 300 mg of clopidogrel. Cardiologists typically use higher doses such as clopidogrel 600 mg, which some neuro-interventionalists also adopt in their practice. IV eptifibatide or Abciximab may be possible agents to quickly provide platelet inhibition until oral medications can be instituted. Doses for stroke treatment are not standardized. Coronary intervention doses provide a frame of reference, although likely higher than ideal for neurological purposes. Qureshi *et al.* described an eptifibatide regimen of 125 µg/kg bolus followed by 0.5 µg/kg/minute infusion for 20 hours in stroke treatment[17]

71

and a regimen of IA reteplase and IV Abciximab of 0.25 µg/kg bolus followed by 0.125 µg/kg/min. [refs. 17,18]. Both are potent glycoprotein IIb/IIIa inhibitors. IV infusions have the benefit of short duration of action, which may be crucial if sICH occurs.

Point of care testing commonly utilized in the angiography suite to assay activated coagulation time may also be used to assay platelet inhibition with various medications. This may have utility in the acute stroke setting to tailor the antiplatelet regimen.

Futile treatment

The possibilities of both unsuccessful treatment and futile treatment should be discussed during the informed consent process. With the introduction of stent-retrievers and good patient selection on the basis of imaging and clinical criteria, the number needed to treat (NNT) to have independent outcome at 90 days is only 4 [refs. 4–7]. Even though rates of recanalization following interventional stroke treatment range from 60 to 86%[1-3], improved functional outcome is not guaranteed despite revascularization. Response to endovascular treatment is more varied in basilar artery occlusions[11]. Chronic disease may also negatively impact outcome after endovascular stroke therapy and, with the other items, has been factored into a proposed scoring system to define patients less likely to improve after IA stroke treatment[19].

Complications secondary to technical error/malfunction

Vessel perforation and dissection

Commercially available stroke devices include the Penumbra system (Penumbra Inc., San Leandro, CA), and stent-retrievers (Trevo®, Stryker neurovascular; Solitaire™, Covidien/Medtronics, USA). Balloon catheters for angioplasty and implantable stents are also used occasionally at times for recalcitrant clots. Non-compliant or semi-compliant balloons may be required. Likewise, the devices must possess a certain amount of tensile strength to accomplish the task of embolectomy. This factor, compounded with blind navigation through occluded vessels, creates risk of vessel dissection and injury. Frank rupture is usually easily noted during angiography (Figure 5.5). The severity depends in part on the vessel size (e.g. M1 rupture may prove fatal whereas a distal M2–3 rupture may be asymptomatic) and the mechanism by which the perforation occurred. Wire perforations are usually self-limited, whereas catheter perforations are less well tolerated. Microcatheters used for stroke treatment are larger than those used for other neuro-interventional procedures and forced catheter advancement through sharp turns can lead to vessel injury. Navigating large bore catheters (e.g. Penumbra 0.054″ or 5 MAX catheters) around the cavernous or ophthalmic carotid region or carotid siphon is often difficult and may lead to dissection if careful technique is not employed. These catheters are oversized to the microwire, typically 0.014″ in size, posing a more traumatic interface against the vessel wall. With increasing force during microcatheter delivery, the catheter builds up momentum against the vessel wall. Frank dissection may not be obvious, but catheter advancement grows more difficult and angiography may demonstrate focal vasospasm. To minimize this risk, advancement over an inner microcatheter of smaller size may allow for smoother transition of size from the Reperfusion catheter to the vessel. This will also vastly ease catheter advancement. Techniques to improve system navigation are discussed below.

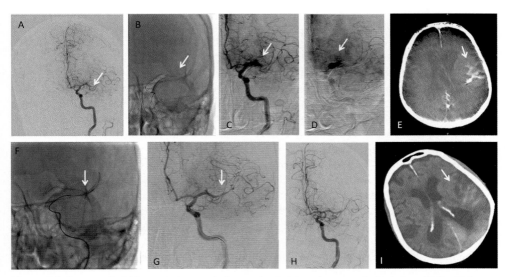

Figure 5.5 Rupture of middle cerebral artery during mechanical thrombectomy. A: Occlusion of left middle cerebral artery superior branch (AP, arrow). B: Stent retriever 4 × 20 mm deployed (AP, arrow). C: Post-retraction contrast extravasation, left middle cerebral artery, early phase angiogram (AP, arrow). D: Post-retraction contrast extravasation, left middle cerebral artery, late phase angiogram (AP, arrow). E: Flat panel intraprocedural CT scan demonstrates hyperdensity in left hemispheric subarachnoid space (arrow). F: A nitinol self-expanding stent 4.5 × 22 mm placed in middle cerebral artery proximal trunk and superior branch (AP, arrow). G: Partial recanalization of superior division of middle cerebral artery (AP, arrow). H: Postprocedural angiogram demonstrates partial recanalization of superior division of middle cerebral artery. I: Postprocedural head CT demonstrates hyperdensity in left hemispheric subarachnoid space and infarction in left middle cerebral artery distribution (arrow).

Device-related perforation is another serious risk. The choice of an appropriate device for the vessel anatomy is paramount here. For instance, at a blind bifurcation point, it may be difficult to deploy a stent-retriever, particularly of large caliber, compared with proximal end aspiration techniques that may be accomplished with aspiration thrombectomy devices (penumbra). However, the overwhelming literature thus far seems to display the safety of using even stent-retrievers here.

In contrast, thrombectomy from distal to proximal aspect of the clot may be preferred with basilar tip occlusions, as there is little room for back and forth maneuvers, such as are necessary with the Penumbra separator. With this anatomy, a straight device may in fact be more dangerous as the tendency will be to penetrate through the basilar tip rather than selecting a (non-visualized) terminal basilar branch. Stent-retrievers that have now become standard-of-care may not pose this challenge as the Penumbra separator would. Newer generations of the Penumbra devices are also softer at the tip and may help to minimize this risk.

Guiding catheters may also dissect the parent vessels, and rushed procedures, often with awake and moving patients with tortuous anatomy, compound this risk. Inflation of the balloon guide catheter may cause vessel injury if the balloon is over-dilated. To avoid this, inflation should follow device prescription. At the very least, such maneuvers undoubtedly result in parent vessel vasospasm, easily documented on angiograms taken immediately after thrombectomy. The tendency for forward migration of the guide catheter during device retraction should be kept in mind during the completion of the pass.

Device fracture

The initial Solitaire device was designed as a detachable adjunct for parent vessel reconstruction during aneurysm embolization. Early detachment or separation of the Solitaire FR revascularization device has been reported in previous studies; most of the reported cases have shown poor outcomes, without successful retrieval of the accidentally detached devices[20]. Detachment of the Solitaire stent during thrombectomy can be due to separation around or inside the proximal marker. Newer devices have been modified not only so that they are not detachable but also to render a "mechanical" unintentional fracture less probable. In none of the recent trials was fracture and retention of a stent-retriever a reported complication. Theoretically, even if this event were to occur, it may in fact be beneficial to bore a new lumen in the occluded vessel. The risk thus becomes the necessity of antiplatelet agents in a patient facing a risk of subsequent reperfusion hemorrhage. Adherence to the manufacturer's instructions for use (IFU) of partial resheathing during retraction and not using the device for more than two passes might decrease the possibility of such device failure.

The MERCI retriever device is no longer recommended for mechanical thrombectomy. Excess torque and counterclockwise torque placed undue strain on the device junction point, resulting in fracture.

Penumbra Separator fracture may be difficult to recognize. The separator is most vulnerable to fracture during to and fro movements in the course of aspiration thrombectomy. Constant fluoroscopy during any Separator maneuver is essential; interventionalists should be careful to recognize any movement of the proximal end which is not translated on X-ray to the distal end. Separator fracture may occur anywhere along the device, but is more difficult to manage if occurring distally. In this case, removal of the Reperfusion catheter with retained Separator fragment under suction may ensure that the fractured tip is aspirated into microcatheter during removal. Flush attachments may be temporarily disconnected from the guide catheter to reduce the chance of the Separator migrating downstream.

While this author has not experienced distal fracture with the Penumbra device, proximal fracture has been noted. In this case, the external portion of the device fractured at the microcatheter hub, leaving no visible segment. A hemostat was applied to the proximal microcatheter just distal to the hub, to pin the Separator within it, and the whole system was then removed together. This is certainly not ideal after attempting to catheterize the target vessel for an hour, but is a far better solution than risking downstream migration of fractured device. Fracture at the distal end may be more common as stress is directly applied here during movements. Interventionalists should proceed with gentle hands when dealing with this system.

Device "stuck"

Inability to retrieve the device after a pass may be encountered. This will usually first be met with the microcatheter and wire. Generally this can be remedied by slight forward advancement of the microcatheter, "resheathing" the stent-retriever while continuing to apply gentle but firm retraction. This phenomenon is not necessarily uncommon and may in fact occur when a thrombus is well engaged within the device, as desired. Inability to retract a Penumbra Separator, on the other hand, may indicate local vessel injury. Extreme caution and avoidance of sudden, forceful moves during removal should be applied in this scenario. Guide catheter angiography may highlight the cause of difficulty. If vessel injury is the culprit, a period of "watchful waiting", leaving the microcatheter and separator in place for a few minutes, can allow temporary cessation of extravasation; meanwhile, reversal agents can be considered if any thrombolytics or other anticoagulants have been administered.

"Benign" vasospasm due to vessel manipulation is more likely to occur in the region of the cavernous–supraclinoid carotid junction (owing to the sharp turn of the anterior genu), compared with hemorrhage related to the device, which is more likely to occur in target vessels.

Balloon dilatation catheters are not commonly first-line agents in acute stroke treatment, but perhaps of all the various devices used, these might hold the highest risk for causing dissection and subsequent inability to withdraw the device. Balloon sizes should be chosen carefully, for example 3–4 mm balloons for MCA occlusions and larger balloons for carotid terminus occlusions. Balloon inflation can be difficult to see under fluoroscopy, and this is the most common reason for their rupture, particularly with compliant balloons that offer less tactile feedback to resistance. Native and subtraction fluoroscopy should be used simultaneously if available. Native images provide optimal visualization of the balloon during inflation, whereas road mapping shows subtraction artifact from vessel movement due to balloon inflation. Some balloons, such as the Hyperform and Hyperglide (eV3), can be deflated by removing the microwire. However, this imbibes blood in the balloon and dilutes the contrast, making it more difficult to see during the next inflation. Precise volume of inflation should be noted and withdrawn before re-inflation to prevent over-inflation. As in any other case of vessel injury, treatment options are limited. If injury occurs distal to the occluded blood vessel, this may prevent significant hemorrhage; hemorrhage in the proximal parent vessel can be severe. Withdrawing the balloon catheter to a point more proximal to the rupture site and re-inflating here may temporarily cause cessation of flow, allowing hemostatic mechanisms to ensue. However, the benefit of this is likely short-lived and minimal.

Distal embolism in same or different vascular territory

Depending on the initial site of occlusion, this may be hard to interpret. For instance, with a scenario of pre-intervention ICA or M1 occlusion, it is difficult to know the state of the distal vasculature. Often in these cases, flow dynamics favor robust filling of the posterior communicator through full posterior cerebral artery (PCA) distribution, or robust filling of the anterior cerebral artery. Once antegrade flow through the MCA is established, however, flow dynamics then may favor flow away from these vessels, if the circle of Willis is complete. Rather than being occluded, unopacified blood from the posterior circulation is likely competing with and washing out contrast injected in the ICA. Investigating the posterior circulation vessels or contralateral ICA, in the case of the anterior cerebral artery (ACA) not filling, will help differentiate whether this is embolization of a new territory or a hemodynamic change due to recanalization of the target vessel (Figure 5.6).

However, exacerbation of thrombus or newly occluded territory may occur in cases of more distal occlusions (e.g. M2, A1–2) if the clot is "lost" during a retrieval process[21]. If this occurs and is recognized, the primary consideration should be the risk–benefit of retargeting the new territory for intervention. Very distal occlusion may be both technically difficult to reach with devices, and not clinically beneficial unless in highly eloquent cortex that has been unaffected clinically *a priori*. The new Mindframe stent retriever (Covidien) is designed for treating M3 branches of 2–3 mm diameter.

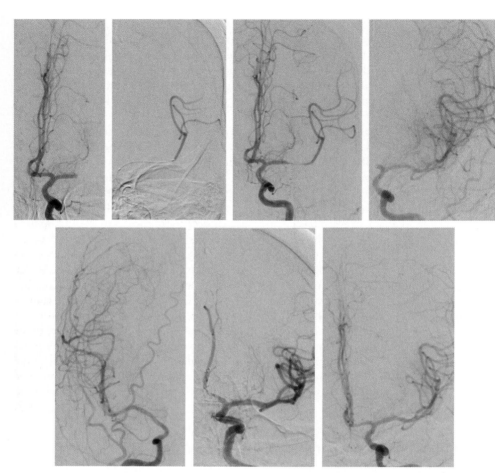

Figure 5.6 A 55-year-old right-handed female with abrupt onset of right homonymous hemianopsia, dense right side hemiplegia with sensory deficit and global aphasia. NIHSS 20 points. Non-contrast head CT, no ICH and ASPECT >7. An 8 Fr concentric catheter was placed in the left internal carotid artery (ICA). A Prowler select plus was then advanced over a Synchro 2 microwire and placed distal to left middle cerebral artery (MCA) M1 segment thrombus. A microcatheter run demonstrated good placement. A Trevo 4 × 20 mm was advanced and placed across the thrombus; a run demonstrated filling of the inferior division. After 5 minutes' wait, the system was removed under fluoroscopic guidance and manual aspiration while the balloon was inflated at the cervical level. A follow-up run demonstrated recanalization of the left MCA, thrombolysis in cerebral infarction (TICI) = 3, but now the presence of a new TICI = 0 in the left anterior cerebral artery (ACA).

Right common carotid artery run demonstrated aplastic right A1 segment. The left ACA was bihemispheric, therefore mechanical thrombectomy was performed with Trevo 4 × 20 mm. After 5 minutes' wait, the system was removed under fluoroscopic guidance and manual aspiration while the balloon was inflated at the cervical level. A follow-up run demonstrated complete recanalization of the left MCA, TICI = 3, and in the left ACA, TICI = 3. At the table the patient was significantly better; the next day she was NIHSS = 0.

Medication errors

Stroke intervention procedures are typically all-consuming mental feats for the operator, with increased reliance on staff for non-technical assistance. The environment may lead to errors in producing the correct medication or the correct dilution for the table. Staff may not be familiar with many routine drugs used, particularly in catheterization labs which

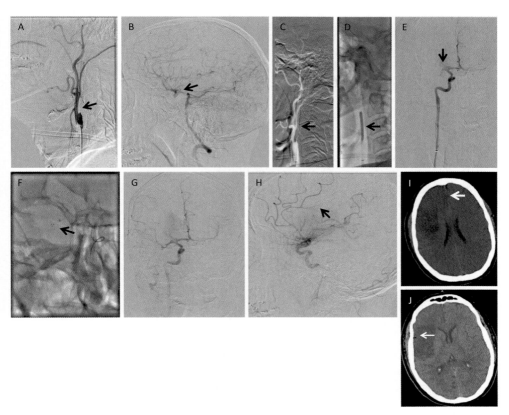

Figure 5.7 Distal embolization during mechanical thrombectomy. **A:** Occlusion of right ICA (lateral view, arrow). **B:** Collateral circulation from posterior cerebral artery (lateral, arrow). **C:** Traversing the occlusion with glide wire (lateral, arrow). **D:** Primary angioplasty right internal carotid artery (lateral, arrow). **E:** Proximal middle cerebral artery occlusion after internal carotid artery recanalization (AP, arrow). **F:** Stent retriever 4 × 20 mm deployed in right middle cerebral artery (AP, arrow). **G:** Partial recanalization right middle cerebral artery (AP). **H:** Occlusion of distal branch of anterior cerebral artery (lateral, arrow). **I:** Early changes of ischemic stroke in right anterior cerebral artery (post-procedure CT scan, arrow). **J:** Air embolism in right middle cerebral artery distribution (postprocedure CT scan, arrow).

only perform emergent (i.e. acute stroke) neuro-interventional cases. Anticipation is imperative here; staff should be adequately trained, by the neuro-interventionalist, in the names, medications, and preparation of drugs. Most suites that perform peripheral interventional cases will be well stocked with Cathflo® (Genentech, San Francisco, CA), the 2 mg vial of tPA, commonly used for catheter declotting, and possibly also larger (usually 50 mg) bottles of tPA. Doses used for neuro-interventional purposes may be significantly less than those used in peripheral cases, and this should also be relayed to the staff. If newer-generation fibrinolytics such as reteplase are used, distinction between this and other agents such as alteplase should be highlighted, particularly as the dosage of one (reteplase) is in units, compared with milligrams for alteplase. Pre-printed protocols with drugs, reconstitution methods, and dilutions (to desired volume) are beneficial; for example, tPA taken from a 2 mg vial should be reconstituted 1:1 with 2 ml of saline solution and further diluted in 8 ml of normal saline to create a 1:5 ml concentration. The amounts in each step may be modified as desired. Other agents that might be utilized, such as verapamil or other anti-hypertensives, for the treatment of vasospasm, may be desired on-table, but unintentionally administered by staff intravenously. The operator and staff should have knowledge and perhaps even codified reversal protocols: calcium for calcium channel blockers, glucagon for beta blockers, etc.

Technical failure
Inability to access occlusion site

The anatomy of patients undergoing acute stroke intervention is rarely favorable. They are usually older, with type 3 aortic arches, and iliofemoral atherosclerosis; the great vessels arise at abrupt right angles from the aortic arch, rendering even diagnostic angiography difficult. On top of this, the catheter systems of acute stroke cases are larger and less navigable than other neuro-interventional microcatheters, requiring guide catheter placement with adequate distal purchase. Long femoral or shuttle sheaths (up to 90 cm with tips placed in descending thoracic aorta) create a straight platform from groin to arch. A diagnostic catheter can be used to select the target great vessel and further guide the sheath closer to the target.

The 6 French Penumbra Neuron MAX delivery catheter (Penumbra Inc, San Leandro, CA) is an excellent guide for acute stroke work. An 0.072" and 0.088" delivery both achieve the same distal vessel purchase. The larger MAX guide catheter requires a larger 8 French femoral sheath (or direct placement in the femoral artery, without a sheath). The larger Reperfusion catheters (e.g. 5 MAX ACE) must be used with the larger Neuron MAX. The Neuron's soft tip enables quite distal placement in parent vessels such as the internal carotid or vertebral artery, but is generally not intended for parent vessel selection. The specially manufactured 5 French Penumbra Select catheters are longer in length than standard diagnostic catheters and are available in a variety of distal tip configurations. These smaller catheters fit coaxially through the Penumbra Neuron as a platform to select the great vessel and then track the guide catheter distally. Navien™ intracranial support catheters (ID 0.058 to 0.072 inches) are also a good option for the Penumbra Neuron catheter.

One difficulty with this coaxial technique is the limited space to reform the shape of the diagnostic catheter Simmons 2 in the aortic arch. It may be easier to select the great vessel with a diagnostic catheter of choice and exchange this for a more suitable guide. The hemostat can also be removed from the diagnostic catheter to provide more working length. Sheath select catheters are also available that can be used to select the vessel (e.g. Shuttle Select catheters for Cook Shuttle sheath).

For microcatheter placement, "coaxial, coaxial, coaxial" is the mantra for successful catheterization. The larger Penumbra aspiration catheters, Navien 0.053" (Covidien), or Concentric DAC (Stryker) offer excellent support for the device delivery microcatheters.

The 3 MAX can be used coaxially with the 5 MAX, and suction can be applied via both. Often, while using a stent-retriever or other smaller inner device through a larger 5 MAX or 5 MAX ACE, during the retrieval, just as with the guide catheter, the intermediate catheter will advance further. This so-called "Solumbra" technique might provide an avenue for further aspiration; after removing the inner microcatheter and device, the ACE or intermediate catheter can be left in place for additional aspiration thrombectomy.

A transbrachial or transradial approach may have to be used to access greater vessels in certain circumstances when the usual approach is unsuccessful, for example difficult aortic

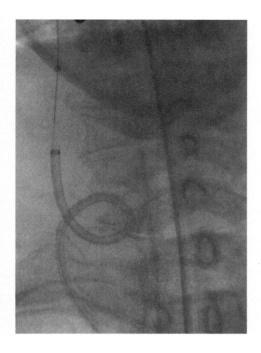

Figure 5.8 Native imaging of the cervical region demonstrates the ease with which the modern guide catheters, in this case the Neuron MAX 0.088", traverse tortuous anatomy (in this case a 360° loop) to allow distal purchase. Care must be taken, however, during multiple passes. It is easy for the guide catheter to move or lose position, and then subsequent (inadvertent) advancement may oppose the catheter tip against the vessel wall, resulting in dissection.

arch anatomy or proximal large vessel stenosis/tortuosity, or occluded femoral arteries. Typically a 6 French sheath may be placed, and the procedure can be performed with a 6 French guide such as a soft-tip Envoy or Neuron catheter (Penumbra, USA). If the 5 French system is considered, there are still various choices of guides such as the Navien™ 058, Envoy, Chaperon, DAC 057, Neuron™ 053, and 5 MAX catheter.

One additional word of caution in utilizing these newer-generation guide catheters in difficult vasculature: Although these catheters are excellent for improving distal purchase, and even can be advanced across 360° loops (Figure 5.8) the catheter tip will at times abut directly against the vessel wall in this type of configuration. Care should be taken to place the catheter in a straight segment either well proximal to, or well beyond such a loop, so that any guide catheter movement will not dissect the vessel at this point.

Unsuccessful thrombectomy

Even after difficult catheterization is accomplished, thrombectomy itself may be unsuccessful. Inadequate time of aspiration is one reason for aspiration thrombectomy failure. Aspiration of 5–15 minutes is reasonable for the Penumbra system, depending on catheter size. Upsizing the device where possible is a reasonable next step. The 5 MAX and ACE device, as stated, is intended for terminal ICA occlusions and large MCA (M1), and possibly even basilar artery occlusions, while the 4 MAX and 3 MAX are designed more for distal occlusions (e.g. M2 and beyond). The 3 MAX specifically is longer than the other catheters, with the specific intent to reach more distal occlusions. Guide catheter and reperfusion catheter compatibility should be checked. It may also be useful to abandon standard convention here, and commence aspiration thrombectomy from the mid-clot position (to ensure that the appropriate target area is covered).

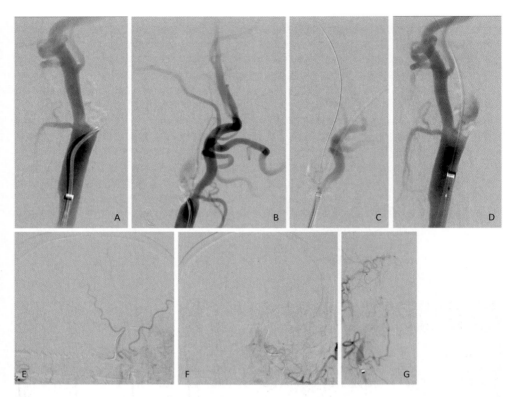

Figure 5.9 A 66-year-old gentleman with NIHSS of 19, no improvement noted with IV alteplase. CT angiogram showed occluded left ICA and MCA. Patient was intubated since could not cooperate during cerebral angiogram. This confirmed occlusion of left ICA (A) with minimal trickle of contrast in carotid bulb, best seen in lateral view (B). Microwire could be advanced, therefore 4 French vertebral artery catheter was placed near origin and exchange length microwire was advanced intracranially into left ICA for support. There is no intracranial filling noted in AP or lateral view (C, D, E, F). A 4 mm Spider distal embolic protection device was advanced into distal left ICA (G) and after performing angioplasty with 5 mm × 30 mm monorail balloon, an Xact stent measuring 9–7 mm × 40 mm was deployed successfully (H). Guide catheter run confirmed terminal left ICA occlusion involving whole supraclinoid segment (I). Microcatheter injection demonstrates thrombus in left MCA extending from M1 to M2 segments (J). Solitaire stent-retriever device was used with distal aspiration through 5 MAX catheter, and complete recanalization was achieved with visualization of left ophthalmic artery, near fetal origin of left posterior cerebral artery, left ACA and TICI 2b filling of left MCA (K, L, M). Follow-up guide catheter injection demonstrates residual 35% stenosis in the stent (N, O). DWI sequence of MRI (P) on following day demonstrated scattered left MCA distribution acute infarct involving the left temporal, frontal, and parietal lobes and left basal ganglia. Patient was discharged to acute rehabilitation and had mild hemiparesis with dysarthria.

In the case of stent-retrievers, there may be variable strategies, for instance making another pass with the same retriever or using a new stent-retriever (same or different company); using direct aspiration with an intermediate catheter such as Neuron 4 MAX or 5 MAX; or using intra-arterial thrombolytics. There is no established dose regimen for IA recombinant tPA, although 22 mg is the maximum dose in the Interventional Management of Stroke 3 trial protocol. In clinical practice, typical IA tPA doses used are much less than this[22].

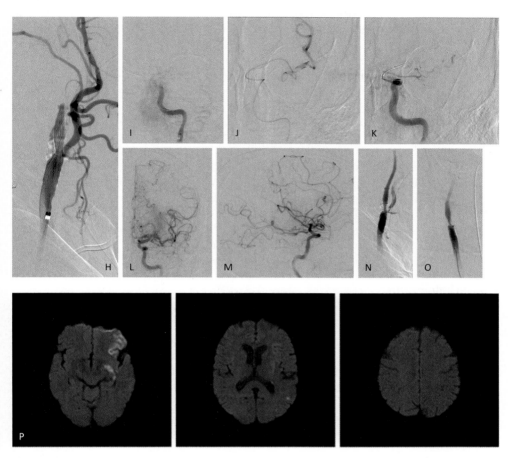

Figure 5.9 *(cont.)*

Tandem stenosis/occlusions

A tandem occlusion is a rare presentation of acute stroke that involves occlusion of the proximal cervical ICA at the bifurcation with an intracranial MCA occlusion, although the distal lesion may also involve the ACA territory. The underlying pathophysiology involves either atherosclerotic disease or a dissection of the proximal vasculature leading to complete occlusion and an embolus causing a distal tandem occlusion. Two approaches exist for the treatment of tandem occlusions, treating either the proximal occlusion or the distal occlusion first; there is no consensus on which approach is more efficacious, but we prefer treating the proximal occlusion first followed by distal occlusion (Figure 5.9).

The concerns for angioplasty and stent placement in acute setting includes the procedure's technical feasibility (e.g. the success of stent insertion under severe stenosis or occlusion and the distal embolization caused by manipulation of highly vulnerable plaque), safety (e.g. the potential risk of developing acute in-stent stenosis due to the lack of antiplatelet premedication), related complications (e.g. cerebral hyperperfusion syndrome (CHS)) and effectiveness for improving patients' neurological deficits and long-term follow-up. It may be difficult to cross the lesion with a distal protection device, and thus a proximal method of protection (e.g. flow reversal or balloon occlusion) may have to be employed. However, with a downstream MCA occlusion, the added step of utilizing a protection device may not confer much additional benefit. In a study of 22 cases that had emergent carotid artery angioplasty and stenting, but had not received dual antiplatelet medications if they had already received IV alteplase, none of these patients developed in-stent thrombosis. In another study of 23 patients, it was concluded that primary stenting of the extracranial carotid artery combined with intracranial mechanical thrombectomy can be an effective treatment for tandem occlusions, can be performed with a high rate of technical success, and can achieve good clinical outcomes in selected patients. However, the incidence of symptomatic intracranial hemorrhage (SICH) may be higher than in other patient populations and may be associated with the use of Abciximab and advanced patient age. Therefore, aggressive antiplatelet use should be avoided in such cases[23]. We are careful about monitoring blood pressure closely and control it to keep it less than 120 mmHg if we achieved good recanalization distally; otherwise, keep between 120 and 140 mmHg.

Conclusions

Interventional stroke therapy presents one of the most difficult procedures in the neuro-endovascular realm. The "need for speed", unfavorable anatomy, recalcitrant clot, and critically ill patients all interact to create a complex treatment scenario. Adequate planning, from medication agents to specific materials, can all help to minimize procedural risks and technical failures.

References

1. Furlan A, Higashida R, Wechsler L, et al. Intra-arterial prourokinase for acute ischemic stroke. The PROACT II study: a randomized controlled trial. Prolyse in Acute Cerebral Thromboembolism. *JAMA* 1999;282:2003–11.

2. Smith WS, Sung G, Saver J, et al. Mechanical thrombectomy for acute ischemic stroke: final results of the Multi MERCI trial. *Stroke* 2008;39:1205–12.

3. PPST Investigators. The Penumbra pivotal stroke trial: safety and effectiveness of a new generation of mechanical devices for clot removal in intracranial large vessel occlusive disease. *Stroke* 2009;40:2761–8.

4. Berkhemer OA, Fransen PS, Beumer D, et al. A randomized trial of intraarterial treatment for acute ischemic stroke. *N Engl J Med* 2015;372:11–20.

5. Campbell BC, Mitchell PJ, Kleinig TJ, et al. Endovascular therapy for ischemic stroke with perfusion-imaging selection. *N Engl J Med* 2015;372:1009–18.

6. Goyal M, Demchuk AM, Menon BK, et al. Randomized assessment of rapid endovascular treatment of ischemic stroke. *N Engl J Med* 2015;372:1019–30.

7. Saver JL, Goyal M, Bonafe A, et al. Solitaire with the Intention for Thrombectomy as Primary Endovascular Treatment for Acute Ischemic Stroke (SWIFT PRIME) trial: protocol for a randomized, controlled, multicenter study comparing the Solitaire revascularization device with IV tPA with IV tPA alone in acute ischemic stroke. *Int J Stroke* 2015;10:439–48.

8. del Zoppo GJ, Higashida RT, Furlan AJ, et al. PROACT: a phase II randomized trial of recombinant pro-urokinase by direct

arterial delivery in acute middle cerebral artery stroke. PROACT Investigators. Prolyse in Acute Cerebral Thromboembolism. *Stroke* 1998;29:4–11.

9. Adams HP, Jr., Effron MB, Torner J, *et al.* Emergency administration of Abciximab for treatment of patients with acute ischemic stroke: results of an international phase III trial: Abciximab in Emergency Treatment of Stroke Trial (AbESTT-II). *Stroke* 2008;39:87–99.

10. Broderick JP, Palesch YY, Demchuk AM, *et al.* Endovascular therapy after intravenous t-PA versus t-PA alone for stroke. *N Engl J Med* 2013;368:893–903.

11. Hussein HM, Georgiadis AL, Vazquez G, *et al.* Occurrence and predictors of futile recanalization following endovascular treatment among patients with acute ischemic stroke: a multicenter study. *AJNR Am J Neuroradiol* 2010;31:454–8.

12. Natarajan SK, Karmon Y, Snyder KV, *et al.* Prospective acute ischemic stroke outcomes after endovascular therapy: a real-world experience. *World Neurosurg* 2010;74:455–64.

13. Janjua N, El-Gengaihy A, Pile-Spellman J, Qureshi AI. Late endovascular revascularization in acute ischemic stroke based on clinical-diffusion mismatch. *AJNR Am J Neuroradiol* 2009;30:1024–7.

14. Levi M, Eerenberg E, Kamphuisen PW. Bleeding risk and reversal strategies for old and new anticoagulants and antiplatelet agents. *J Thromb Haemost* 2011;9:1705–12.

15. Cooper ES, Bracey AW, Horvath AE, *et al.* Practice parameter for the use of fresh-frozen plasma, cryoprecipitate, and platelets. Fresh-Frozen Plasma, Cryoprecipitate, and Platelets Administration Practice Guidelines Development Task Force of the College of American Pathologists. *JAMA* 1994;271:777–81.

16. Yoon W, Seo JJ, Kim JK, *et al.* Contrast enhancement and contrast extravasation on computed tomography after intra-arterial thrombolysis in patients with acute ischemic stroke. *Stroke* 2004;35:876–81.

17. Qureshi AI, Hussein HM, Janjua N, Harris-Lane P, Ezzeddine MA. Postprocedure intravenous eptifibatide following intra-arterial reteplase in patients with acute ischemic stroke. *J Neuroimaging* 2008;18:50–5.

18. Qureshi AI, Harris-Lane P, Kirmani JF, *et al.* Intra-arterial reteplase and intravenous Abciximab in patients with acute ischemic stroke: an open-label, dose-ranging, phase I study. *Neurosurgery* 2006;59:789–96; discussion 96–7.

19. Flint AC, Cullen SP, Faigeles BS, Rao VA. Predicting long-term outcome after endovascular stroke treatment: the totaled health risks in vascular events score. *AJNR Am J Neuroradiol* 2010;31:1192–6.

20. Kwon HJ, Chueh JY, Puri AS, Koh HS. Early detachment of the Solitaire stent during thrombectomy retrieval: an in vitro investigation. *J Neurointerv Surg* 2015;7:114–17.

21. Kurre W, Vorlaender K, Aguilar-Perez M, *et al.* Frequency and relevance of anterior cerebral artery embolism caused by mechanical thrombectomy of middle cerebral artery occlusion. *AJNR Am J Neuroradiol* 2013;34:1606–11.

22. Khatri P, Hill MD, Palesch YY, *et al.* Methodology of the Interventional Management of Stroke III Trial. *Int J Stroke* 2008;3:130–7.

23. Heck DV, Brown MD. Carotid stenting and intracranial thrombectomy for treatment of acute stroke due to tandem occlusions with aggressive antiplatelet therapy may be associated with a high incidence of intracranial hemorrhage. *J Neurointerv Surg* 2015;7:170–5.

Carotid angioplasty and stenting: complication avoidance and management

Ramachandra P. Tummala

Introduction

From the ongoing debate and trials addressing the indications for and relative efficacy of carotid angioplasty and stenting (CAS) versus carotid endarterectomy (CEA) in stroke prevention, a key message emerges: both CAS and CEA are durable treatments when carried out successfully, with the bulk of strokes occurring periprocedurally in head-to-head trials[1]. Meticulous attention to complication avoidance and management during CAS is fundamental to its overall success in stroke prophylaxis. While CAS is generally straightforward, certain patients continue to pose technical challenges during various stages of the procedure.

Table 6.1 summarizes the major randomized clinical trials regarding CAS. The following techniques are the result of experience with these technical difficulties and complications. The purpose of the present chapter is not to discuss the merits or disadvantages of carotid stenting, nor is it to compare carotid stenting with CEA. The risks of endovascular therapy must always be weighed against the risks of surgery or medical therapy in the individual patient. It is with the anticipation that an increased number of complex cases will be referred for endovascular therapy that the described techniques may be germane. Some of these technical "pearls" are already used at other centers; undoubtedly many more are unknown to our group but already used by other experienced interventionalists. The following techniques have allowed the expansion of the endovascular limits of treating carotid artery disease, and we believe they are useful for complication avoidance and management.

Standard technique for carotid angioplasty and stenting

The approach for routine CAS is fairly standardized with minor institutional variations (Figure 6.1). We perform almost all of these procedures through a transfemoral approach. Through a groin sheath, we advance a 5 French diagnostic catheter (often a Simmons 2 configuration catheter) into the mid common carotid artery (CCA) and obtain a diagnostic angiogram, including baseline intracranial runs. Under normal conditions, we advance a stiff exchange length wire into the distal external carotid artery (ECA) and exchange the diagnostic catheter and groin sheath for a long introducer sheath (often a 90 cm long 6 French Cook Shuttle, Cook Incorporated, Bloomington, IN). Alternatively with tortuous anatomy, various other guide catheters can be used. After positioning the tip of the introducer or guide catheter (for simplicity we will refer to these devices as guide

Complications of Neuroendovascular Procedures and Bailout Techniques, ed. Rakesh Khatri, Gustavo J. Rodriguez, Jean Raymond and Adnan I. Qureshi. Published by Cambridge University Press.
© Cambridge University Press 2016.

Table 6.1 Summary of randomized clinical trials of carotid angioplasty and stenting (CAS) versus carotid endarterectomy (CAE)

	CAVATAS[8]	Wallstent[9]	SAPPHIRE[10]	EVA-3S[11]	SPACE[12]	CREST[13]
Year published	2001	2001	2004	2006	2006	2010
Period of enrollment	May 1992 to July 1997	January 1997 to June 1999	August 2000 to July 2002	September 2000 to September 2005	March 2001 to March 2006	December 2000 through July 2008
Country	Europe, Australia, and Canada	United States	United States	France	Germany, Austria, and Switzerland	United States and Canada
Inclusion criteria	Presence of clinically important stenosis determined by local criteria	Symptomatic ICA stenosis ≥60%	Symptomatic ICA stenosis ≥50%, asymptomatic ICA stenosis ≥80%, and ≥1 high-risk surgical criteria	Symptomatic ICA stenosis ≥60%	Symptomatic ICA stenosis ≥50% according to NASCET criteria or ≥70% according to ECST criteria	Symptomatic ICA stenosis ≥50% on angiography, ≥70% on US, on CTA or MRA if the stenosis on US was 50–69%. In 2005 extended to asymptomatic stenosis of ≥60% or angiography, ≥70% US, or ≥80% on CTA or MRA if the stenosis on US was 50–69%.
Determination of eligibility	Non-invasive techniques or angiography	Angiography	Doppler ultrasound or angiography	Conventional angiography or Doppler plus MRA	Duplex ultrasound or angiography	Angiography, CTA, MRA, US

Table 6.1 (cont.)

	CAVATAS[8]		Wallstent[9]		SAPPHIRE[10]		EVA-3S[11]		SPACE[12]		CREST[13]	
Requirements for interventionalists	Not specified		Not specified		Required to submit experience and results		Performed at least 12 carotid stenting procedures or at least 35 stent placement procedures in the supra-aortic trunks, of which at least 5 were in the carotid artery		Performed at least 25 successful consecutive percutaneous carotid angioplasties or stent procedures		More than 12 procedures per year, with complication and death rate <3% for asymptomatic and <5% among symptomatic patients	
Primary end point	30-day rate of disabling stroke or death		Ipsilateral stroke or procedure-related or vascular death at 1 year		A composite of death, stroke, or MI within 30 days after the intervention or death or ipsilateral stroke between 31 days and 1 year		Any stroke or death within 30 days after treatment		Ipsilateral ischemic stroke or death from randomization to 30 days after procedure		The primary end point was the composite of any stroke, myocardial infarction, or death during the periprocedural period or ipsilateral stroke within 4 years after randomization.	

Intervention	CEA	CAS	CEA	CAS	CEA	CAS	CEA	CAS	CEA	CAS	CEA	CAS
Patients treated, n	246	240	112	107	151	159	259	261	565	567	1240	1262
Mean age, y	67	67	70	67	72	72	70	69	68	68	69	69
Symptomatic	91%	88%	100%	100%	29%	30%	100%	100%	100%	100%	53%	53%
Men	70%	69%	62%	66%	68%	68%	78%	72%	72%	72%	66%	64%
CAD	37%	39%			74%	85%			24%	21%		
Angina			29%	37%								

86

MI	17%	19%	28%	19%			13%	11%				
Previous CEA					24%	29%						
CHF			4%	7%	18%	18%						
History of stroke	39%	37%	37%	40%	24%	27%	20%	13%	43%	44%		
History of TIA	26%	25%	62%	65%	32%	31%	23%	25%	31%	30%		
Hypertension	58%	53%	82%	69%	85%	86%	72%	73%	76%	75%	86%	86%
Diabetes mellitus	13%	14%	28%	34%	27%	26%	26%	22%	28%	26%	30%	31%
Hyperlipidemia	32%	34%	58%	55%	79%	80%	56%	58%	86%	83%		
Stenosis (mean)	77%	75%	75%	76%								
Contralateral occlusion	8%	10%					1%	5%			3%	2%
Technical success	89%			97%		89%		93%			89%	
Primary end point rates	5.9%	6.4%	3.6%	12.1%	20.1%	12%	3.9%	9.6%	6.3%	6.8%		7.2%
30-day combined periprocedural complication rate	9.9%	10%	4.5%	12.1%	5.4%	4.8%	3.9%	9.6%	6.5%	7.7%	4.5%	5.2%

CAD: coronary artery disease; CHF, congestive heart failure; ECST, European Carotid Surgery Trial; CTA: computed tomography angiography; MI: myocardial infarction; MRA: magnetic resonance angiography, NASCET, North American Symptomatic Carotid Endarterectomy Trial; TIA, transient ischemic attack; US: ultrasound.

Table 6.2 Common devices in a typical carotid stent placement procedure

Closed cell carotid stent	Wallstent and NexStent (Boston Scientific Natick, MA) Xact (Abbott Vascular, IL)
Open cell carotid stent	Acculink (Abbott Vascular, IL) Precise (Cordis, NJ) Exponent (Medtronic, MN) Protégé (Covidien, CA) Zilver 518® RX (Cook Medical, IN)
Distal embolic protection device	Angioguard (Cordis, NJ) Emboshield (Abbott Vascular, IL) Accunet (Abbott Vascular, IL) Spider (Covidien, CA) Gore Embolic Filter (Gore, DE) FilterWire EZ (Boston Scientific, MA) FiberNet (Medtronic, MN)
Proximal embolization protection devices	Gore Flow Reversal System (Gore, AZ) Mo.Ma (Medtronic, MN)

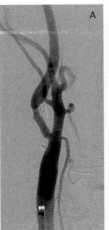 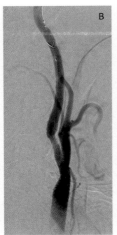 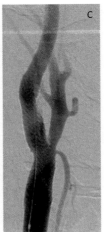

Figure 6.1 A 68-year-old gentleman with symptomatic right ICA stenosis. **A:** AP view demonstrates right ICA stenosis measuring about 60%. A 6 French Cook shuttle guide is also visualized. **B:** A 7 mm to 10 mm × 40 mm Acculink stent deployed across stenosis. Distal embolic protection device is also visualized in distal cervical ICA. **C:** Post angioplasty, improved lumen with residual stenosis of about 25%.

devices) in the distal CCA, the patient is anticoagulated with intravenous heparin to achieve an activated clotting time of greater than 250 seconds. Using roadmap guidance, we cross the stenotic lesion with a distal embolic protection device that is deployed in a straight segment of the distal cervical internal carotid artery (ICA). We only perform pre-stenting angioplasty (predilatation) if the lesion is too stenotic to cross with the stent delivery system. After stent deployment, a post-stenting angioplasty (postdilatation) is performed. If the patient's baseline heart rate is less than 80, we administer 0.2 mg of intravenous glycopyrrholate or 0.4 mg atropine, prior to angioplasty. Final angiographic images including intracranial runs are reviewed prior to retrieval of the distal embolic protection device. At the conclusion of the procedure, we use most of the various commercially available devices for percutaneous closure if the common femoral artery access is suitable. Routine carotid stenting can be performed relatively quickly with minimal blood loss. Usual devices in routine practice are provided in Table 6.2.

The following sections will address potential problems as they arise at various stages of the procedure.

I. Vascular access

Stable guide device positioning is mandatory before proceeding with any carotid intervention. Guide device access can be difficult if the CCA is tortuous, if the angle of the origin of the brachiocephalic artery or left CCA off the aortic arch is very acute, or if the aortic arch is diseased or heavily calcified. These anatomic factors may not be an issue during a diagnostic angiogram; however, they can be far more problematic during an intervention, owing to the inherent stiffness of the large guide device needed for most carotid interventions. Advancing the guide device usually requires stable placement of the exchange length wire in a distal ECA branch, ideally the occipital artery or internal maxillary. One would normally obtain very distal purchase in the ECA to facilitate a stable exchange for the guide catheter in an unfavorable arch. Gaining distal access in the ECA helps overcome the acute angulation of the left CCA or brachiocephalic artery; otherwise the entire system may prolapse back into the ascending aorta or arch during the exchange maneuvers. In the following discussion, several situations are presented in which the standard maneuvers cannot be performed or are unusually difficult.

Distal CCA stenosis or ECA occlusion

In the case of an ECA occlusion or a stenotic distal CCA, the plaque should not be disrupted during vascular access, because of the possibility of distal embolization. Therefore, the standard exchange technique for the guide device cannot be performed safely because the exchange wire must cross the plaque before advancing into the ECA. Provided that the angle and length of the target CCA are favorable, we will exchange the diagnostic catheter over a stiff J-shaped wire. The J-shaped end of the wire is positioned just proximal to the CCA stenosis, and a standard exchange is performed. Care must be taken not to allow the J-wire to migrate distally and potentially disturb the plaque.

Sometimes, in our experience, an Amplatz superstiff with 1 cm soft tip can be helpful (usually exchange length Amplatz superstiff is 7 cm long) as long as the wire can be advanced without diagnostic catheter herniation.

Distal CCA stenosis or ECA occlusion in addition to an unfavorable aortic arch

As noted in the previous section, distal wire purchase in the ECA is not feasible. However, a J-wire in the CCA will not be stable enough to allow for a standard exchange maneuver. In this situation, we have several options available. A telescoping technique in which the guide device is advanced over a smaller catheter which has been previously advanced over the J-wire may provide sufficient stability to allow placement of the guiding system. A 125 cm long, 5 Fr JR4 or Vitek catheter (Cook, Bloomington, IN) is inserted through a 90 cm long, 6 Fr Cook Shuttle sheath or an 8 Fr guide (Cordis, Miami Lakes, FL) This relatively stiff 5 French 125 cm long catheter has a distal curve configuration which we have occasionally found useful for accessing the great vessels. In combination with a stiff J-wire, this catheter may be stiff enough to maintain a stable configuration while the guide device is advanced.

When the configuration of the aortic arch or the origins of the great vessels is so unfavorable that the telescoping technique fails, our recourse is a 6 French or 8 French

Simmons 2 configuration guide catheter. Since most carotid stent delivery systems require a larger introducing system, we generally use the 8 French Simmons 2 guide catheter. Unlike a diagnostic Simmons 2 catheter, the 8 French version cannot be reconstituted easily. It usually must be advanced into the contralateral external iliac artery or into the left subclavian artery in order to safely assume its reconstituted shape. The reconstituted 8 French Simmons 2 guide catheter can then be manipulated into the brachiocephalic artery or left CCA without using a wire. Its shape is ideal for an acutely angled left CCA. Like all the Simmons catheters, the 8 French is meant for proximal catheterization of the great vessels. This is sufficient for most carotid interventions since distal access is usually unnecessary. This catheter is particularly useful if there is a "kink" in the CCA that would prohibit advancement of a guide catheter. The large Simmons guide catheter is generally stable and usually will not herniate into the aortic arch as the stent delivery system is advanced[2]. If we anticipate that the aortic arch will not be amenable to standard or telescoping techniques, we avoid them altogether and use the 8 French Simmons 2 catheter primarily.

Before the 8 French Simmons 2 configuration guide catheter was available to us, our salvage maneuver for gaining vascular access was the telescoping technique with balloon assistance. If the telescoping construct described above is not successful, one can consider advancing a balloon catheter into the CCA and inflating the balloon to firmly appose the vessel wall. This may provide the counter-resistance necessary to advance the guide device into the CCA. This maneuver obviously carries risk of injury to the vessel and should be performed only as a last resort to gain access to the CCA. Keep in mind that if one has this much difficulty accessing the CCA, the access necessary to repair any potential vessel injury may not be available.

The "coronary technique" uses an Amplatz AL1 guiding catheter to engage the origin of the CCA, permitting delivery of protection device and stent[3].

An alternative would be to try a transbrachial approach to access the left CCA with a 6 French shuttle or 8 French guide catheter.

Aorto-iliac occlusion

Since many patients with carotid stenosis also have peripheral arterial occlusive disease, a simple transfemoral approach may not be possible in some. A significant stenosis of the common femoral, external iliac, or common iliac artery may be treated with angioplasty or stenting to allow insertion of the large guide catheters needed for carotid intervention. An experienced operator may be able to cross even a long aorto-iliac occlusion, sometimes extending cephalad as far as the renal arteries, and gain access for the carotid intervention. When a long occlusion is navigated, we generally advise stent recanalization of the occluded segment prior to removal of the introducer. For many operators, an aorto-iliac occlusion prohibits a transfemoral approach. In this setting, carotid interventions can be performed via the radial or brachial artery. Because of the size restrictions with many stent delivery systems, transradial or brachial approach is less practical. Although we have used the radial and brachial artery approaches successfully, they can be cumbersome and are far less attractive than the transfemoral route. If the stent delivery system is small enough, a 6 French Simmons 2 guide catheter is a useful device to gain access to the tortuous great vessels when using an upper extremity approach. This catheter is much easier to reconstitute than its 8 French analog. As an

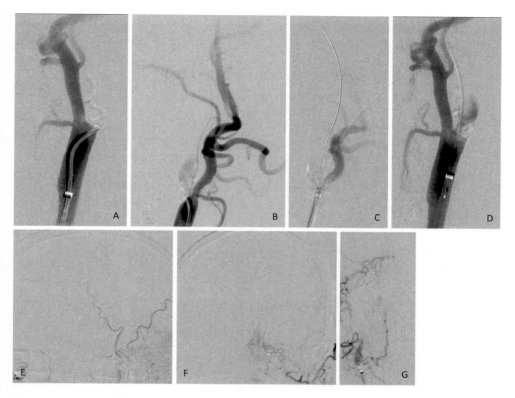

Figure 6.2 A 66-year-old gentleman with National Institute of Health stroke scale (NIHSS) of 19, no improvement noted with IV alteplase. See also Figure 5.9. CT angiogram showed occluded left internal carotid artery(ICA) and middle cerebral artery (MCA). Patient was intubated since could not cooperate during cerebral angiogram. It confirmed occlusion of left ICA (A) with minimal trickle of contrast in carotid bulb best seen in lateral view (B). Microwire could be advanced; therefore 4 French vertebral artery catheter was placed near origin and exchange length microwire was advanced intracranially into left ICA for support. There is no intracranial filling noted in AP or lateral view (C, D, E, F). 4 mm Spider distal embolic protection device was advanced into distal left ICA (G) and after performing angioplasty with 5 mm × 30 mm monorail balloon, Xact stent measuring 9–7 mm × 40 mm was deployed successfully (H). Guide catheter run confirmed terminal left ICA occlusion involving whole supraclinoid segment (I). Microcatheter injection demonstrates thrombus in left Middle cerebral artery extending from M1 to M2 segments (J). Solitaire stent-retriever device was used with distal aspiration through 5 Max catheter, and complete recanalization was achieved with visualization of left ophthalmic artery, near fetal origin of left posterior cerebral artery, left anterior cerebral artery, and TICI 2b filling of left middle cerebral artery (K, L, M). Follow up guide catheter injection demonstrates residual 35% stenosis in the stent (N, O). DWI sequence of MRI (P) following day demonstrated scattered left MCA distribution acute infarct involving the left temporal, frontal, and parietal lobes and left basal ganglia. Patient was discharged to acute rehabilitation and had mild hemiparesis with dysarthria.

additional note, the operator usually receives more radiation exposure when using an upper extremity approach.

II Approaching and crossing the lesion

In this section, we shall discuss endovascular management of difficult carotid plaques. We use embolic protection in almost every carotid intervention. The approved, commercially available distal embolic protection devices are mounted on a 0.014 inch shapeable wire. The two most basic principles of crossing the carotid stenosis smoothly are to have the proper

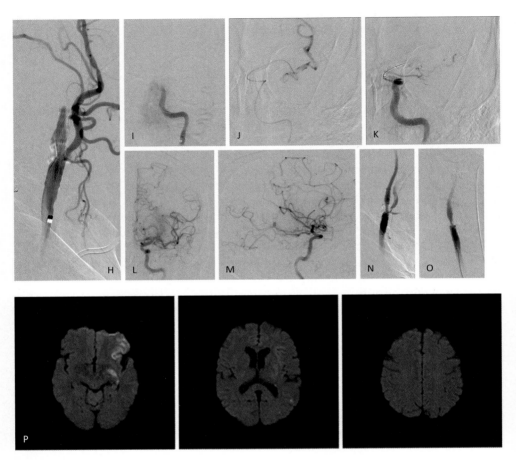

Figure 6.2 (*cont.*)

view of the lesion and the proper shape on the wire. To this end, prior three-dimensional rotational angiography or multiple oblique views may be helpful to identify the best working view.

Crossing high grade and irregular stenosis

A very severe or irregular stenosis may be difficult to cross. Positioning the tip of the guide device as close as possible to the stenosis without disturbing the lesion may provide enough support for the wire to cross the lesion. A 5 French angled multipurpose catheter can be inserted through the guide device to provide the proper angle to engage the lesion as well as offer enough support to allow advancement of the distal embolic protection device across the stenosis. This technique may be particularly useful in the case of a pseudo-occlusion or an acute occlusion. Alternatively, a microcatheter with distal curve or a steerable microcatheter may be used to gain access to a tiny angulated residual lumen (Figure 6.2). One can also advance the curved wire into the ECA and then slowly pull it back while aiming the curve towards the ICA to allow it to fall into the ICA and to engage the stenosis. However, it is important not to force the wire or the distal embolic protection device across the lesion since this can result in procedural complications including distal embolism.

Difficulty with crossing distal embolic protection device

Rarely, a distal embolic protection device will not cross the lesion. One endovascular option in this situation is to use proximal instead of distal embolic protection. The other option is to cross the stenosis with a microcatheter and microwire, exchanging the microcatheter for a small balloon, and performing a modest angioplasty. The angioplasty should be sufficient to allow passage of the distal protection device. We typically use a 2 or 2.5 mm balloon for this purpose. With some systems, the original microwire may be used to support the embolic protection filter. Otherwise, the microwire used initially to navigate across the lesion is kept in place until the distal protection device has also crossed the stenosis and is deployed in the distal cervical ICA (Figure 6.2). Although this sequence requires crossing the lesion twice before deployment of the distal embolic protection device, we have found it to be relatively benign. Deployment of the stent and angioplasty following stent placement, the two events which are believed to be the most likely to produce significant emboli, are still performed using embolic protection.

Uncommonly, the anatomy of the ICA may preclude safe placement of a distal embolic protection device. Most filters require a straight distal ICA segment for optimal wall apposition and such a segment may not be available. A severe "kink", tortuosity or a distal, tandem stenosis may prevent navigation of these devices into a safe segment of the distal ICA (Figure 6.3). Some patients with fibromuscular dysplastic changes in the ICA

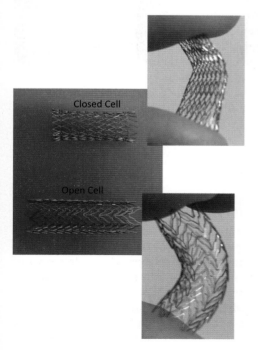

Figure 6.3 When an attempt is made to bend the closed cell design stent, it kinks with sharp bends compared with open cell design.

Closed Cell

Open Cell

represent a higher risk for dissection when using a distal protection device. In such situations, one also might consider performing the intervention using a proximal embolic protection device. A final consideration is to perform the procedure without distal embolic protection, the risk of which should be weighed against non-endovascular treatment options.

III Deployment of stent

Deployment of the stent can be challenging in the presence of significant ICA tortuosity. Stent positioning may be especially critical if the stenosis involves a curve or if there is a "kink" in the ICA just distal to the stenosis. Many times, the distal embolic protection wire or the stent delivery catheter will straighten a curve in the ICA. Therefore, angiographic assessment is necessary just before stent deployment to confirm optimal positioning of the stent. It is equally important to select the proper stent based on the patient's anatomy and the suspected morphology of the lesion. There is no single stent that is appropriate for all lesions. For example, a stenosis involving a tortuous segment of the ICA may be best treated with an open cell stent whereas a closed cell stent may be better for a heavily calcified lesion (Figure 6.3). The interventionalist must be familiar with the different stent designs. At a minimum, one should be aware of the merits and disadvantages of open versus closed cell designs and high versus low porosity designs. Given the shortcomings of current stent technology, a neuroendovascular center should be supplied with more than one type of stent.

It is best to avoid a "kink" that lies immediately distal to the lesion. In these cases, placement of the stent proximal to the sharp turn in the ICA is optimal. Otherwise, the stent may accentuate the kink. The length of the tip (nosecone) of the delivery system should also be considered during stent selection since a long nosecone may engage the kink.

Owing to its inherent, stored mechanical energy, the stent delivery system may advance distally as the stent is deployed; consequently, the stent may overshoot the stenosis. Occasionally, even when the stent delivery system is stable, the stent can move proximally or distally (colloquially known as "watermelon seeding") when deployed. This movement of the stent may result in incomplete coverage of the lesion and occurs more commonly when a stent is deployed off center across a severe stenosis, particularly a severe densely calcified stenosis. Slightly pulling or pushing on the stent delivery catheter as soon as a small segment of stent is seen to emerge during stent deployment (prior to stent apposition to the artery wall) facilitates accurate stent positioning. Failure to position the stent properly may lead to a second, overlapping stent.

Difficulty with removal of the stent delivery system

In our experience, the smoother the leading and trailing edges of the tip of the obturator segment of the catheter, the less frequently this problem occurs. This problem is more likely to develop if the stent is deployed across a severe stenosis without adequate pre-dilatation, if the stenosis is at a curve, and when the edges of the stenosis are abrupt rather than tapered (this can lead to buckling of portions of a stent cell into the lumen). Obviously, most of these situations can be avoided with proper planning. Though uncommon, this problem seems to occur more often with open cell than closed cell stents. If the stent delivery catheter gets stuck on the deployed stent, first, when possible, try to resheath the distal end of the stent deployment catheter. This may allow the catheter to be removed without difficulty. If this fails, careful advancement of the guide device into the stent may provide better support of the stent deployment catheter and hopefully center the catheter within the stent lumen. Careful fluoroscopic monitoring is required during these maneuvers to assure that the stent is not displaced or deformed. If these techniques are not successful, one may use a balloon to further dilate the stent, hopefully freeing the stent deployment catheter. A better solution to avoid this trouble altogether may be to predilate extremely stenotic concentrically calcified stenoses with a cutting balloon. A closed cell stent is a better choice with this type of lesion as the delivery system is less likely to get caught in the stent.

IV Retrieval of distal embolic protection device

Difficulty with retrieval of distal embolic protection device

One can easily be lulled into believing that the procedure is finished once the carotid stent has been deployed and the post-stenting angioplasty has been done. However, retrieval of the distal embolic filter will occasionally be the most challenging part of the entire intervention. Therefore, this step should not be performed with a relaxed attitude. Most of the commercially available distal protection devices are designed to be retrieved using a special catheter or sheath. These retrieval catheters are relatively large, and navigating them through a stent can be difficult. A curved segment of the stented ICA may impede advancement of the retrieval device. The proximal tines of the stent may prevent the catheter from entering the stent lumen, particularly if the proximal end of the stent is in an angulated portion of the artery. Occasionally, the struts of the stent can catch the retrieval catheter. The retrieval of the filter may be successful, but the stent may trap the catheter as it is pulled back through the stent. These problems tend to occur more frequently with stents having an open cell or high porosity architecture. One of the problems with the retrieval catheters lies in their relative inflexibility which alone can make it difficult to advance them across a newly stented vessel. The most obvious way to overcome this obstacle is to advance the guide device over the filterwire until its tip is within the stent. This will usually provide the support needed to navigate the retrieval catheter through the stent. In particularly difficult cases, we will advance the guide device through the stent until it abuts the filter device. The filter can then be retrieved directly into the guide device if the retrieval catheter still cannot be advanced.

If the guide device cannot be advanced, we attempt to insert a smaller curved guide catheter over the wire. We may be able to advance the tip of this second catheter up to the distal embolic protection device. The second guide catheter may provide sufficient support to allow us to advance our initial guide device, and then we may be able to remove the second guide catheter and insert the filter retrieval catheter. Even if we cannot reinsert the filter retrieval catheter, we may be able to attempt retrieval of the distal embolic protection device into the smaller curved guide catheter. In the most extreme cases, one can retrieve the filter directly into the guide device.

Occasionally a distal embolic protection device will be trapped because of vasospasm. When vasospasm interferes with removal of the distal embolic protection device, the vasospasm will usually improve following an intra-arterial injection of 50–200 μg of nitroglycerine. Other vasodilators, such as verapamil or nicardipine, can also be used. Careful imaging is necessary to assure that there is no underlying dissection.

If removal of the distal embolic protection device is inhibited due to the presence of a dissection induced by the device itself, it may be possible to collapse the device enough in its retrieval catheter to allow it to be redeployed further distally. This may enable treatment of the dissection with a stent. One can also partially collapse the filter and place a second wire in parallel prior to removal of the filter. Otherwise, one can remove the filter and attempt to recross the lesion as needed. More proximal dissections, such as those induced by the stent or angioplasty catheter, should be carefully evaluated. Small non-flow limiting dissections might be left untreated and observed. Usually we repair dissections with a second self-expanding stent.

Overload of distal embolic protection device with embolic debris

Rarely, complete or partial occlusion of the ICA will occur as a result of overload of the distal embolic protection device. This is a dangerous situation associated with a significant risk of stroke. In some cases, one may be able to aspirate enough material from the filter through the guide device to allow safe removal of the filter. If the initial CCA access was straightforward, replacing the guide device with a balloon occlusion system can be considered to allow for proximal flow arrest and aspiration during filter removal. Finally, as with retrieval of the stent delivery system, the final recourse may be surgical removal.

V Miscellaneous tips

We cannot easily categorize the strategies in this section. They are maneuvers that we find useful in specific troublesome situations.

Management of adverse hemodynamic events

Following routine practice patterns, we perform carotid interventions under continuous hemodynamic surveillance that includes telemetry and blood pressure monitoring. Carotid angioplasty can induce transient bradycardia and hypotension, both of which may be profound[4]. In our experience, this tends to occur more frequently when treating densely calcified lesions at the CCA bifurcation. Occasionally, arrhythmias, even asystole, may occur. Simply having the patient cough forcefully several times often will induce a return to a regular cardiac rhythm. Premedication with 0.5 to 1.0 mg atropine or 0.2 mg glycopyrrholate intravenously 10 minutes prior to the anticipated angioplasty can be useful but not always effective in preventing these adverse events. While the bradycardia usually resolves within seconds, the hypotension may persist for hours or even days. When this occurs, we immediately start the patient on a dopamine infusion and administer colloids. Since the dopamine is rarely necessary for more than 24 hours, a peripheral infusion of dopamine is adequate. In addition to withholding the patient's routine antihypertensive medications, volume repletion with colloids and early mobilization are the best methods to avoid prolonged hospitalization. The patient usually resumes antihypertensive medications 2 to 3 days later.

Patients with symptomatic coronary artery disease are managed very conservatively. We typically avoid aggressive angioplasty in these patients. A stent having relatively high radial force may be sufficient to provide a satisfactory result without additional angioplasty. If a significant stenosis remains after stenting, we will perform a modest angioplasty (i.e. undersize the balloon or inflate it well below nominal pressure). Complete resolution of the carotid stenosis is unnecessary in these patients, and "angiographic greed" may result in unwelcome cardiac complications.

Guide catheter instability

If the guide device has been successfully placed in the distal CCA but its position is tenuous owing to angulation more proximally, it may herniate toward the aortic arch when trying to advance the distal embolic protection device or the stent delivery system. We may gain extra stability by placing a "buddy" support wire in the ECA. An 0.018 inch relatively stiff shapeable wire placed in the ECA usually provides enough stability. Using a low profile, flexible stent system also helps.

Perforation of ECA branches

In routine carotid interventions, the ECA branches serve as sites for wire placement during exchange maneuvers, particularly during placement of the guide device into the CCA. The stiff 0.035 inch wires can perforate the small ECA branches, and life-threatening neck hematomas may result. If this rare complication occurs, the first step is to assess and secure the patient's airway. We favor elective intubation while the patient remains stable. If no immediate neck hematoma is seen, the patient may be observed for neck hematoma and extubated after 1 or 2 days.

If extravasation of blood and contrast from one of the branch arteries is noted, several options exist to occlude the injured vessel. First, if possible, anticoagulation should be reversed. Anticoagulation with heparin should be reversed with protamine if there are no plans to proceed with the carotid intervention immediately afterwards, or if a significant neck hematoma develops. Even if extravasation of contrast from the perforated branch is minimal, one tends to underestimate the time needed to secure the bleeding point. Often a microcatheter is advanced over a microwire into the perforated artery and positioned as close to the perforation site as possible. In our experience with this complication, we have used platinum coils and N-butyl-2-cyanoacrylate to embolize the ruptured vessel. A plug of absorbent gelatin may also be used. The possibility of a lower cranial nerve injury or embolization through a dangerous anastomosis must be considered when occluding ECA branches. After embolization of the perforated artery, an injection of the ipsilateral sub-clavian artery is prudent to assess for additional extravasation through costocervical or thyrocervical collaterals.

Trapping of a wire by the stent

Similar to the above description of trapped catheters, the distal embolic protection device wire, or even a plain guidewire, may become entangled with the stent. Any attempts to advance a device over the wire may result in longitudinal movement or buckling of the stent. If a wire is entrapped by the stent, we can attempt to free it using a balloon. We advance a low profile balloon as close as possible to the attachment point between the stent and wire. Inflation of the balloon frequently will detach the wire from the stent and return it to a central position within the vessel lumen. This step can be repeated several times, and it may be necessary to push or pull the wire slightly while the balloon is inflated to free it from the stent.

Management of unexpected intraluminal thrombus, ruptured plaque and other foreign bodies

On rare occasions, a thrombus or ruptured plaque fragment may be seen within the stent or within the ICA proximal to the filter. This finding is identified much more frequently if intravascular ultrasonography (IVUS) is routinely employed. The significance of this finding has not been thoroughly studied, particularly when the intraluminal object is only seen on IVUS and not on the angiogram. Although the best therapy for this problem is unknown, our experience indicates that leaving these intraluminal objects untreated can be dangerous. As long as the distal protection device is in place, various strategies can be attempted without much concern of disrupting the intraluminal material. If portions of the atheromatous plaque are identified prolapsing through the stent struts into the vessel lumen, one may dislodge the intraluminal mass into the distal embolic protection device using the tip of the guide device.

Another strategy is advancement of the guide device over the wire until its tip is just proximal to the intraluminal object and then attempting a suction thrombectomy. Local infusion of thrombolytics or glycoprotein IIb/IIIa inhibitors may clear an intraluminal thrombus. If this fails, one can consider inflating a balloon past the object and attempting a Fogarty maneuver by dragging the material back into the guide catheter. Of course, care must be taken not to disrupt the stent with these techniques. If the intraluminal lesion remains, then we do not hesitate to deploy a second stent to trap the thrombus or plaque against the vessel wall. The second stent should ideally have a closed cell, low porosity design and have the same diameter as the initial stent. One must be satisfied that the intraluminal material has been cleared from the lumen before retrieving the distal embolic protection device. We often will place these patients on a glycoprotein IIb/IIIa inhibitor for 12 to 24 hours afterwards.

Very rarely a device will fracture, resulting in a retained fragment within the vessel lumen. When this occurs, proximal flow arrest and later flow reversal may be helpful. Various retrieval devices, such as snares, are commercially available to attempt removal of the foreign body. If the foreign body cannot be retrieved, it may be necessary to place a stent to trap the object against the vessel wall.

Extension wires

Most devices currently used during carotid interventions have a monorail (rapid exchange) design. Consequently, the wire attached to most distal embolic protection devices are less than 200 cm in length. If the only available balloon or stent does not have a monorail design, the length of the wire will be insufficient for an exchange maneuver. In this event, one usually does not have to retrieve the filter and recross the lesion with an exchange length wire. Often, the addition of an extension wire to the existing monorail length wire will be sufficient. The extension wire has a hollow bore that slides over the end of the existing wire. This is a useful salvage technique that carries the annoyance of over-the-wire exchanging of devices but little additional risk.

Thromboembolic complications

At most institutions, including ours, carotid interventions are usually performed with the patient awake but sedated mildly. Consequently, the patient can be examined periodically

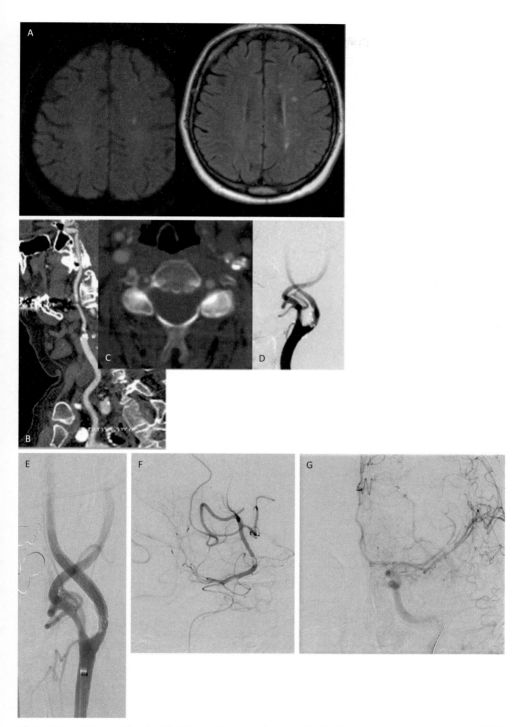

Figure 6.4 A 67-year-old male with history of hypertension, hyperlipidemia, alcohol abuse, symptomatic left ICA stenosis. A: magnetic resonance imaging diffusion-weighted imaging (MRI DWI) demonstrates tiny acute left frontal parietal subcortical watershed infarcts and fluid-attenuated inversion recovery (FLAIR) sequence demonstrating old

during the procedure. We examine the patient before the procedure, after obtaining vascular access with the guide device, after the post-stenting angioplasty, and at the conclusion of the procedure. A neurological change may be the first sign of a distal embolism or other problem. It is mandatory to obtain frontal and lateral images of the intracranial circulation as part of the baseline angiogram. These images are then available for comparison with the final intracranial angiogram. Evaluation of the capillary phase of the angiogram is important in order to detect subtle perfusion defects.

If an alteration of the patient's neurological status is detected, one must consider the differential diagnosis of **hypoperfusion, embolism, hemorrhage, or hypotension**. If an alteration of the patient's neurological status is detected, the operator should complete the current maneuver such as deployment of the stent, inflation of the balloon, etc. Then, after a brief neurological examination, the etiology of the neurological deficit can be sought. An immediate angiogram should be performed to evaluate the carotid artery and the intracranial circulation. In addition to perfusion defects, the angiogram should be evaluated for vessel displacement and other signs of mass effect. Acute vessel displacement is likely to be due to intracranial hemorrhage.

If a neurological change is highly suspicious for an embolism but there is no angiographic evidence of vascular occlusion, we immediately obtain a cerebral CT scan to evaluate for hemorrhage. If no hemorrhage is identified, the degree of neurological deficit determines how aggressive we are in treating the patient. We generally treat significant neurological deficits (i.e. moderate to severe weakness, dysphasia) with an intravenous or intra-arterial bolus of a glycoprotein IIb/IIIa inhibitor. We do not treat mild deficits (i.e. pronator drift, dysarthria) as the prognosis is very favorable with conservative management.

If an intracranial arterial occlusion is noted, the patient's neurological condition and the location of the occlusion determine how aggressively we attempt to achieve revascularization. Thus, an intraprocedural embolism is generally managed using the same endovascular techniques which we would apply for acute stroke. Such maneuvers include retrieval of the thrombus or the intra-arterial administration of thrombolytics. Typically, the occlusion occurs in distal branches such as the angular artery. The distal embolic protection device is retrieved, and we advance a navigable guide catheter through the stent and into the distal cervical ICA. Selective microcatheterization of the occluded branch is performed when possible. Since most occlusions in this setting involve smaller branches, thrombolysis with local intra-arterial thrombolytics or glycoprotein IIb/IIIa inhibitors, or mechanical disruption of the embolus with the microcatheter is performed. We attempt thrombectomy when we are trying to remove a large embolus in a proximal artery. As with many intra-arterial stroke interventions, a combination of strategies may be necessary. Care must be taken to retrieve a stent-retriever device before it crosses through the carotid stent to prevent

Figure 6.4 (cont.) small watershed infarcts between cortex and deep white matter. B, C: CT angiogram demonstrates heavily calcified plaque with severe stenosis. D: Lateral angiogram demonstrates 90% stenosis with calcified plaque with possible ulceration. E: Post-angioplasty and stenting lateral angiogram demonstrated patent left ICA with no significant residual stenosis. However, within a few minutes, patient was noted to have aphasia and right hemiparesis. F: Cerebral angiogram demonstrated left middle cerebral artery (distal M2 branch filling defect and several distal M3 and M4 branches occlusions) thromboembolism treated with intra-arterial Eptifibatide infusion through microcatheter and intravenous bolus, with some improvement in overall contrast clearance and improved recanalization in follow-up angiogram. G: Patient deteriorated further requiring intubation. Non-enhanced head CT scan demonstrated large basal ganglia hematoma with intraventricular hemorrhage requiring reversal of heparin, platelet transfusion, decompression craniectomy and external ventricular drainage placement.

entanglement of carotid stent migration. If that is not possible than mechanical aspiration may be used.

Cerebral hyperperfusion syndrome

The cerebral hyperperfusion syndrome (CHS) is a rare complication after revascularization of the carotid artery. It is characterized by ipsilateral headache, seizure activity, focal neurological deficit, and ipsilateral intracerebral edema or hemorrhage. A high clinical suspicion and early diagnosis will allow early initiation of therapy and preventing fatal brain swelling or bleeding in patients with peri- and postinterventional CHS. It is accompanied by postoperative or postinterventional hypertension in almost all patients. Risk factors include perioperative hypertension, high grade stenosis of ICA with poor collateral flow, contralateral carotid occlusion or high grade stenosis, periprocedural ischemia, presence of cerebral microangiopathy, and decreased cerebrovascular reactivity (Figure 6.5).

Early recognition is very important to prevent cerebral edema and hemorrhage. It carries very high morbidity and mortality. Careful monitoring and control of blood pressure in the intensive care unit is imperative. The prognosis following intracerebral bleeding is very poor, with mortality over 50% and significant morbidity of 80% in the survivors[5–7]. The prognosis of CHS in patients without cerebral edema or hemorrhage is clearly better, especially when they are identified and treated early. The most important aspects in preventing and treating this syndrome are early identification, careful monitoring, and control of blood pressure, ideally in a high-dependency unit setting.

Extracranial carotid pseudoaneurysms

Several etiologies have been documented, including blunt trauma, radiation necrosis, mycotic infection, iatrogenic insult, or neoplastic invasion of the vessel wall. If untreated,

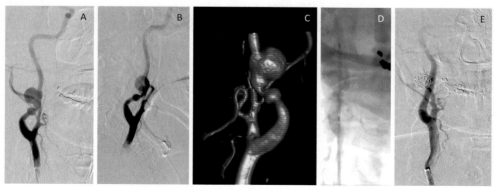

Figure 6.5 A 69-year-old female with previous history of right hemispheric stroke and enlarging right internal carotid artery pseudoaneurysm. It demonstrated aneurysmal dilatation of ICA 6.4 mm × 6.3 mm followed by focal stenosis (60%) and then dysplastic appearance of the artery with a pseudoaneurysm measuring about 13.2 mm × 13 mm incorporating the lumen of ICA with a wide neck measuring about 11.5 mm (A, B, C). An Xact stent measuring 8–6 mm × 40 mm was advanced and deployed successfully across the aneurysm after jailing the microcatheter into the aneurysm. This was chosen as the stent has close cell design (D). A total of five microcoils were advanced and deployed successfully into the aneurysm with near-complete obliteration (E).

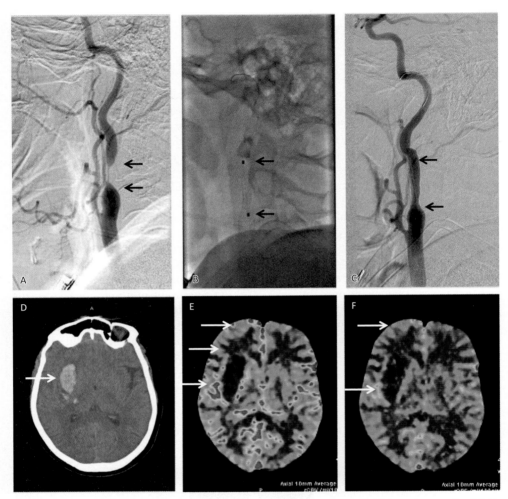

Figure 6.6 Post carotid angioplasty/stent placement hyperperfusion syndrome. **A:** High grade stenosis of right internal carotid artery cervical region (lateral view, arrow). **B:** Deployment of Cordis PRECISE® PRO RX® carotid stent system 7 × 40 mm in right ICA cervical region (lateral view, arrows); **C:** Minimal residual stenosis after stent deployment in right ICA cervical region (lateral, arrows). **D:** Right basal ganglionic intracerebral hemorrhage on CT scan 2 days after stent deployment (arrow). **E:** Increase in regional cerebral blood volume in ipsilateral hemisphere on CT perfusion 2 days after stent deployment (arrows). **F:** Increase in regional cerebral blood flow in ipsilateral hemisphere on CT perfusion 2 days after stent deployment (arrows).

they may enlarge, causing progressive occlusion of the parent vessel or symptoms related to local mass effect such as dysphagia, neck swelling, and pain. Carotid pseudoaneurysms may also serve as a source of emboli, resulting in cerebral infarction. Usually these are treated by endovascular methods including stent assisted coiling or covered stents and have relatively low complication rates (Figure 6.6) The major complication associated with stenting a pseudoaneurysm is a thromboembolism or stenting a false lumen. Therefore they should be crossed with a microcatheter over microwire and, after confirming true lumen, a stent is placed across the pseudoaneurysm. Other complications include endoleaks, stent occlusion, stent migration, infection, and late stroke. If asymptomatic and relatively small, then they are treated medically.

Conclusions

If the procedure is too difficult, particularly during the early vascular access stages, one must consider aborting and pursuing other treatment options. Before performing carotid artery interventions, the operator must ensure the availability of appropriate devices, including those that might be needed to treat complications. The use of minimal sedation allows for a thorough, reproducible neurological examination during the procedure. The operator should prepare devices in advance as much as possible while waiting for the patient to be fully heparinized. When a problem occurs, we advise systematic evaluation of the situation. The operator should look for proximal herniation of the devices, dissections (proximal or distal), distal migration of devices, hemorrhage (intra- or extracranial), vasospasm, and distal embolism.

Increased experience and technological advancements have made difficult carotid cases more amenable to endovascular treatment. However, some patients remain high risk for carotid stenting owing to mainly anatomic factors, and CAE may be a better choice in these cases. Some patients are high risk for both endovascular and open surgical procedures. In these cases, the risks of both procedures must be weighed before treatment. As with any procedure, careful patient selection is the best way to avoid complications in endovascular carotid interventions. With the increased prevalence of endovascular therapy for carotid disease, operators must be familiar with management of unexpected complications and salvage techniques. We anticipate a growing need for these techniques with the increasing number of complex cases referred for endovascular therapy.

References

1. Naylor AR. Stenting versus endarterectomy: the debate continues. *The Lancet Neurology* 2008;7:862–4.

2. Chang FC, Tummala RP, Jahromi BS, *et al.* Use of the 8 French Simmons-2 guide catheter for carotid artery stent placement in patients with difficult aortic arch anatomy. *Journal of Neurosurgery* 2009;110:437–41.

3. Solomon B, Berland T, Cayne N, *et al.* The coronary technique for complex carotid artery stenting in the setting of complex aortic arch anatomy. *Vascular and Endovascular Surgery* 2010;44:572–5.

4. Niesen WD, Rosenkranz M, Eckert B, *et al.* Hemodynamic changes of the cerebral circulation after stent-protected carotid angioplasty. *AJNR American Journal of Neuroradiology* 2004;25:1162–7.

5. Nikolsky E, Patil CV, Beyar R. Ipsilateral intracerebral hemorrhage following carotid stent-assisted angioplasty: a manifestation of hyperperfusion syndrome – a case report. *Angiology* 2002;53:217–23.

6. Phatouros CC, Meyers PM, Higashida RT, *et al.* Intracranial hemorrhage and cerebral hyperperfusion syndrome after extracranial carotid artery angioplasty and stent placement. *AJNR American Journal of Neuroradiology* 2002;23:503–4.

7. Knur R. Cerebral hyperperfusion syndrome following protected carotid artery stenting. *Case Reports in Vascular Medicine* 2013;2013:207602.

8. Endovascular versus surgical treatment in patients with carotid stenosis in the Carotid and Vertebral Artery Transluminal Angioplasty Study (CAVATAS): a randomised trial. *Lancet* 2001;357:1729–37.

9. Alberts MJ. Results of a multicentre prospective randomised trial of carotid artery stenting versus carotid endarterectomy. *Stroke* 2001;32:325-d.

10. Yadav JS, Wholey MH, Kuntz RE, *et al.* Protected carotid-artery stenting versus endarterectomy in high-risk patients. *The New England Journal of Medicine* 2004;351:1493–501.

11. Mas JL, Chatellier G, Beyssen B, *et al.* Endarterectomy versus stenting in patients with symptomatic severe carotid stenosis. *The New England Journal of Medicine* 2006;355:1660–71.

12. Ringleb PA, Allenberg J, Bruckmann H, *et al.* 30 day results from the SPACE trial of stent-protected angioplasty versus carotid endarterectomy in symptomatic patients: a randomised non-inferiority trial. *Lancet* 2006;368:1239–47.

13. Brott TG, Hobson RW 2nd, Howard G, *et al.* Stenting versus endarterectomy for treatment of carotid-artery stenosis. *The New England Journal of Medicine* 2010;363:11–23.

Complications with extracranial stenting other than carotid stenting

Rakesh Khatri

Vertebral artery angioplasty and stent placement

Approximately 80% of strokes are ischemic in origin, of which 20% to 25% are located in the posterior circulation involving the vertebrobasilar system (VBS). According to American Heart Association (AHA) guidelines, it is recommended that non-invasive imaging by computed tomography (CT) angiography or magnetic resonance (MR) angiography for detection of vertebral artery disease should be part of the initial evaluation of patients with neurological symptoms referable to the posterior circulation and those with subclavian steal syndrome. In patients with posterior cerebral or cerebellar ischemic symptoms who may be candidates for revascularization, catheter-based contrast angiography can be useful to define vertebral artery pathology and anatomy when non-invasive imaging fails to define the location or severity of stenosis. Small studies looking at medical therapy versus stent placement, and stent placement versus endarterectomy, have been published, but more data are required in order to provide the necessary level of evidence[1,2].

The vertebral artery (VA) is divided into extracranial (V1 to V3) and intracranial (V4) segments (Figure 7.1). The first segment (V1) begins from the origin of the VA and extends between the longus colli and scalenus anterior muscles to where it enters the transverse foramina at the fifth or sixth cervical vertebra. The second segment (V2) begins from the level of the fifth or sixth cervical vertebra and extends to the second cervical vertebra, travelling through the transverse foramina at each vertebral level, with an alternating intra- and interosseous course. The third segment (V3) extends between the C2 transverse process and base of the skull where it enters the foramen magnum. The last segment (V4) extends from the point at which the arteries enter the dura to the termination of both VAs at the vertebrobasilar junction.

The most common complications seen with VA angioplasty and stent placement are cerebrovascular events, stent fracture, and vessel rupture[3-6]. The rate of ischemic stroke was found to be between 0 and 5% at variable follow-up times[2,5-7].

Typical steps involved in angioplasty and stent placement of the VA are summarized below. Clinical cases of V1 and V2 segment angioplasty and stent placement are shown in Figure 7.2 and Figure 7.4. Figure 7.4 also shows in-stent stenosis management with angioplasty.

Preprocedural management

Patients are administered aspirin (325 mg daily) and clopidogrel (75 mg daily) orally starting 3 days before the procedure. If clopidogrel cannot be initiated 3 days before

Complications of Neuroendovascular Procedures and Bailout Techniques, ed. Rakesh Khatri,
Gustavo J. Rodriguez, Jean Raymond and Adnan I. Qureshi. Published by Cambridge University Press.
© Cambridge University Press 2016.

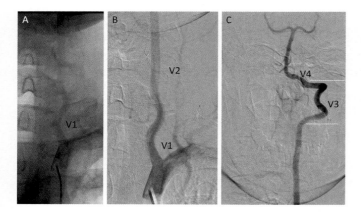

Figure 7.1 Non-subtracted (A) and subtracted left subclavian angiography demonstrates the vertebral artery origin, the three extracranial segments (V1–3), and one intracranial segment (V4).

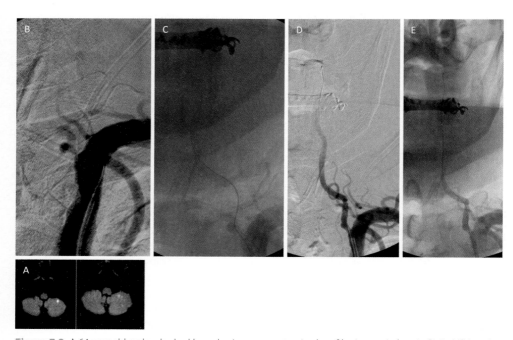

Figure 7.2 A 64-year-old male who had been having recurrent episodes of brainstem ischemia. Brain MR imaging (MRI) demonstrated left cerebellar stroke. Patient had significant atherosclerotic disease in the posterior circulation with occlusion of the mid basilar artery. He had filling of posterior cerebral artery from anterior circulation. There was 75–80% stenosis at the origin of the left VA with delayed contrast clearance in the left VA suggestive of hemodynamically significant stenosis. Right VA was hypoplastic. **A:** MRI, diffusion-weighted imaging (DWI) sequence showing scattered cerebellar strokes. **B:** Left VA origin stenosis measuring about 75–80%. **C:** AP subtracted view; a monorail Integrity balloon-expandable stent (3 mm × 18 mm; Coronary Stent System, Medtronic) was advanced over a Transcend (Stryker) microwire. **D, E:** Subtracted and non-subtracted AP angiography showing patent VA origin with stent.

the procedure, a loading dose of 300–600 mg is administered. If dysphagia is present, antiplatelet medications can be administered by using a nasogastric or pre-existing percutaneous gastrostomy feeding tube. Patients should have laboratory testing for platelet, hematocrit, basic metabolic profile, and a coagulation profile.

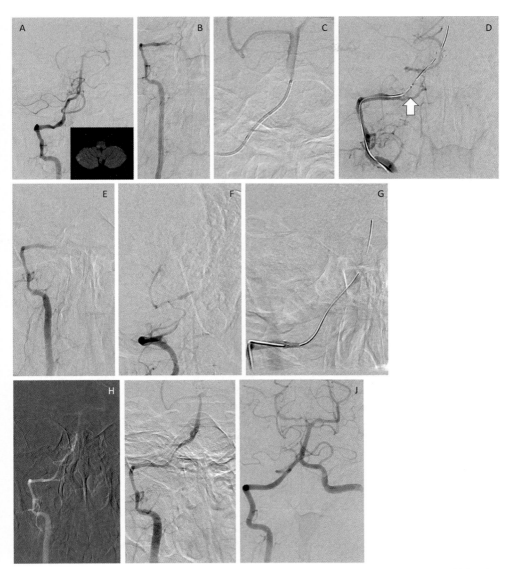

Figure 7.3 Failure of proximal end of Enterprise stent to open in VA dissection/occlusion. A 35-year-old female presented with right cerebellar and medullary minor stroke. Cerebral angiogram demonstrated right VA luminal irregularity at C2–C3 vertebral level with maximal luminal narrowing of about 45% (A). She was started on anticoagulation, but presented with repeat stroke 3 weeks later, with occluded right VA (B). The distal stent was deployed successfully in the proximal basilar artery, but the proximal tines did not open (D). The delivery wire could not be withdrawn, and this was considered to be due to significant compression by proximal stent lines. A Prowler Select Plus microcatheter was advanced over the wire and the Enterprise stent could then be resheathed.

A: Right VA luminal irregularity noted at C2–C3 vertebral level, with maximal luminal narrowing measuring about 45%. B: Occluded right VA. C: Microcatheter angiogram showing patent basilar artery. D: Enterprise stent (4.5 mm × 22 mm) placement; proximal tines did not open, therefore it was sheathed. E, F: AP and lateral view of persistent occlusion of occluded right VA after stent removal. G: Enterprise stent placement, 4.5 mm × 37 mm. H, I: Recanalization of right VA with residual moderate narrowing and luminal irregularity. J: Follow-up after 4 weeks, showing complete recanalization of right VA.

If the patient is using long-term warfarin, warfarin should be discontinued 3 days prior to the procedure. A repeat coagulation profile should be performed and a complete neurological examination should be documented before the procedure.

Periprocedural management

After arterial access through the femoral or radial artery has been established, a 50–70 U/kg bolus of heparin is administered intravenously and activated clotting time (ACT) is followed per institution protocol. Typically a 6 French guide catheter (Envoy; Cordis/Johnson & Johnson, Miami Lakes, FL) is placed in the ipsilateral subclavian artery. If necessary, the guide catheter is stabilized by coaxial placement of a 0.014 to 0.018 inch microwire into the distal subclavian artery. Stenosis at the origin can be crossed by using a 0.014 inch microwire, either directly with a balloon catheter (monorail system versus conventional length) or microcatheter over an exchange length 0.014 inch, 300 cm microwire. We typically use a Transcend ES microwire (Stryker Neurovascular, Mountain View, CA). A distal embolic protection device may be used if desired by the operator, but we do not typically use it. Bare metal stents (balloon-expandable) are typically used for treatment of stenosis. Angioplasty before or after stent can be performed in selected situations for optimal results.

The use of coronary balloon-expandable stents to treat stenosis of VA origin (Figure 7.2) is more common than use of the self-expanding stents. The balloon-expandable stents have a good combination of adequate radial force, low crossing profile, and limited foreshortening. Drug-eluting stents (DES) (sirolimus or paclitaxel coating) have been used, but there is very limited data on the use of DES in the VA. The expectation from DES is a decrease in restenosis through inhibition of smooth muscle and endothelial proliferation. Although experience described in the coronary literature largely supports such a practice, DES in cardiac procedures have recently been found to be associated with clot formation in some cases[8,9], resulting in thrombosis at the stent site. The alternative is to use self-expanding stents, but they suffer from size limitations of currently available stent diameter and also from occasional misplacement, requiring placement of an additional stent. The choice of monorail or over-the-wire systems depends on the experience and comfort level of the operator. Therefore, in patients with severe tortuosity of the vessel in whom support may be an issue, a coronary stent may be preferred. The stent length should be enough to extend proximally 1 mm to 2 mm into the lumen of the ipsilateral subclavian artery and at least 3 mm into the normal distal VA, covering the entire lesion. Either the coronary balloon-expandable stents or self-expanding stents can be chosen to treat stenosis involving the V2 segment. For stenosis involving the V3 segment, a nitinol self-expanding stent is suitable because of vessel tortuosity (Figure 7.3). For the case shown in Figure 7.3 we discuss not only the usual self-expanding stent placement but also the rare complication when the stent tines do not expand completely. This may be due to a device defect, although external compression from mural thrombus should also be considered. Fortunately we were able to resheath the stent; otherwise a low-profile balloon could be advanced into the stent and inflated cautiously to help the stent expand.

After positioning of the stent, an angiogram is performed in the working projection (used to deploy the stent) to document the technical result of the procedure. The final angiogram is compared with the initial preprocedure angiogram.

Postprocedural management

No further heparin is administered after the procedure.

A complete neurological examination is performed immediately after and 24 hours after the procedure. Aspirin (325 mg daily) and clopidogrel (75 mg daily) should be prescribed at discharge.

Potential complications

There are many complications similar to those that have already been discussed for carotid angioplasty and stenting, such as access phase difficulty, aorto-iliac atherosclerotic stenosis or occlusion, in-stent thrombus, and thromboembolic complications. Here, we will emphasize some of the other issues not already fully covered; to avoid repetition, we will only briefly mention those that have been covered already.

Below, we list some of the most important points for angioplasty and stenting at the origin of the VA. Even though some may be obvious, in our experience they are worth mentioning.

(1) Always spend time to obtain the best working projection that demonstrates the origin of the vertebral artery.

(2) If a lesion represents a very high grade stenosis, it should be crossed only with microwire. Avoid crossing it with guidewire, and avoid abutting the guide catheter to the calcified origin. This lessens the chances of plaque disturbance and also avoids complete occlusion of the VA lumen by the guide catheter tip.

(3) A distal embolic protection device may be used if preferred by the operator and if the VA anatomy would allow. Most operators typically do not use a distal embolic protection device[7].

(4) If there is moderate to severe stenosis, angioplasty should be performed prior to stent deployment in order to prevent stent herniation.

(5) Over-inflation of the balloon must be avoided, to prevent dissection or balloon rupture.

(6) Ensure that air is removed from the stent delivery system and balloon for optimal visualization and to prevent complications from balloon rupture.

Bailout techniques

Significant proximal tortuosity

- A buddy 0.014 inch microguidewire can be used to stabilize the 6 French guide catheter in the ipsilateral subclavian artery. With this technique it is still possible to advance the balloon as well as the stent, despite the presence of a small microwire within the guide catheter[10,11].

- A larger guide catheter (7 French to 10 French) may be used. This technique, however, may produce more groin complications including hematoma, vasospasm, catheter-induced vasospasm or dissection and embolization, and formation of thrombi around the larger surface of these catheters.

- Radial artery access can be attempted if the patient passes Allen's test confirming patency of the palmar arterial arch.

- Direct puncture of the VA should be avoided and only performed under surgical exposure. However, this technique increases the possibility of puncture-related vasospasm with or without thrombus formation and cervical hematoma.

Traversing high grade stenosis

Arterial dissection may occur when traversing high grade stenosis and may create a false lumen. Advancing and deploying a stent within the false lumen can be disastrous since it may occlude the artery completely. Crossing a high grade lesion with Synchro 2 microwire and a microcatheter, such as an Excelsior SL-10 (Stryker Neurovascular, Fremont, CA), may help prevent this. If in any doubt, microcatheter injection can be performed after traversing the lesion to ensure that the catheter tip is in the true lumen.

Ensuring accurate placement of the stent

The VA origin moves during breathing. Therefore, prior to deployment of the stent, the operator should determine the best timing for stent placement. If the patient is cooperative, guide catheter injection can be performed after stent placement across the lesion but prior to deployment in either the expiration or inspiration phase. The patient may be asked to stop breathing while the stent is being deployed. In addition, calcified plaque at the lesion as well as bony landmarks such as rib or clavicle should be used to accurately place a stent. Sometimes, the unsubtracted images may provide the best information.

Preventing stent herniation during deployment

The "watermelon seed" phenomenon can sometimes be observed for tight lesions during balloon angioplasty. The balloon may herniate upward or downward during angioplasty in relation to the lesion. Usually a longer balloon may avoid the watermelon seed effect. Pre-stent angioplasty is usually performed to prevent the herniation of the stent during the deployment in tight lesions.

Distal embolic protection device cannot be retrieved using standard technique

A 4 French 125 cm angle-tip catheter can be used to retrieve the distal embolic protection device since the angle tip may help in navigating through the sharp angulation and protruding struts of the stent.

Dissection of the vertebral artery

This may need additional stents depending on the degree of flow limitation. If minor and not flow-limiting, then the lesion can be observed with antiplatelet medications on board.

In-stent thrombus

Ensure that ACT is at least 250 seconds. The situation may need local infusion of thrombolytics or glycoprotein IIb/IIIa inhibitors. If this strategy fails, one can consider inflating a balloon past the thrombus and attempting a Fogarty maneuver by dragging the material back into the guide catheter. Of course, care must be taken not to disrupt the stent with these techniques. If the intraluminal lesion remains, then deploying a second stent to trap the thrombus or plaque against the vessel wall may be considered on a case by case basis. We often will place these patients on a glycoprotein IIb/IIIa inhibitor for 12 to 24 hours afterwards.

Platelet function assays for aspirin and Plavix responsiveness should also be sent to ensure the patient is responsive to these medications.

Vertebral artery spasm

The V3 and V4 segments of the VA may develop vasospasm due to straightening by microwire and stent delivery devices. Such vasospasm is temporary and will resolve as soon as the microwire and stent delivery devices are removed. A more sustained vasospasm may develop at the distal end of the deployed stent due to realignment and radial distension of the VA, particularly if the treated segment is very tortuous. Intra-arterial vasodilator infusion may be necessary.

Change in neurological status

At most institutions, similar to carotid interventions, VA angioplasty and stenting are usually performed with the patient awake but with minimal sedation. Consequently, the patient can be examined periodically during the procedure. We examine the patient before the procedure, after obtaining vascular access with the guide device, immediately after angioplasty and stenting, and at the conclusion of the procedure.

If an alteration of the patient's neurological status is detected, one must consider the differential diagnosis of hypoperfusion, embolism, hemorrhage, or hypotension. The operator should complete the current maneuver (such as deployment of the stent, inflation of the balloon, etc.). Then, after a brief neurological examination, the etiology of the neurological deficit can be sought. An immediate frontal and lateral angiogram should be performed to evaluate the patency of the vertebral and basilar arteries. In addition to perfusion defects, the angiogram should be reviewed for vessel displacement and other signs of mass effect. Acute vessel displacement is likely to be a result of intracranial hemorrhage. Evaluation of the capillary phase of the angiogram is important in order to detect subtle perfusion defects and microvascular compromise due to microemboli. If there is no angiographic evidence of vascular occlusion, we immediately obtain a cerebral CT scan to evaluate for intracerebral hemorrhage. If no hemorrhage is identified, the degree of neurological deficit determines how aggressive we are in treating the patient. We generally treat significant neurological deficits (i.e. moderate to severe weakness, dysphasia) with an intravenous or intra-arterial bolus of a glycoprotein IIb/IIIa inhibitors.

If an intracranial arterial occlusion is noted, the patient's neurological condition and the location of the occlusion determine how aggressively we attempt to achieve revascularization. Thus, an intraprocedural embolism is generally managed using the same endovascular techniques that we would apply for acute ischemic stroke. Such maneuvers include retrieval of the thrombus or the intra-arterial administration of thrombolytics. Selective microcatheterization of the occluded branch is performed when possible. Since most occlusions in this setting involve smaller branches, we perform thrombolysis with local intra-arterial thrombolytics or glycoprotein IIb/IIIa inhibitors, or mechanical disruption of the embolus with the microcatheter. We attempt thrombectomy when we are trying to remove a large embolus in a proximal artery. As with many intra-arterial stroke interventions, a combination of strategies may be necessary.

In-stent restenosis

In-stent restenosis (ISR) is reported at variable rates, ranging from 16% to 66% (Figure 7.4). This large variation in ISR rate may be due to the reports being small case series, or due to variable regimens of antiplatelet medication after the procedure, ISR definition, and types of stent being used. A study based on vertebral ostium stenting showed that ISR is not

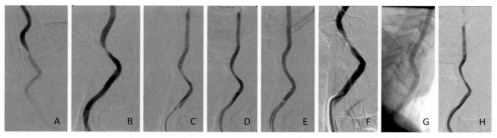

Figure 7.4 V2 segment angioplasty and stent placement and in-stent stenosis in left VA on follow-up. The patient is a 55-year-old gentleman who has history of neck radiation for his dorsal sarcoma. Patient has right VA occlusion with dominant left VA stenosis measuring almost 90% at C5–C6 vertebral level in the V2 segment (A: lateral view; B: AP view). Successful left VA angioplasty and stenting was performed using 4 × 20 mm balloon and 5 × 30 mm Precise stent (C and D). Post-stent angioplasty was performed with 5 × 20 mm balloon (E) with no residual stenosis. In-stent stenosis was noted measuring about 70% at 15 month follow-up (F and G), requiring angioplasty with 5 × 20 mm balloon. Moderate residual stenosis, about 45%, was noted (H). Aggressive angioplasty was not performed, to prevent risk of dissection and clinically asymptomatic status.

always clinically benign, as 10% of patients presented with ischemic symptoms. In one reported review, 23% developed restenosis and 9% required reintervention.

Subclavian and innominate artery stent placement

Endovascular approaches to supra-aortic lesions are now the preferred treatment for occlusion or stenoses in the brachiocephalic vessels. Treatment is offered for presumed symptomatic lesions. Please refer to the sections on preprocedural, periprocedural, and postprocedural management above, since the overall principles of management are similar to VA stenting except for the larger sizes of balloons and stents.

Typically balloon-mounted stents are used at ostial lesions. In subclavian artery stenosis, typically the flow in the VA is retrograde, thereby giving some protection from cerebral embolism. Use of a distal embolic protection device for innominate artery stenosis is not so well established; however, in our opinion, it should be considered if technically feasible, to prevent cerebral embolism[12].

In addition to the points mentioned above for VA stenting, there are a few points worth considering for subclavian artery and innominate artery stenting procedures.

(1) The operator should study the images from any non-invasive tests that have already been performed (such as CT angiogram) to understand arch anatomy and plan the access. Dual access may be used in complex lesions, combining a transradial/transbrachial with a transfemoral approach to define the lesion length. Simultaneous roadmapping may be used to cross the lesion. Pigtail catheter injection and aortogram should be performed to evaluate the stenosis at the origin of the innominate artery.

(2) Stent size should be 1 to 2 mm wider than the parent vessel and long enough to cover the entire lesion with a single stent. The stent should extend 1 to 2 mm into the aorta with minimal overlap of the carotid artery origin. If the whole diseased segment cannot be covered by a single stent, then plan on stenting the distal segment first and then the proximal segment, to avoid difficulty with crossing an already deployed stent.

Angioplasty can be done with the same balloon if better wall apposition is warranted or if there is significant stenosis within the stent prior to removal of the balloon catheter. If ineffective, then a different, larger balloon can be used, remembering to avoid

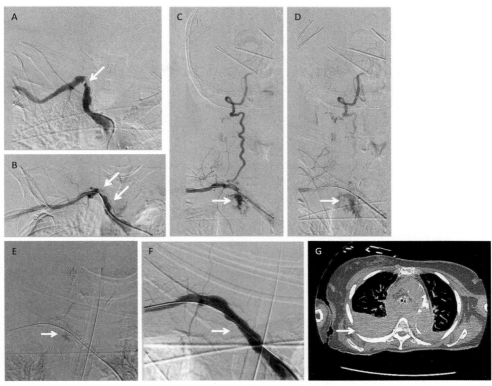

Figure 7.5 Post-angioplasty rupture of subclavian artery. **A:** High grade stenosis of right subclavian artery (AP, arrow). **B:** Placement of Fox Plus 9.0 × 20 mm angioplasty balloon across the lesion (AP, arrows). **C:** Contrast extravasation at site of angioplasty after angioplasty (at 8 atmospheres) in early arterial phase (AP, arrows). **D:** Contrast extravasation at site of angioplasty after angioplasty in late arterial phase (AP, arrows). **E:** Small amount of extravasation after placement of Gore Viabran endoprosthesis 9.0 × 50 mm stent (AP, arrows). **F:** Complete resolution of extravasation after post stent angioplasty using Fox Plus 9.0 × 20 mm angioplasty balloon inflated to 5 atmospheres (AP, arrows). **G:** CT scan of chest demonstrating hemothorax with maximum collection at site of angioplasty (arrow).

over-inflation to prevent rupture or dissection of the native vessel or stent fracture. Angioplasty of atherosclerotic vessels requires use of non-compliant balloons that have the potential to cause rupture or tearing of the target vessel (see Figure 7.4). This complication is uncommon and rarely reported. Consequently, there is little available data to guide management decisions when it does occur. Management alternatives for these injuries include surgical repair, endovascular placement of a stent or graft, temporary balloon tamponade, or conservative therapy with hemodynamic monitoring and follow-up imaging, depending on the scenario. We favor placement of a covered stent if contrast extravasation is noted after angioplasty and conservative follow-up, or placement of an additional stent if noted after post-stent angioplasty[3].

(3) In a recent Cochrane review for endovascular treatment of subclavian stenosis, there is currently insufficient evidence to determine whether stenting is more effective than angioplasty alone for stenosis of the subclavian artery.

(4) Infrequently, the innominate or subclavian artery may rupture during angioplasty (Figure 7.5). Contrast extravasation is seen initially, followed by hypotension and

dyspnea due to hemothorax. Temporary occlusion of the proximal artery may be possible by submaximal inflation of the balloon used for the initial angioplasty. The bleeding may stop because of proximal occlusion. The operator must consider intravenous fluids and red blood cell (RBC) transfusions, and reverse heparin using protamine. Such lesions usually require a covered stent graft, e.g. Viabahn covered stent (Gore, Flagstaff, AZ). After deployment, post-stent angioplasty may be required to ensure adequate opposition of the stent to the arterial segment proximal and distal to the lesion. It may be necessary to remove the guide catheter or guide sheath and advance the stent graft delivery catheter over the wire. Otherwise, a large diameter catheter is required to accommodate the large outer diameter of the stent graft delivery catheter; the existing guide catheter or guide sheath may be too small for such advancement.

There are some unique scenarios for innominate artery lesions and their bailout that have been reported and are worth mentioning.

Use of two-wire technique for innominate artery stent placement under embolic protection

In this report, operators had a case with a high grade innominate artery stenosis that blocked passage of a 0.035 inch stent delivery system from the femoral approach. A 0.018 inch guidewire was advanced in retrograde fashion via the right radial artery and captured via the femoral approach, establishing right radial–femoral through-and-through access. The 0.018 inch guidewire provided excellent support for positioning an 8 French hydrophilic sheath at the origin of the innominate artery. A 0.035 inch catheter was used to cross the lesion from the femoral approach, and a 0.014 inch buddy wire was introduced into the right common carotid artery. A 7 mm SpideRX filter was then deployed over the 0.014 inch guidewire. The two-wire combination was used to load a 0.035-inch-compatible balloon-expandable stent system, which was deployed in the innominate artery and flared proximally, with excellent angiographic result[13].

Post-traumatic pseudoaneurysm/dissection of the innominate artery

Aortic arch injuries are rare, even more so with no physical evidence of chest trauma. The innominate artery is the second most commonly injured branch of the mediastinal vessels, after the isthmus of the thoracic aorta, with the proximal segment most commonly involved. All post-traumatic innominate artery pseudoaneurysms need to be corrected to prevent complications such as rupture, thrombosis, embolism and enlargement causing compression of other vital thoracic structures. In trained hands, endovascular repair can be performed promptly and efficiently. A stent graft (e.g. Viabahn covered stent; Gore, Flagstaff, AZ) can be used in these cases if the patient is clinically stable.

References

1. Ederle J, Bonati LH, Dobson J, et al. Endovascular treatment with angioplasty or stenting versus endarterectomy in patients with carotid artery stenosis in the Carotid and Vertebral Artery Transluminal Angioplasty Study (CAVATAS): long-term follow-up of a randomised trial. The Lancet Neurology 2009;8:898–907.

2. Compter A, van der Worp HB, Schonewille WJ, et al. Stenting versus medical treatment in patients with symptomatic vertebral artery stenosis: a randomised open-label

phase 2 trial. *The Lancet Neurology* 2015; 14:606–14.

3. Broadbent LP, Moran CJ, Cross DT 3rd, Derdeyn CP. Management of ruptures complicating angioplasty and stenting of supraaortic arteries: report of two cases and a review of the literature. *AJNR American Journal of Neuroradiology* 2003;24:2057–61.

4. Jenkins JS, Patel SN, White CJ, *et al.* Endovascular stenting for vertebral artery stenosis. *Journal of the American College of Cardiology* 2010;55:538–42.

5. Kocak B, Korkmazer B, Islak C, Kocer N, Kizilkilic O. Endovascular treatment of extracranial vertebral artery stenosis. *World Journal of Radiology* 2012;4:391–400.

6. Sun X, Ma N, Wang B, *et al.* The long term results of vertebral artery ostium stenting in a single center. *Journal of Neurointerventional Surgery* 2014; 7:888–91.

7. Qureshi AI, Kirmani JF, Harris-Lane P, *et al.* Vertebral artery origin stent placement with distal protection: technical and clinical results. *AJNR American Journal of Neuroradiology* 2006;27:1140–5.

8. Luscher TF, Steffel J, Eberli FR, *et al.* Drug-eluting stent and coronary thrombosis: biological mechanisms and clinical implications. *Circulation* 2007;115:1051–8.

9. Schulz S, Schuster T, Mehilli J, *et al.* Stent thrombosis after drug-eluting stent implantation: incidence, timing, and relation to discontinuation of clopidogrel therapy over a 4-year period. *European Heart Journal* 2009;30:2714–21.

10. Kizilkilic O. Vertebral artery origin stenting with buddy wire technique in tortuous subclavian artery. *European Journal of Radiology* 2007;61:120–3.

11. Uysal E, Caliskan C, Caymaz I, Orken DN, Basak M. Stenting of vertebral artery origin with the buddy wire technique in tortuous subclavian artery. A case report. *Interventional Neuroradiology: Journal of Peritherapeutic Neuroradiology, Surgical Procedures and Related Neurosciences* 2010;16:175–8.

12. Sakamoto S, Kiura Y, Kajihara Y, Mukada K, Kurisu K. Endovascular stenting of symptomatic innominate artery stenosis under distal balloon protection of the internal carotid and vertebral artery for cerebral protection: a technical case report. *Acta Neurochirurgica* 2013;155:277–80.

13. Ryer EJ, Oderich GS. Two-wire (0.014 & 0.018-inch) technique to facilitate innominate artery stenting under embolic protection. *Journal of Endovascular Therapy: An Official Journal of the International Society of Endovascular Specialists* 2010;17:652–6.

Chapter 8

Complications during head and neck embolization

Asif Khan, Rakesh Khatri, and Jefferson T. Miley

Head and neck embolization procedures are typically associated with less risk than intracranial embolization, but potentially disabling major complications are known to occur through inadvertent embolization into retinal or intracranial circulation via anastomotic pathways, and by involving the blood supply of cranial nerves.

Table 8.1 summarizes indications for external carotid artery (ECA) embolization.

The most common complications associated with embolization within the tributaries of the ECA include cranial nerve palsies, skin or mucosal necrosis, and unintended vascular occlusions[1]. Ipsilateral temporofacial pain and facial edema[2] have also been described after embolization for epistaxis.

Skin or mucosal necrosis: Necrosis of the skin at the tip of the nose[3], alar skin and cartilage, mucosa of the hard palate[4] and facial skin[5] may occur.

Cranial nerve palsies: This may affect cranial nerves VII, XI, and XII. Facial nerve palsy appears to be the most frequent nerve palsy (approximately 5% of patients with ECA embolization for glomus tumor), and near-complete recovery may be seen over 6 months in a majority of patients[6-9]. The relevant arterial supply is highlighted in Table 8.2[10]. The tympanic and mastoid segments of the facial nerve receive an overlapping blood supply from the stylomastoid artery and the petrosal branch of the middle meningeal artery. In 60% of patients, the stylomastoid artery arises from the occipital artery, and in 40% of patients, it arises from the postauricular artery. The chances of palsy are higher if branches of the occipital, postauricular, and middle meningeal arteries are all embolized, because of overlapping sources of blood supply to the facial nerve. Lower cranial nerve palsy is very infrequent after jugular foramen tumor embolization. The glossopharyngeal, vagus, and spinal accessory nerves receive their blood supply from the jugular branch of the neuromeningeal trunk of the ascending pharyngeal artery[11]. The hypoglossal branch of the ascending pharyngeal artery supplies the hypoglossal nerve.

Unintended vascular occlusions: Retinal artery occlusion and visual loss can rarely occur through the anastomosis between external (sphenopalatine and greater palatine branches of the internal maxillary artery (IMAX)) and internal carotid artery (ICA, anterior and posterior branches of the ophthalmic artery)[12,13]. Transient ischemic attack or minor ischemic strokes have been reported rarely after embolization into the ECA branches[14,15]. These occur because of passage of embolic material into the intracranial circulation through external–internal carotid arterial anastomotic pathways.

Complications of Neuroendovascular Procedures and Bailout Techniques, ed. Rakesh Khatri,
Gustavo J. Rodriguez, Jean Raymond and Adnan I. Qureshi. Published by Cambridge University Press.
© Cambridge University Press 2016.

Table 8.1 Head and neck embolization procedures via the external carotid artery and its branches

Head and neck vascular tumors

- Paraganglioma
- Carotid body tumor/chemodectoma
- Lymphangioma
- Glomus jugularae
- Carcinoma of mouth, tongue, pharynx, larynx

Meningeal tumors

- Meningioma
- Schwannoma

Sinonasal neoplasms

- Juvenile nasopharyngeal angiofibromas
- Hemangioma
- Hemangiopericytoma
- Pyogenic granuloma gravidarum
- Nasopharyngeal carcinoma-related complications

Aneurysms and arteriovenous malformations

- Head and neck arteriovenous malformation
- Aneurysm/pseudoaneurysm
- Dural arteriovenous fistula
- Hereditary hemorrhagic telangiectasia (Osler–Weber–Rendu syndrome)

Posterior epistaxis

- Idiopathic (10%)
- Trauma
- Postoperative/surgical trauma

Trauma

- Multifocal small size arterial injury
- Medium size arterial rupture

Table 8.2 Blood supply of cranial nerves

Nerve	Blood supply
Facial nerve (VII)	Petrosal branch of middle meningeal artery, stylomastoid branch of occipital artery OR postauricular artery
Glossopharyngeal nerve (IX)	Jugular branch of neuromeningeal trunk of ascending pharyngeal artery
Vagus nerve (X)	Jugular branch of neuromeningeal trunk of ascending pharyngeal artery
Spinal accessory nerve (XI)	Jugular branch of neuromeningeal trunk of ascending pharyngeal artery
Hypoglossal nerve (XII)	Hypoglossal branch of neuromeningeal trunk of ascending pharyngeal artery

(From ref. 10: Gartrell BC *et al. Otol Neurotol.* 2012 Sep;33(7):1270–5. With permission.)

It is imperative to the neurointerventionalist to have full knowledge of the dangerous anastomosis between branches of the ECA, ICA, and vertebral artery[1], as well as blood supply to lower cranial nerves.

Major extracranial–intracranial anastomotic pathways

See Figure 8.1.

Cervical anastomosis

Thyrocervical trunk–vertebral artery anastomosis: The ascending cervical artery and the deep cervical artery, which are both branches of the subclavian artery, can anastomose with the vertebral artery between the C2–C4 vertebral levels by augmentation of anastomoses within the paravertebral muscles.

Ascending pharyngeal artery–vertebral artery anastomosis: The musculospinal branch, which is the most proximal branch of the ascending pharyngeal artery, anastomoses laterally with the C3 radicular branch of the vertebral artery. More distally, the prevertebral branch anastomoses with vertebral artery at C1 vertebral level.

Occipital artery–vertebral artery anastomosis: Posterior radicular branches arise from the horizontal portion of the occipital artery at the C1 and C2 vertebral levels and anastomose with the vertebral artery. The stylomastoid artery, which supplies the meninges of the posterior fossa, arises from either the occipital artery or the posterior auricular artery and forms anastomosis with the infereolateal trunk, meningohypophyseal trunk, and the posterior meningeal artery from the vertebral artery and other external carotid branches as well.

Orbital region anastomosis

The ophthalmic artery acts as an interface between the IMAX and the ICA. During embolization within the distribution of IMAX tributaries, embolization of the central

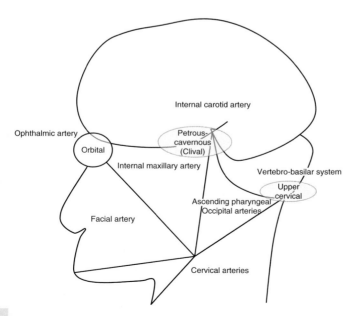

Figure 8.1 Diagram of the functional vascular anatomy of the head and neck with the three major extracranial–intracranial anastomotic pathway regions: the orbital, petrous–cavernous–clival, and upper cervical regions. From ref. 16: S. Geibprasert *et al. Am J Neuroradiol.* 2009 30(8):1459–68, with permission.

retinal artery via ophthalmic artery can result in monocular blindness. The most common variant is the meningo-ophthalmic artery which is derived from embryologic stapedial artery and supplies retina instead of the central retinal artery. In such an occurrence, there is non-visualization of the ophthalmic artery from the ICA injection and opacification of choroidal blush on ECA contrast injection. In this setting, middle meningeal artery embolization has a high risk of embolic occlusion of the distal ophthalmic artery. The distal IMAX can also have another anastomosis with the inferior branch of the lacrimal artery, which is one of the largest branches of the ophthalmic artery. The anastomosis involves the anterior deep temporal artery and the infraorbital artery. An infrequent anastomosis can be seen between the frontal branches of the superficial temporal artery and the distal portion of the ophthalmic artery.

Petrous–cavernous region anastomoses

Several anastomoses can exist between the ascending pharyngeal artery and either the petrous or cavernous segment of the ICA. These channels are too small to be visualized on cerebral angiography but may become more prominent in the setting of ICA stenosis or occlusion to allow blood flow via the ECA into the petrous ICA. The anteriorly located pharyngeal trunk has three branches: the inferior, middle, and superior pharyngeal arteries. The latter has the most important anastomotic routes, including the eustachian tube anastomotic circle that connects with the mandibular artery from the petrous ICA, and an anastomosis with the accessory meningeal artery (AMA) and pterygovaginal artery from the distal IMAX. There is also a carotid canal branch which anastomoses with branches of the cavernous ICA. The inferolateral trunk, along with the meningohypophyseal trunk, is a branch of the C4 segment of the ICA. The middle meningeal and anterior meningeal arteries can anastomose with the cavernous ICA through the infereolateal trunk.

Standard endovascular access and embolization of head and neck tumors

Hypervascular head and neck tumors are embolized preoperatively primarily to help the surgeon to decrease the surgery time, reduce blood loss, and reduce morbidity.

Basic characteristics of embolic agents, principles of treatment, and techniques related to embolization procedure have already been discussed in Chapter 3. Please refer to that chapter for details; these are not repeated here, to avoid duplication. Please refer to Figure 8.2 for a case discussion.

In cases in which feeding arteries are too small to access, a direct tumor puncture may be performed since it would have better penetration of the tumor vascular bed than intra-arterial embolization (Figure 8.3). Other scenarios may include multiple feeders, where direct access to the tumor and embolization by percutaneous method may obviate the need for multiple catheterization, decrease procedure time, offer better penetration of the tumor vascular bed, and potentially decrease the risk of stroke.

Once sterilized, a selective angiogram should be performed, and the operator should mark the surface skin over the target vessel to be punctured. Using constant fluoroscopic guidance, a dimethyl sulfoxide (DMSO)- or nBCA-compatible 21 gauge spinal needle can be used to puncture the surface skin and can be advanced into the target vessel of the tumor under biplane roadmap guidance until a constant steady ooze of blood is appreciated. Some authors fix a microcatheter (e.g. Echelon 10) to the tip of the spinal needle with glue so that

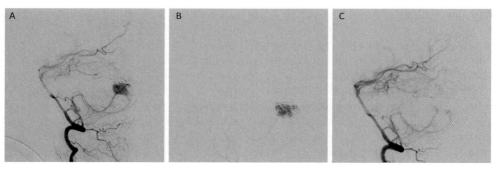

Figure 8.2 A 62-year-old man presented to the hospital with a 6-month history of progressive ataxia and nausea; more recently he had been experiencing frequent falls. The patient was found to have a posterior fossa tumor suggestive of a vascular tumor such as a cerebellar hemangioblastoma. Post embolization, the tumor was easily resected by the surgeon. **A:** Prominent tumor blush that measures 2 × 1 cm, arising from the distal left posterior-inferior cerebellar artery, cortical branches, mainly the medial hemispheric branch. **B:** Microcatheter tumor embolization using Onyx 18. **C:** A follow-up run was performed and demonstrated significant reduction of the tumor blush.

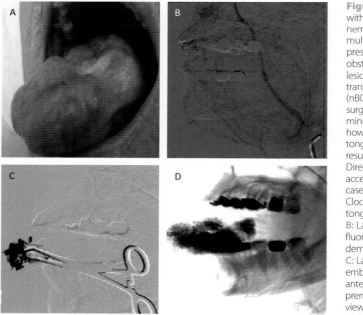

Figure 8.3 A 62-year-old man with a known tongue hemangioma, who had received multiple previous treatments, presented with symptoms of obstructive sleep apnea (OSA). The lesion was embolized via transmucosal n-butyl cyanoacrylate (nBCA) injection before being surgically excised. There was minimal bleeding after the surgery; however, there was significant tongue swelling after embolization, resulting in prolonged intubation. Direct regional nBCA injection is an acceptable choice for selective cases of tongue hemangiomas. Clockwise from top left: **A:** Baseline tongue with hemangioma visible. **B:** Lateral view pre-embolization fluoroscopy of tongue demonstrating parenchymal blush. **C:** Lateral view percutaneous embolization phase with needle in anterior one-third of tongue (glue premixed with contrast). **D:** Lateral view post-embolization with nBCA cast.

they can use it to inject the embolic agent. A 20 cm Luer lock extension tubing, which is DMSO-compatible, can be used as an alternative. Angiogram is performed with a 5 ml syringe, and after confirming placement, embolization is performed. The spinal needle can then be repositioned multiple times to fill other intra-tumoral vessels or the tumor bed until satisfactory tumor embolization is achieved.

Some cautions are advised.

- Always use biplane blank roadmap for the embolization phase.
- When the embolizing agent is reaching the edges of the tumor, pay extra attention to the margins, since the embolizing material may advance into a large artery, including the ICA in the case of extracranial tumors, such as glomus tumor. If there is concern, then use a compliant balloon and inflate during embolization to prevent cerebral embolism. The operator must evaluate collateral flow from prior angiogram to ensure that the patient has adequate reserve. Some operators also use electroencephalogram (EEG)/ somatosensory evoked potentials (SSEP) during embolization.
- Use lead gloves when performing the direct puncture technique to decrease radiation exposure.

Endovascular tips in head and neck trauma

For the purpose of this chapter, injuries will be classified into blunt and penetrating injuries. Treatment will be classified into flow restoration and embolization (small and large vessels).

There exists a vast literature on stroke caused by blunt cervical vascular injuries, often involving the vertebral artery, carotid artery or both. Very well established screening guidelines, medical awareness, and rapid non-invasive access to angiographic evaluation have resulted in an "increase" in injuries. The medical management of such condition is controversial regarding "best therapy".

On the other hand, penetrating injuries commonly involve the cervical vessels because of their anatomic "exposure". Vessel injuries often involve the artery and vein. The likelihood of which cervical vessel is affected is proportional to the diameter of the vascular structure. Intracranial vascular injuries are rare, but certainly not uncommon. These often involve traumatic dissections resulting in the creation of an intimal flap or development of a traumatic intracranial aneurysm.

The ultimate goal in treatment is to prevent further morbidity and mortality. The decision of endovascular treatment can be clear, such as in a massive traumatic epistaxis, or controversial, as in traumatic dissection where medical therapy is often preferred. Therefore in the treatment decision, variables such as clinical stability, active stroke symptoms, published data (limited except for blunt cervical vascular injuries) and natural history should be considered.

Trauma: hemorrhage
Approach

In trauma, the side in which the injury has occurred is often unknown, and injuries may also be bilateral. In the event of shock from massive hemorrhage, the authors use bilateral transfemoral arterial approaches using 6 Fr multipurpose guide catheters for diagnostic and immediate therapeutic reasons.

Small vessel occlusion (epistaxis)

(1) Solid embolic agents such as polyvinyl alcohol (PVA) of 250 to 500 µm in size are most often used. Liquid embolic materials, mainly n-butyl-cyanoacrylate (nBCA) and Onyx (Micro Therapeutics, Irvine, CA), can also be used depending on the operator's experience and comfort.

(2) Coils: Pushable coils or detachable coils (must use two marker microcatheters) are occasionally used. Their disadvantage includes loss of future access through the same pedicle, which may become pertinent since collaterals may develop from other arteries into the same area and result in future epistaxis.

(3) Gelfoam may also be used after particle embolization.

- Safety: The anticipated complication of using embolic agents depends on the location of the microcatheter. Multiple anastomoses exist in between branches of the internal maxillary with the ophthalmic artery and petrous/cavernous ICA or between the occipital, deep cervical, ascending cervical arteries and vertebral artery. Therefore in the treatment of epistaxis it is **recommended to be as superselective as possible**.

- Tip: Connect a 10 ml particle syringe to a 3 cc high-pressure syringe to constantly mix the particles, in order to avoid sedimentation and to deliver the particles. It is useful to have additional 3 cc syringes filled with saline to help "flush" forward the microcatheter while delivering particles. If the microcatheter becomes clogged, this microcatheter should be removed.

Large vessel occlusion

(1) Vascular plug: A vascular plug can be used as a rapid and easy to navigate device to achieve immediate homeostasis. The preferred device is the AMPLATZER™ vascular plug (St. Jude Medical)

(2) Coils: These are generally reserved to slow flow in vascular segments or venous structures since they carry a high risk of anterograde migration. Operator should choose a relatively long coil, and if high flow state such as the ICA, try to achieve proximal occlusion with a balloon guide catheter or compliant balloons in order to minimize the risk of antegrade migration.

(3) Detachable balloons: This device is now rarely available, but has been used in such conditions[5].

- Safety: When planning a large vessel occlusion (for instance of the common carotid artery or the ICA), an iatrogenic infarct should be considered imminent. Also, if a vessel occlusion is performed far from the hemorrhagic site, hemorrhage may not be controlled due to existing collaterals.

- Tip: If the hemorrhage arises from a distal segment of a large vessel (e.g. intracranial carotid artery laceration in transphenoidal pituitary surgery), consider navigating a balloon guide catheter into the vessel of interest in attempt to arrest or minimize blood loss temporarily until a permanent therapy is completed. Typical angiographic features of iatrogenic ICA injury after transphenoidal pituitary surgery may include the following: contrast media extravasation within the sphenoid sinus, carotid artery occlusion and/or stenosis, pseudo/dissecting aneurysm within the carotid artery, and carotid cavernous fistula. If time allows and patient stable, then check on collateral supply with emphasis on venous filling delay. When cross circulation is adequate, sacrificing the ICA may be an option. Occluding the artery at the site of tear is of paramount importance to prevent retrograde leak. However, if cross circulation is inadequate, preserving the ICA is of absolute necessity. In these circumstances, use of a stent graft would be a viable option[17-19].

Flow restoration

Covered stent: Used for flow restoration when it is considered that vessel occlusion carries a high risk of morbidity/mortality. Different device properties make them suitable for extracranial or intracranial vessel placement.

Safety: Owing to the high thrombogenic properties of covered stents, antiplatelets are strongly recommended along with parenteral agents to prevent acute stent thrombosis until oral agents are considered therapeutic.

> Tip: A number of covered stents are available, e.g. GORE®, VIABAHN®.
> Endoprosthesis, Fluency® (Bard peripheral vascular), but these are considered relatively "stiff" to navigate since they use a 0.035 inch wire platform, and therefore can be used in relatively straight vessels such as the extracranial carotid and vertebral arteries.

When attempting to use a covered stent intracranially, the Jostent coronary stent graft (Jomed GmbH, Rangendingen, Germany) is more trackable than the previously mentioned stents, but a solid guide catheter foundation should still be considered (i.e. Cook Shuttle and Envoy). Jostent uses a 0.014 inch wire platform.

Following proper covered stent placement, evaluate for an endoleak. If present, this should be treated accordingly[20].

Trauma: dissection

Flow restoration

When clinically indicated, self-expanding stents are used to achieve intimal flap apposition. Depending on the vessel diameter, most carotid artery stents can be used, but the Neuroform (Stryker Neurovascular), Cordis Enterprise, or XPERT (Abbott Vascular) stents can also be used in small caliber vessels, depending on the location of the vessel damage.

Large vessel occlusion

See Figures 8.4 and 8.5. Once again, this treatment should only be carried out in an already occluded vessel and in a patient in whom it is considered that the occlusion will not add further morbidity. The vessel commonly occluded in the setting of trauma is the vertebral artery, where surgical manipulation increases the risk of intraoperative hemorrhage or thrombus migration. This should be considered only after consultation with the surgeon and only if it assists the surgeon in decreasing the risk of stroke.

The complications of external carotid artery intervention

General

These complications can be seen with any wire or catheter manipulation in the ECA and its branches.

Arterial spasm

See Figure 8.6. Branches of the ECA are of small diameter (1–2 mm) and have tortuous courses. Therefore, both distension by catheters within the arteries and straightening of arterial branches by wire or catheter can lead to arterial spasm. Arterial spasm can prevent further advancement of wire or catheter and impede the injection of medication or embolic material. The most effective treatment is withdrawal of the inciting wire or catheter.

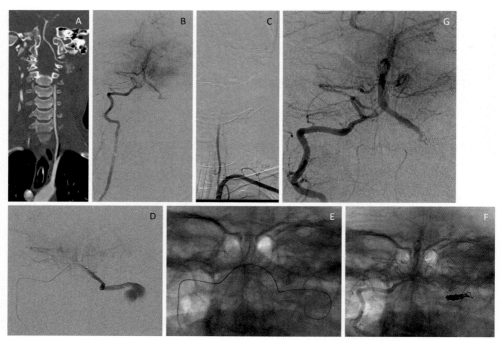

Figure 8.4 Left vertebral artery (VA) transection after gunshot wound. **A:** Computed tomography (CT) angiogram showing left VA contrast extravsation near horizontal segment and C1 complex fracture. **B:** Right VA injection demonstrating reflux into left VA and occlusion at horizontal segment. **C:** Left VA injection demonstrates occluded distal V2 segment. **D:** Microcatheter injection demonstrates contrast extravasation, confirming transection. **E:** Microcatheter advanced beyond the horizontal segment in retrograde manner. **F:** Coil embolization of the dissected VA segment. **G:** Right VA injection demonstrating flow in left intracranial segment of VA but no filling in the horizontal segment.

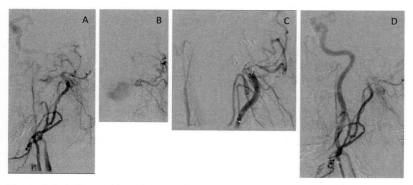

Figure 8.5 A 70-year-old gentleman with uncontrolled bleeding from oral cavity and neck region. Patient has infiltrating squamous cell carcinoma in the neck. Conservative measures had failed and the patient was hemodynamically unstable. Angiogram demonstrates active contrast extravasation from left IMAX by 5 French guide and microcatheter injection (**A** and **B**). Endovascular coiling was performed at the site of extravasation. The microcatheter was brought inside the left ECA near the site of IMAX origin, and coil embolization performed (**C**). Guide catheter injection does not demonstrate any further extravasation (**D**). Patient was also clinically noted to have cessation of bleeding.

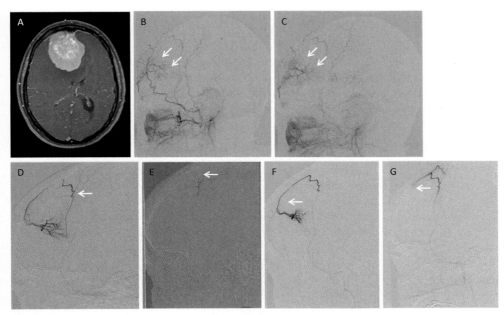

Figure 8.6 Severe vasospasm of branches of middle meningeal artery during tumor embolization.
A: Right frontal meningioma with contrast enhancement on T1 weighted image on magnetic resonance imaging (MRI) (arrow). B: Arterial supply of tumor from frontal branches of middle meningeal artery in early phase (lateral, arrow). C: Arterial supply of tumor from frontal branches of middle meningeal artery in late phase (lateral, arrow). D: Microcatheter position in distal branch of middle meningeal artery (lateral, arrow). E: Spasm of branch supplying the tumor after injection of Embosphere microspheres (150–300 μm; Merit Medical Systems) falsely appearing as obliteration of tumor vascularity (lateral, arrow). F: Visualization of tumor vascularity after injection of 1 mg of nicardipine (1 ml) (lateral, arrow). G: Actual obliteration of tumor vascularity after injection of Embospheres (300–500 μm) (lateral, arrow).

The resolution of arterial spasm occurs within the next several minutes. Infusion of vasodilators such as nicardipine, verapamil, or nitroglycerin may be considered.

Arterial dissection and thrombosis

Arterial distension by catheters and straightening of arterial branches by wire or catheter can lead to arterial dissection and thrombosis. Arterial dissection and thrombosis are usually asymptomatic because of extensive anastomotic arterial supply within the ECA vasculature. However, such events can prevent further advancement of wire or catheter and impede injection of medication or embolic material. The most effective treatment is withdrawal of inciting wire or catheter. Antiplatelet agents such as aspirin or clopidogrel may be used to prevent propagation of thrombosis.

Arterial rupture

Rapidly progressive arterial dissection or perforation due to mechanical trauma induced by wire or catheter can lead to arterial rupture. The first manifestation may be contrast extravasation and collection outside the silhouette of the ECA or branches. Local rapidly progressive swelling in the face or oropharynx may be seen. Most rupture episodes are self-contained owing to severe arterial spasm in the ruptured artery. External compression may be possible over the site of arterial rupture. Reversal of any anticoagulation with protamine sulfate is recommended. If initial efforts are unsuccessful in preventing ongoing bleeding, coil embolization of the branch of the ECA should be considered. Obliteration of the branch or main trunk of the ECA is well tolerated owing to extensive anastomotic arterial supply within the ECA vasculature. However, obliteration of the ruptured artery must be close to the site of arterial rupture to prevent retrograde/alternate filling into the ruptured segment from anastomotic arterial supply. The main trunk and branches of the ECA are too small for strategies such as covered stent placement.

Related to embolization of external carotid artery branches

Distal vasculature ischemic injury

The extensive anastomotic arterial supply within the ECA vasculature allows adequate perfusion subsequent to obliteration of the branch or main trunk of the ECA. However, the anastomosis in certain vascular beds such as nasal mucosa or nasal tip depends upon patency of the small arteries and arterioles. Very small particles that lodge in distal microvasculature such as capillaries may result in occlusion distal to the anastomotic network. Similarly, embolization of multiple branches of the ECA may result in ischemic injury. Liquid embolic agents with high penetration may also pose a risk of extensive distal embolization. The ischemic injury manifests as pain with pallor of external skin region. Subsequent necrotic changes may manifest as inflammatory changes such as swelling, ulceration, and gangrene. When ischemic injury is suspected, cutaneous application of vasodilators such as nitro paste may increase regional flow through collateral arteries and arterioles. Local vasodilation may also result in clearance of some of the embolic particles from the distal microvasculature. However, if necrosis occurs, tissue debridement and skin grafting may be necessary. There are certain branches of the ECA which are devoid of anastomotic networks, such as the inferior alveolar artery, and occlusion can result in periosteal necrosis of the mandible.

Inadvertent embolization of extracranial arteries

During embolization procedures, an effort is made to advance the microcatheter to a point in the artery that excludes all the tributaries that supply the normal tissue of the face, tongue, and oropharynx. However, as the embolic material occludes the distal microvasculature, the outflow resistance to blood flow and embolic material increases. The outflow resistance can increase to a point where there is complete stasis of contrast injected through the microcatheter. Retrograde flow of embolic material may lead to embolization of branches that were proximal to the distal end of the microcatheter. Prevention of such embolization requires intermittent assessment of flow pattern through the target vasculature. Retrograde flow and stasis must be recognized at an early stage. Identification of retrograde flow around the distal end of the microcatheter requires selection of an angiographic view that allows adequate visualization of the distal end of the microcatheter in the longitudinal axis and, in particular, avoids end-on views. If retrograde flow is recognized, the injection of the embolic material must be discontinued. Manual suction and retraction of the microcatheter under suction may be necessary. Such suction prevents dispersion of embolic material that is still within the lumen of the microcatheter. If occlusion is seen of an artery by liquid embolic material with diameter greater than 1 mm, mechanical manipulation using snare or balloon catheters may create an orifice through the embolic material cast. In smaller arteries or arteries occluded with embolic particles, injection of vasodilators through a new micro-catheter in the vicinity of the occlusion may improve perfusion in the affected vascular territory.

The dura mater receives arterial supply from branches of the IMAX, ascending pharyn-geal artery, and occipital artery. The middle meningeal artery from the IMAX is the major supply to the dura. The extensive vascularization from various intracranial and extracranial arteries prevents any ischemic changes within the dura.

Inadvertent embolization of intracranial arteries

The ECA branches can form anastomoses with intracranial arteries which may be angio-graphically visible or occult. A description of such anastomotic pathways was provided in an earlier section. As the embolic material occludes the distal microvasculature, the outflow resistance increases, resulting in activation of latent anastomotic channels between branches of the ECA and intracranial arteries. Embolic material tends to move into the path of least resistance, and such channels provide a low-resistance efflux into the large intracranial arteries. Prevention of such embolization requires intermittent assessment of the flow pattern through and around the target vasculature. New arterial anastomotic channels must be recognized at an early stage. Embolic material, once it enters the intracranial arteries, disperses very quickly into distal intracranial vasculature. Parent artery occlusion is uncom-mon, and distal microvascular failure manifesting as regional delay in contrast outflow is common. Once intracranial involvement is suspected, two issues require immediate assessment:

(1) Has the patient developed any new cerebral ischemic symptoms?

(2) Is there any occlusion or abnormal flow pattern visualized in the intracranial artery in question?

Selective microcatheter placement into the intracranial artery in question with subsequent microcatheter injection of thrombolytics may improve flow through dissolution of second-ary thrombi. Intra-arterial vasodilators in the vicinity of occlusion may improve perfusion in the affected vascular territory through collateral channels and result in efflux of some of the particles through the dilated microvasculature. On rare occasions, the liquid embolic material may precipitate within the anastomotic channels and partly protrude within the lumen of the intracranial artery. An intracranial stent placed across the protruding liquid embolic material may trap the precipitated embolic material and prevent fragmentation within the intracranial artery.

References

1. Duffis EJ, Gandhi CD, Prestigiacomo CJ, et al. Head, neck, and brain tumor embolization guidelines. *J Neurointerv Surg.* 2012;4:251–255

2. Shah QA. Bilateral tri-arterial embolization for the treatment of epistaxis. *J Vasc Interv Neurol.* 2008;1:102–105

3. Andersen PJ, Kjeldsen AD, Nepper-Rasmussen J. Selective embolization in the treatment of intractable epistaxis. *Acta Otolaryngol.* 2005;125:293–297

4. Sadri M, Midwinter K, Ahmed A, Parker A. Assessment of safety and efficacy of arterial embolisation in the management of intractable epistaxis. *Eur Arch Otorhinolaryngol.* 2006;263:560–566

5. Grandhi R, Panczykowski D, Zwagerman NT, et al. Facial necrosis after endovascular onyx-18 embolization for epistaxis. *Surg Neurol Int.* 2013;4:95

6. Kalani MY, Ducruet AF, Crowley RW, *et al.* Transfemoral transarterial onyx embolization of carotid body paragangliomas: Technical considerations, results, and strategies for complication avoidance. *Neurosurgery.* 2013;72:9–15; discussion 15

7. Marangos N, Schumacher M. Facial palsy after glomus jugulare tumour embolization. *J Laryngol Otol.* 1999;113:268–270

8. Bentson J, Rand R, Calcaterra T, Lasjaunias P. Unexpected complications following therapeutic embolization. *Neuroradiology.* 1978;16:420–423

9. Valavanis A. Preoperative embolization of the head and neck: Indications, patient selection, goals, and precautions. *AJNR Am J Neuroradiol.* 1986;7:943–952

10. Gartrell BC, Hansen MR, Gantz BJ, *et al.* Facial and lower cranial neuropathies after preoperative embolization of jugular foramen lesions with ethylene vinyl alcohol. *Otol Neurotol.* 2012;33:1270–1275

11. Ozanne A, Pereira V, Krings T, Toulgoat F, Lasjaunias P. Arterial vascularization of the cranial nerves. *Neuroimaging Clin N Am.* 2008;18:431–439, xii

12. Mames RN, Snady-McCoy L, Guy J. Central retinal and posterior ciliary artery occlusion after particle embolization of the external carotid artery system. *Ophthalmology.* 1991;98:527–531

13. Krajina A, Chrobok V. Radiological diagnosis and management of epistaxis. *Cardiovasc Intervent Radiol.* 2014; 37:26–36

14. Strach K, Schrock A, Wilhelm K, *et al.* Endovascular treatment of epistaxis: Indications, management, and outcome. *Cardiovasc Intervent Radiol.* 2011;34:1190–1198

15. Gottumukkala R, Kadkhodayan Y, Moran CJ, Cross de WT, 3rd, Derdeyn CP. Impact of vessel choice on outcomes of polyvinyl alcohol embolization for intractable idiopathic epistaxis. *J Vasc Interv Radiol.* 2013;24:234–239.

16. Geibprasert S, Pongpech S, Armstrong D, Krings T. Dangerous extracranial-intracranial anastomoses and supply to the cranial nerves: vessels the neurointerventionalist needs to know. *AJNR Am J Neuroradiol.* 2009;30:1459–1468.

17. Ghatge SB, Modi DB. Treatment of ruptured ICA during transsphenoidal surgery. Two different endovascular strategies in two cases. *Interv Neuroradiol.* 2010;16:31–37.

18. Kocer N, Kizilkilic O, Albayram S, *et al.* Treatment of iatrogenic internal carotid artery laceration and carotid cavernous fistula with endovascular stent-graft placement. *AJNR Am J Neuroradiol.* 2002;23:442–446.

19. Park YS, Jung JY, Ahn JY, Kim DJ, Kim SH. Emergency endovascular stent graft and coil placement for internal carotid artery injury during transsphenoidal surgery. *Surg Neurol.* 2009;72:741–746.

20. Stavropoulos SW, Charagundla SR. Imaging techniques for detection and management of endoleaks after endovascular aortic aneurysm repair. *Radiology.* 2007;243:641–655.

Complications during endovascular provocative testing and bilateral inferior petrosal sinus sampling

Ameer E. Hassan, Haralabos Zacharatos, Gustavo J. Rodriguez, and Ricardo Hanel

Provocative testing

The purpose of provocative testing in neurointervention is to simulate what the consequences would be if a blood vessel were occluded, or if part of the nervous system vascularized by a specific blood vessel were challenged, prior to a definitive treatment, usually endovascular embolization or surgical resection. The administration of a short-acting anesthetic agent or temporary mechanical occlusion in the vascular distribution of interest is followed by a neurological examination to assess for clinical changes. These procedures, if performed by experienced operators, carry a low risk of complications. However, we believe that the key to a successful provocative test is the knowledge of its intricacies and diligence in the steps taken, as well as correct interpretation to avoid false readings. Here we cover the most common provocative tests used in neurointervention and common complications of which the operator needs to be aware.

The Wada test

Despite the advent of functional magnetic resonance imaging (fMRI), magnetoencephalography (MEG), and high-density electroencephalography (EEG) recordings, the Wada test is still the gold standard test in the presurgical evaluation of epilepsy patients that are surgical candidates[1]. The conventional Wada test consists of an injection of a $GABA_A$-agonist agent (usually amobarbital, a short-acting barbiturate) into the internal carotid arteries, one side at a time, followed by neuropsychological assessment[2]. Time should be allowed for the patient to recover fully from the anesthetic effects before the other hemisphere is tested. The neurological assessment evaluates the non-anesthetized hemisphere. The purpose is to identify the language and memory lateralization. Caution with sedatives is recommended, so as not to mask the evaluation. Simulation of the surgical resection of the temporal lobe would predict postoperative memory and language dysfunction.

Some patients suffering from intractable mesial temporal lobe epilepsy who are candidates for temporal lobectomy traditionally undergo the intracarotid artery amobarbital (Wada) test. Patients with right-handedness, right temporal lesions, and strong verbal memory may not need to undergo the Wada test, given the low risk for failing the test[3].

Intracarotid Wada procedures at times have been shown to have inconsistencies in their results and have led to difficulty in localization of memory, language, and neuro-behavioral functional areas. Possible reasons for these inconsistencies are that the Wada testing does

Complications of Neuroendovascular Procedures and Bailout Techniques, ed. Rakesh Khatri, Gustavo J. Rodriguez, Jean Raymond and Adnan I. Qureshi. Published by Cambridge University Press.
© Cambridge University Press 2016.

not inhibit the specific arterial territory supplying the lesion but inhibits the entire hemisphere, making it hard to precisely study the targeted area; in addition, $GABA_A$-agonists (such as amobarbital) only inhibit gray matter and not white matter structures.

Superselective Wada testing

As a result of inactivating widespread hemispheric structures, memory testing is confounded by simultaneous inhibition of multiple areas (Table 9.1).

Superselective Wada techniques enable inhibition of an arterial territory supplying a more specific location in the brain, therefore allowing reliable prediction of postoperative residual deficits. The major components of the limbic system (located within the mesial temporal lobe) are the amygdala, the hippocampal formation (the structure most widely identified with memory encoding), and the parahippocampal gyrus. The internal carotid artery perfuses directly or through its branches irrigates its major portion, but not the posterior two-thirds of the hippocampus, which is supplied by the posterior cerebral artery in the majority of patients.

The delivery of amobarbital to specific regions of the brain avoids the confounding effects of inhibiting a large portion of the cerebral hemisphere. Examples of supraselective Wada testing include the selective injection of sodium amobarbital into the posterior cerebral artery, the anterior choroidal artery, or the internal carotid artery during temporary balloon occlusion distal to the origin of the anterior choroidal artery (Figure 9.1). The indication would be for patients who failed intracarotid amobarbital testing or had acute drug reactions that interfered with subsequent memory testing, or in cases when the standard Wada testing is inaccurate or the anterior cross-flow of blood is present[4].

Table 9.1 Undesired side effects of conventional Wada procedure

Phantom limb movements

Euphoria

Agitation/aggression

Crying

Behavioral disturbances: fear, verbal/physical disinhibition

Attentional disturbances

Aphasia

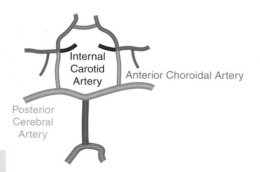

Internal Carotid Artery

Anterior Choroidal Artery

Posterior Cerebral Artery

Figure 9.1 Arterial sites for selective Wada testing. Blue: internal carotid artery; red: anterior choroidal artery; peach: posterior cerebral artery.

With superselective injection in the anterior choroidal artery, the following deficits are expected to be found: motor deficits, language disturbance, cranial nerve VII palsy, somatosensory disturbances, miosis, visual field defects, and ptosis[5].

The selective posterior cerebral artery injection is more time-consuming than the nonselective internal carotid artery amobarbital procedure. The presence of increased tortuosity of both vertebral arteries at the C1 and C2 level will limit the catheter control. The tip of the microcatheter should be placed in the mid to distal peduncular (P1) segment of the posterior cerebral artery, which will enable amobarbital perfusion of the vascular bed distal to the peduncular (P1) segment, including the following structures: subiculum, dentate, gyrus, hippocampus, and associated white matter tracts. The following findings are expected: contralateral hand weakness, contralateral hemisensory symptoms, such as dysesthesia with decreased sensation of touch, and contralateral hemianopsia. Contralateral hemianopsia and hemisensory impairment last for approximately 3–5 minutes and rarely interfere with the memory testing if the testing items are properly presented in the preserved visual field.

Superselective pre-embolization provocative testing

The additional use of lidocaine in superselective provocative testing can increase the sensitivity and predictive value of pre-surgical or pre-embolization testing, potentially reducing the frequency of treatment-related morbidity[6]. The co-administration of the local anesthetic lidocaine, a voltage-gated sodium channel blocker, is known to inhibit white matter tracts in the central nervous system as well as the cranial nerves. It helps detect eloquent brain function not revealed by the individual administration of the gray-matter-specific brevital or amobarbital. While GABA agents block neurons, lidocaine blocks axons. All the studies using sequential administration of $GABA_A$-agonists for gray matter and lidocaine for inhibition of white matter have been with superselective injection and have been shown to be safe, feasible, and effective in treatment planning[6].

The combination of the two agents increases the sensitivity and specificity of the Wada test, and it has been used prior to brain arteriovenous malformation (AVM) embolization[6], spinal embolization, and embolization of external carotid artery branches at risk for vasa nervorum accidental embolization.

In spinal angiography, prior to embolization, the microcatheter should be placed in close proximity to the nidus or fistula point. If this is not possible and if the lesion is close to the anterior or posterior spinal arteries, the Wada test should be considered. Most patients are under general anesthesia, and the spinal Wada testing requires surrogate tests such as somatosensory evoked potentials (SSEPs) and motor evoked potentials (MEPs) to substitute for the neuroexam[7–9].

During embolization of lesions with blood supply from external carotid branches, anastomoses with the internal carotid or vertebral artery are initially ruled out angiographically. Amytal can be then used followed by neurological examination to assess the presence of non-angiographically visible vascular connections (<200 μm). In the case of absent deficits with amytal, lidocaine can be used to assess the presence of vasa nervorum: if there are neurological deficits pertaining to cranial nerves, then large particles (300–500 μm) can be used for embolization to avoid post-treatment cranial neuropathies[10].

Complications

Complications can be classified into those inherent to the cerebral angiography and those related to the injection of the anesthetic agents. They can also be classified according to temporal profile, as temporary or permanent. Not many reports are available pertaining to complication rates. Most reports available are about the Wada test, and while the overall risk of the Wada procedure may be 11%, the risk of permanent neurological complications is less than 1%[11]. Complications related to the diagnostic angiography include but are not limited to: headaches, nausea, vomiting; thromboembolism during vessel catheterization owing to difficult access or thrombosis related to devices; or dissection with subsequent risk of cerebrovascular events. An institution performing large volumes of Wada testing reported a risk of 0.7% of carotid dissection[12].

The risks associated with catheter manipulation in the intracranial vasculature are greater than when performing Wada in the internal carotid. In addition to the previous complications, there is a risk of vessel perforation and cerebral hemorrhage.

Different anesthetic agents have been used in the Wada test, amobarbital being the most common. Other agents have been pentobarbital and methohexital. Common side effects derived from their use are encephalopathy and seizures[11]. While ongoing seizures can occasionally develop that require additional medical therapy, these complications are usually self-limited. Pentobarbital is the antielpilipetic that is least likely to cause encephalopathy, and methohexital is more likely to cause seizures[1,13].

A serious complication that must also be considered is the possibility of accidental reflux of an anesthetic agent into the basilar artery during the selective posterior cerebral artery test, leading to unconsciousness and respiratory failure (requiring ventilatory support). Brain-stem inactivation can also theoretically impair cardiovascular centers, leading to hypotension. Cerebral edema can occur if the drugs are not mixed correctly.

Balloon test occlusion

Mechanical occlusion of a vessel has been shown to be a safe way to estimate the effect of occlusion of the vascular supply by embolization or surgical ligation. Balloon test occlusion (BTO) is performed to predict the negative hemodynamic consequences of vessel occlusion that could result with cerebral infarct and permanent functional deficits.

The purpose is to study the potential adverse outcome of sacrificing a vascular territory as part of the treatment for tumors, mainly skull base tumors, or the treatment of internal carotid artery aneuryms. It is also used to test the outcome of vessel sacrifice or to guide treatment during vessel sacrifice in traumatic injury of the carotid artery.

Balloon test occlusion: the classical approach

Certain conditions must be met to ensure proper test results. The proper site and level of expected vessel sacrifice must be tested to predict the outcomes of the permanent occlusion. Test occlusion will take into account collateral vasculature in case of permanent vascular occlusion[14]. The site of occlusion should be distal to any collateral feeder that may supply blood to the territory of interest. To prevent thrombosis related to catheterization, heparin should be infused before the devices are advanced. Routine administration of 70–100 IU/kg of heparin is performed as an intravenous bolus prior to the test. In addition, heparin (2000 to 5000 IU/l) can be used via continuous infusion flush, to irrigate the guide catheter and the femoral artery sheath in the meantime. If the procedure is taking a significant time (>1 hour), it is recommended to monitor anticoagulation, aiming for an activated clotting time (ACT) >250 seconds.

Perform a baseline neurological examination and a diagnostic four-vessel cerebral angiogram before balloon inflation in order to study possible collateral flow and anatomical variants. Balloons must be sized to the vessel being temporarily occluded. A BTO of a vessel should always have the balloon inflation at the same level as the predicted vessel size. The occlusion is confirmed with angiography, and recurrent checks may be necessary to ensure persistent occlusion. Compliant balloons decrease the chance of complications but significantly elevate the costs. Always confirm occlusion by injecting contrast through the guide catheter lumen.

Clinical evaluation: Always clinically test the patient for any neurological deficits and pay specific attention to deficits pertaining to the supplied vascular territory.

Keep the vessel occluded for about 15–30 minutes if the patient tolerates, and then consider a hypotensive challenge. If at any time the patient develops symptoms, then the patient has failed the test occlusion. If the patient passes the test clinically, however, this does not guarantee that the patient will not develop symptoms once the vessel is occluded permanently.

False and incomplete tests

It is important to recognize that there is the possibility of a false positive or negative test and to know the reasons behind it. The consequences of having a false test should clearly be explained to the patient prior to the definitive treatment. It is known that despite having passed the BTO, there is still the risk of brain ischemia in up to 10% of patients when the definitive occlusion is performed[15]. Explanations for these false negatives may be related to the lack of sensitivity of the BTO, delayed thromboembolism, or the site of permanent occlusion being different from the site of the BTO[16].

In some instances the test will be incomplete, either because the patient develops symptoms not related to the hemodynamic challenge but to a thromboembolic event, or because of patient intolerance to the test. Different ancillary tests, described below, have been developed to decrease the risks of having a false test or to substitute for an incomplete test. Neurophysiological monitoring (NPM) can directly assess the functional state of specific cerebral regions and provides an indirect measure of regional ischemia produced in the cerebral circulation. It typically includes continuous EEG, SSEPs, hypotension challenge, measurement of stump pressures, computed tomography (xenon computed tomography, single-photon emission computed tomography, or positron emission tomography) or magnetic resonance (MR) perfusion with or without acetazolamide challenge. Methods based on quantitative analyses are less likely to end in a false negative test than those based on qualitative analysis, since occlusion of an artery often entails hemodynamic changes in the contralateral site[17]. Special attention is given in the text below to emerging techniques, such as transcranial Doppler as a screening tool, and the venous phase of cerebral angiography.

Hypotension challenge: Early case series showed that temporary balloon occlusion of a vessel could challenge the blood flow to that vascular territory but, because of collateral flow, not lead to demonstrable neurological deficits, and yet still lead to a significant amount of stroke risk along the line[18]. This led to additional testing with a hypotensive challenge because this magnifies the hemodynamic effects of the vascular occlusion. When no deficit is appreciated during BTO, the blood pressure can be lowered to a target pressure of 66% of the mean arterial pressure baseline. If the patient develops neurological symptoms at any point, the test should be aborted, and the patient has failed the test occlusion. Agents used for lowering blood pressure should be short-acting (nitroprusside, nicardipine, or fenoldopam[19]) and used in infusions. Agents should be started at the lowest dose possible

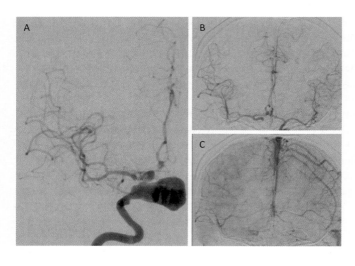

Figure 9.2 A 40-year-old woman with a giant, 28 mm wide neck aneurysm arising from the intracranial right internal carotid artery and causing compression of the right optic nerve, pituitary stalk, and hypothalamic region (A). The patient underwent a balloon test occlusion of the right internal carotid artery in preparation for definitive treatment. The main collateralization was via the anterior communicating artery (B). The venous phase showed no delay in the venous filling of the right hemisphere when the balloon was inflated in the right internal carotid artery and an injection was performed in the left internal carotid artery (C). The patient passed the test.

and increased every few minutes if no new neurological deficits are appreciated. Patients may get severe headaches, nausea, and vomiting if the doses are increased too fast or too frequently. Additional hypertensive agents (labetolol or hydralazine) may be added when unable to reach target pressure.

Transcranial Doppler: A good screening tool to assess the carotid artery is the transcranial Doppler. Prior to a BTO, if there is a decrease in the velocity of the ipsilateral middle cerebral artery to <30% of the baseline during carotid compression, this is predictive of BTO failure. This concept is not valid if there is a carotid–cavernous fistula or other vascular tumors[20].

Angiographic evaluation: Careful interpretation of the arterial and venous phases may also predict the outcome of a vessel sacrifice. Angiographic surrogates are increasingly used and allow a shorter BTO with theoretical lower risks and the possibility of using general anesthesia. While the balloon is inflated, initially, there is visualization of cross-flow to the contralateral middle cerebral artery via an anterior or posterior communicating artery. Using the best collateral, evaluation of the venous phase is performed. The venous-phase BTO positive predictive value ranges from 98% to 100%, and requires less than 2 minutes' evaluation. Venous-phase BTO does, however, require simultaneous carotid catheterization. The synchronicity of venous filling between the occluded and non-occluded hemispheres is evaluated, and a delay of <0.5 seconds allows a safe permanent vessel occlusion (Figure 9.2). Meanwhile a delay of 3 seconds or more may predispose to ischemia[21,22].

In the posterior circulation, more evidence exists that in the presence of two vertebral arteries that fill the basilar artery, the sacrifice of one does not require a BTO. Instead, the BTO is reserved to evaluate the circle of Willis. For such purposes, test occlusion of the bilateral vertebrobasilar junction is required. No angiographic surrogate exists, requiring the classical approach of 15 to 30 minutes of occlusion with a neurological evaluation[23].

Complications

Apart from the risks related to the diagnostic angiography, there are others linked to the balloon inflation and/or the hypotension challenge. Few reports exist on complications during BTO. In the largest series, the absolute risk of complications has been quoted as less than 4%, and most complications were transient. And while the risk of neurological complications was around 2%, the risk of permanent neurological complications was less than 0.5% when BTO was performed in the internal carotid artery[24,25]. Most neurological complications were related to damage of the vessel wall during balloon inflation, causing a dissection with or without pseudoaneurysm formation and/or embolism. Therefore we emphasize the importance of using anticoagulation during the test and the importance of matching the balloon size to the size of the vessel. Prior to the balloon inflation, we recommend checking for stability of the system to avoid migration of the balloon during inflation, as the migration could favor the tearing of the vessel. During inflation, also avoid using supranominal pressures when using a non-compliant balloon, to avoid its rupture. Balloon rupture can lead to air embolism. Super-compliant balloons also may pose a risk of vessel wall damage, since they exert the main radial force in a smaller area. The risk of complications can be higher when there is an underlying pathology in the wall of internal carotid artery such as atheromatous disease, or wall vulnerability due to a collagen disorder such as Ehlers–Danlos syndrome. The operator must always evaluate for thrombosis, dissection, and vasospasm after removing the balloon. If the patient develops neurological deficits during the test, deflate the balloon and perform an angiogram to exclude local thrombosis or vasospasm. If there is distal embolization, treat if necessary (thrombolytics or GpIIb/IIIa inhibitors). Give a fluid bolus and consider IV vasopressors if the blood pressure is significantly low. The duration of the test may also affect the risk of complications.

The risks associated with wire and balloon manipulation are greater in intracranial vessels than in extracranial arteries. Other, usually transient, complications related to the medications or hypotension challenge include vagal response, headache, nausea, and vomiting.

Venous sampling

Invasive central venous sampling diagnostic tests have been used to evaluate the hormonal composition of the venous environment in the cavernous sinus, inferior petrosal sinus, or internal jugular vein. By sampling the blood in the venous environment surrounding the pituitary gland, the systemic dilution effect is minimized, allowing more accurate measurement of pituitary specific hormones. Bilateral internal jugular venous sampling, bilateral cavernous sinus sampling, and bilateral inferior petrosal sinus sampling are the diagnostic tests that have been used to study the unilateral concentration of pituitary hormones. The venous sampling is used for detecting pituitary origin of Cushing's disease and for identifying the laterality of the tumor.

In a typical case of bilateral inferior petrosal sinus sampling (Figure 9.3), an 18-year-old woman presented with Cushing's syndrome: further work-up demonstrated suppression with cortisol, and an MRI of the pituitary showed a small (4 mm) hypoenhancing lesion suspicious for a microadenoma. Bilateral inferior petrosal sinus sampling was performed with results shown in Table 9.2.

At baseline, the ratio of the right petrosal sample to the peripheral sample is increased (>2). After intravenous administration of corticotropin-releasing hormone (CRH), there is a greater increase in adrenocorticotropin hormone (ACTH) levels in the petrosal samples compared with the peripheral sample, which is marked in the right side. Multiple samples are obtained; one of the reasons is to demonstrate consistency of the recordings and trends, as this helps in case of mislabeling of the samples.

Table 9.2 Results of inferior petrosal sinus (PS) sampling for patient with Cushing's syndrome

Time	Location Right PS ACTH (pg/ml)	Left PS ACTH (pg/ml)	Peripheral ACTH (pg/ml)
−15 minutes	39	16	13
−10 minutes	29	14	14
−5 minutes	56	16	13
CRH injection	41	23	14
+5 minutes	5077	156	26
+10 minutes	1718	95	55
+15 minutes	1410	101	57

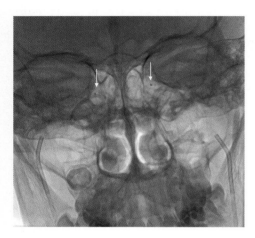

Figure 9.3 Bilateral inferior petrosal sinus sampling. AP view demonstrates guide catheters in bilateral internal jugular veins, and microcatheters are visualized distally in inferior petrosal sinuses near cavernous sinus.

Anatomy of venous drainage of the pituitary gland

On the surface of the pituitary gland, there are two plexiform venous networks that drain laterally either into the intercavernous sinuses or directly into the cavernous sinuses. Ipsilateral drainage of each half of the anterior lobe occurs into the corresponding cavernous sinus and ultimately into the inferior petrosal sinus. The inferior petrosal sinus is a dural sinus that extends from the posterior aspect of the cavernous sinus approximately 23–28 mm laterally and posteriorly to the internal jugular vein (Figure 9.4). In the majority of individuals, the inferior petrosal sinus becomes a vein, approximately 2 mm in diameter, as it enters the jugular foramen, prior to draining into the internal jugular vein. The inferior petrosal sinus decreases in diameter from 7–10 mm at the cavernous sinus to 2–4 mm as it approaches the jugular foramen, indicating that blood flow in the inferior petrosal sinus seems to be directed mainly to the vertebral venous plexus.

Anatomic variants

There is a substantial variability at the rostrocaudal level at which the inferior petrosal sinus enters the internal jugular vein. Shiu et al.[41] described the appearance and relative frequency

Table 9.3 Venous drainage patterns of the inferior petrosal sinus

Types	Prevalence	Characteristics
Type I	45%	Inferior petrosal sinus drains directly into the internal jugular bulb
Type II	24%	The sinus, either directly or through a communicating vein, anastomoses with the anterior condylar vein, which extends from the marginal sinus around the foramen magnum to the vertebral venous plexus
Type III	24%	Inferior petrosal sinus exists as a plexus of veins rather than as a single vessel. The inferior petrosal sinus drains into the internal jugular vein and (via the marginal sinus and the anterior condylar vein) into the vertebral venous plexus, which also anastomoses extensively with the basilar venous plexus coursing along the surface of the clivus
Type IV	7%	Inferior petrosal sinus drains directly into the vertebral venous plexus. There is no connection between the inferior petrosal sinus and the internal jugular vein in a true type IV pattern; instead, the inferior petrosal sinus drains directly into the anterior condylar vein

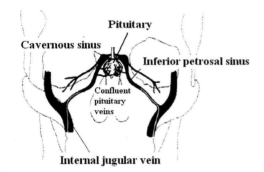

Figure 9.4 Pituitary venous drainage.

of four separate and distinct types of venous drainage of the inferior petrosal sinus (types I–IV) (Table 9.3; Figure 9.5).

Inferior petrosal sinus sampling

Bilateral inferior petrosal sinus sampling is the gold standard method of the venous sampling techniques used in the differentiation of Cushing's disease from an ectopic source of ACTH[26,27]. Bilateral inferior petrosal sinus sampling provides a higher sensitivity and better specificity than other available biochemical testing strategies in patients who do not have a pituitary lesion greater than 1 cm in size on MRI[28].

Data collected during the procedure enables the pituitary microadenoma to be lateralized, providing the neurosurgeon with information needed to select the treatment approach appropriately (Figure 9.6). The procedure has also been used in the evaluation of patients with pituitary microadenomas secreting growth hormone. The pre-test probability of a pituitary source of ACTH (Cushing's disease) is estimated to be approximately 90% in unselected patients presenting with ACTH-dependent Cushing's syndrome[29] (Table 9.4). The challenge of differentiating between Cushing's disease and ectopic ACTH

Table 9.4 Endogenous Cushing's syndrome summary

Endogenous Cushing's syndrome

ACTH-dependent Cushing's syndrome (70–80%)
- A. ACTH-secreting pituitary adenomas: Cushing's disease (80–90%)
- B. ACTH-producing ectopic tumors (10–20%)

Bronchial carcinoids: most common source of ACTH ectopic production outside of the brain

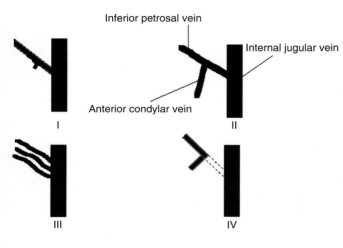

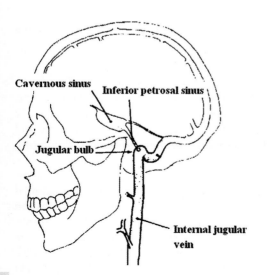

Figure 9.5 A: Venous anatomy, types I–IV. Type I: Anastomosis between the inferior petrosal sinus and the internal jugular vein; the anterior condylar vein is small or absent. Type II: A prominent anastomosis is present between the large anterior condylar vein and the inferior petrosal sinus. Type III: The inferior petrosal sinus exists as several small channels, which may form a plexus. Type IV: The inferior petrosal sinus empties directly into the anterior condylar vein, never anastomosing with the internal jugular vein. Bilateral inferior petrosal sinus sampling is anatomically possible in 99% of people, with no connection between the inferior petrosal sinus and the internal jugular vein observed in approximately 1% of the patients[23].

B: Lateral view of the skull outlining the ipsilateral cavernous sinus, inferior petrosal sinus and internal jugular vein. The anteromedial aspect of the jugular bulb is where the inferior petrosal sinus enters the internal jugular vein. Reproduced with permission from ref. 42: Qureshi, A.I. (2011) *Textbook of Interventional Neurology.*

Table 9.5 Descending order of prevalence of neoplastic causes of excess ACTH secretion

Pituitary corticotroph adenomas

Ectopic ACTH-secreting tumors

Ectopic CRH-secreting tumors (very rare)

ACTH: adrenocorticotropin hormone, CRH: corticotropin releasing hormone

Table 9.6 Non-invasive biochemical tests used to distinguish between pituitary and ectopic ACTH-dependent Cushing's syndrome

Dexamethasone suppressed CRH stimulation test

High dose dexamethasone suppression test

Low dose dexamethasone suppression test

Peripheral metyrapone stimulation test

Peripheral CRH test

Peripheral desmopressin stimulation test

Plasma ACTH concentration

ACTH: adrenocorticotropin hormone, CRH: corticotropin releasing hormone

syndrome requires the measurement of plasma ACTH levels, non-invasive dynamic tests and imaging studies such as MRI (Tables 9.4, 9.5). A combination of these tests is usually necessary as none has 100% specificity (Table 9.6).

Technical aspects of inferior petrosal sinus catheterization

The bilateral inferior sinus sampling procedure is performed with posteroanterior fluoroscopy and with the patient's head held in a neutral position. The origin of the inferior petrosal sinus is best identified in the lateral plane; concomitant antero-posterior images identify reflux into the opposite inferior petrosal sinus[30]. Once the catheter is in the internal jugular vein, the catheter tip is rotated so that it is directed medially and anteriorly. The catheter tip is held several centimeters below the expected level of the inferior petrosal sinus. While the catheter is in this position the guidewire (only a guidewire coated with hydrophilic material should be used) is advanced until it enters a medially directed vein. The trajectory of guidewire movement can indicate its position. Miller and Doppman suggested that guidewire movement superiorly and medially, or medially and then superiorly, is indicative of placement within the inferior petrosal sinus[30]. Miller and Doppman cautioned against advancing the catheter more than 1 to 1.5 cm into the inferior petrosal sinus. If the guidewire continues to advance medially, almost to the midline, or starts to head inferiorly instead of superiorly, the wire may have entered the anterior condylar vein. In the event of a rare, true type IV drainage pattern (no connection between the internal jugular vein and the inferior petrosal sinus), Miller and Doppman attempted, but failed, to access the inferior petrosal

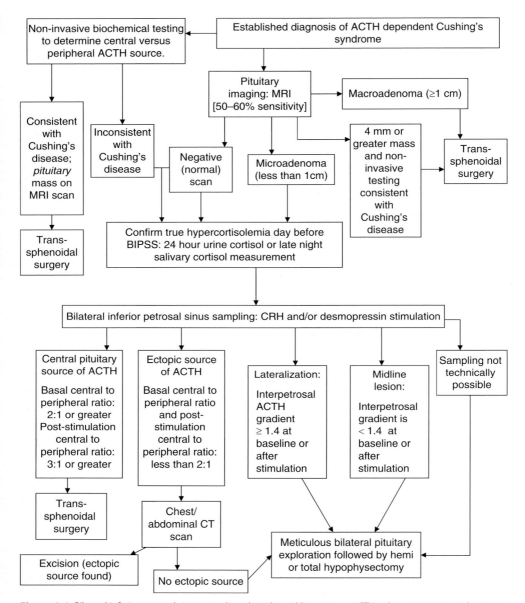

Figure 9.6 Bilateral inferior petrosal sinus sampling algorithm. Abbreviations: ACTH: adrenocorticotropin hormone; CRH: corticotropin releasing hormone; BIPSS: bilateral inferior petrosal sinus sampling; CT: computed tomography; MRI: magnetic resonance. From ref. 42: Qureshi, A.I. (2011) *Textbook of Interventional Neurology*, Figure 17.3.

sinus using the vertebral vein[30]. On the other hand, Landolt *et al.*[43] were able to successfully navigate the catheter into the inferior petrosal sinus via the vertebral vein. In this situation, the catheter tip should be withdrawn slightly and the guidewire should be re-advanced with its tip directed superiorly to engage and enter the anterior portion of the inferior petrosal sinus. The side-to-side variability in the venous anatomy of the inferior petrosal sinuses will determine how difficult it is to catheterize them. It has been shown that a small inferior petrosal sinus on one side is associated with a larger sinus on the contralateral side. Similarly, a variable junction between the inferior petrosal sinus and the internal jugular vein according to its type of venous drainage pattern (type I–IV) will also contribute to the level of difficulty of the procedure. When faced with a situation where one inferior petrosal sinus is extremely difficult to catheterize, the operator is encouraged to catheterize the contralateral inferior petrosal sinus in order to visualize the anatomy of the other inferior petrosal sinus through contrast reflux.

Direct percutaneous internal jugular vein access may be necessary in the case of femoral vein occlusion, such as the presence of an inferior vena cava filter, or aberrant anatomy of the great veins. The operator should cannulate the internal jugular vein using direct ultrasound-guided puncture of the internal jugular veins as inferiorly as possible in the neck, because most Cushing's syndrome patients have short, thick necks.

Comparison of bilateral inferior petrosal sinus and internal jugular venous sampling

Bilateral inferior petrosal sinus sampling is more sensitive than bilateral internal jugular venous sampling with or without CRH stimulation, with a sensitivity of 80%[31,32].

Central to peripheral adrenocorticotropin hormone ratio: basal and post-stimulation results

The ratio of central (inferior petrosal sinus) to peripheral ACTH concentration is used to distinguish between pituitary Cushing's disease and the occult ectopic ACTH syndrome. Simultaneous measurements of ACTH levels are taken from each inferior petrosal sinus and from a peripheral vein. The central to peripheral ratios are calculated at baseline (pre-stimulation) and at various time points after intravenous peripheral CRH and/or desmopressin injection (see for example Figure 9.3; Table 9.2). The inferior petrosal sinus time point with the highest central to peripheral ACTH ratio is used for interpretation. A central pituitary source of ACTH overproduction is presumed if the inferior petrosal sinus to peripheral (central to peripheral) ratio is 2:1 or greater at baseline, or if the ratio is 3:1 or greater at any time after the peripheral administration of CRH and/or desmopressin.

If the threshold criterion is not met, a peripheral (ectopic) source can be presumed. In most patients who have occult ectopic ACTH syndrome, a central to peripheral ratio of less than 2 is found before and after CRH and/or desmopressin administration. The central to peripheral ratio that has the highest diagnostic sensitivity for Cushing's disease has been found to occur at 5 minutes post-stimulation. Serial sampling is important, owing to the pituitary gland's transient secretion of ACTH pre- and post-stimulation.

Corticotropin releasing hormone

Ovine and human CRH stimulation have been used, with no clear superiority of one over the other.

Desmopressin

A significant subgroup (4–15%) of patients with Cushing's disease fail to demonstrate diagnostic gradients during bilateral inferior petrosal sinus sampling after CRH stimulation. In an effort to improve the diagnostic sensitivity of stimulation testing, CRH and desmopressin may be used alone or sequentially. Desmopressin is a long-acting vasopressin analog with a high affinity for the V2 vasopressin receptor, but a relatively low affinity for the V3 receptor that predominates in the normal pituitary gland. It increases ACTH secretion in 80–90% of patients with Cushing's disease, but only rarely in normal individuals or patients with pseudo-Cushing's syndrome. Some ectopic ACTH-secreting tumors (20–50%) may respond to desmopressin, limiting its usefulness in distinguishing the source of ACTH. The doses studied previously are of 10 mg, at which dose the ACTH response is most exaggerated[33]. Handling of the sample is done in a similar way as with CRH. Offering a similar sensitivity and specificity to CRH, it has been also suggested an increase in sensitivity when they are used in combination[34].

False positive results

Table 9.7 False positive etiologies

Asymmetric pituitary venous drainage

Pseudo-Cushing's syndrome

Pituitary corticotroph hyperplasia secondary to ectopic neuroendocrine CRH secretion

Cyclic Cushing's syndrome (cyclic secretion of ACTH) during eucortisolemic phase

Cortisol blocking drugs: ketoconazole, metyrapone, mitotane, and aminoglutethamide

Adrenal Cushing's syndrome (intermittent cortisol producing adrenal tumors)

Bilateral adrenalectomy

Intermittent ectopic ACTH-secreting adenoma

Normal individuals with high pulsatile pituitary ACTH secretion

Extrasellar location of ACTH microadenoma

ACTH: adrenocorticotropin hormone; CRH: corticotropin releasing hormone

False negative results

Table 9.8 False negative etiologies

Asymmetric/aberrant pituitary venous drainage

Inability to pass the catheter into position owing to jugular occlusion

Anatomical abnormalities: inability to sample bilateral inferior petrosal sinuses

Anomalous venous drainage: hypoplastic inferior petrosal sinus

Lack of inferior petrosal sinus drainage of pituitary

Human error: lack of experience

Human error: wrong positioning of catheter tip, wrong venous sample obtained

Table 9.8 (*cont.*)

Human error: inadequate CRH and/or desmopressin stimulation dosage administered

Pituitary adenoma minimally responsive to CRH and/or desmopressin stimulation

Unilateral central venous sampling

History of previous pituitary surgery leading to altered venous drainage pattern

Pituitary corticotroph adenoma originating ectopically in the sphenoid sinus

Cyclical ACTH-producing pituitary adenomas (off phase)

Poor handling of the ACTH assay

Poor sample processing technique (failure to chill samples appropriately)

ACTH: adrenocorticotropin hormone; CRH: corticotropin releasing hormone

Table 9.9 Pseudo-Cushing's syndrome etiologies

Adrenal disorders that autonomously secrete glucocorticoids

Alcoholism

Anorexia nervosa

Depression

Generalized resistance to glucocorticoids

Iatrogenic or exogenous hypercortisolism

Pregnancy

Hypercortisolism can be seen with these conditions. Iatrogenic or exogenous hypercortisolism must be excluded in order for a true endogenous Cushing's syndrome to be diagnosed.

Technical points to increase the accuracy of the technique
Preprocedure assessment

For the bilateral inferior petrosal sinus sampling procedure, the patient must be confirmed to be hypercortisolemic by measuring a 24 hour urine sample for free cortisol concluding on the morning of the sampling procedure, or taking a late-night salivary cortisol measurement the night before the procedure. The patient should not be taking any medication that may block cortisol production at the time of the procedure or have had an adrenalectomy. Iatrogenic or exogenous hypercortisolism and pseudo-Cushing's syndrome must be excluded in order for a true endogenous Cushing's syndrome to be diagnosed. (Table 9.9)

Stimulation and sampling technique

Simultaneous blood samples can be obtained from each of the three ports: left inferior petrosal sinus, right inferior petrosal sinus, and peripheral vein via the femoral vein sheath. Typically, two sets of simultaneous baseline samples are drawn and then three sets of stimulated (CRH and/or desmopressin) samples are drawn. Subsequently, stimulation is

Table 9.10 Summary of bilateral inferior petrosal sinus procedure

Conscious sedation

Sterile preparation of bilateral femoral veins at the groin with insertion of venous sheaths

Heparin infusion

Fluoroscopically guided placement of catheters into the bilateral inferior petrosal sinuses

Venography to determine symmetrical or asymmetrical venous flow

Contrast-enhanced fluoroscopy to confirm reflux into ipsilateral cavernous sinus

Baseline blood samples

CRH and/or desmopressin stimulation

Post-stimulation blood samples

Catheter removal and groin pressure until venous hemostasis

CRH: corticotropin releasing hormone

achieved with a peripheral, slow (over 1 minute) intravenous bolus of CRH at a dose of 1 μg/kg (maximum 100 μg) and/or desmopressin (10 μg/kg).

The general schedule of sampling following stimulation is usually on the following time schedule: -5 minutes (pre-stimulation), -1 minute (pre-stimulation), +3–5 minutes (post-stimulation), +8–10 minutes (post-stimulation) and +13–15 minutes (post-stimulation). A sample collection takes approximately 20–40 seconds. A variety of sample volumes ranging from 3 ml to 10 ml have been recommended by investigators for measurement of ACTH.

Sample handling and hormone assay technique

Prior to sampling, an appropriate number of labeled lavender-top tubes, with ethylenediaminetetra-acetic acid, should have been placed in an ice water bath. Mislabeling of the samples is a common cause of misinterpretation. After successfully drawing each sample into a syringe, it is then transferred to the appropriately labeled and numbered lavender-top tube using a 16 gauge needle.

These samples can either be processed by the investigators or the hospital's laboratory. All samples should be centrifuged within 1 hour of collection in a refrigerated centrifuge for 10 minutes at 1500g and 4–5°C.

The plasma is decanted into polypropylene tubes and placed on dry ice in an insulated container. These specimens are then sent for ACTH assay at 1:1, 1:10, and 1:100 dilutions.

Intraprocedural heparin

To prevent sinus thrombosis related to catheterization, heparin should be infused before catheters are advanced. Routine administration of 3000–4000 IU of heparin should be made as an intravenous bolus through the femoral vein sheath before the catheters are advanced into the internal jugular veins. In addition to the routine administration, we add heparin (2000 IU/l) to the flush solution and use this solution, via continuous drip, to irrigate both petrosal sinus catheters and the femoral vein sheath whenever they are not being manipulated. Pre- and postprocedure assessment of the coagulation system, platelets, and hematocrit is recommended.

Complications associated with inferior petrosal sinus sampling

Bilateral inferior petrosal sinus sampling is generally a safe outpatient procedure with minimal morbidity and mortality. Miller and Doppman.[30] reported no deaths or serious complications in 335 procedures. Serious complications have, however, been reported: in a series of more than 500 patients, the risk of major neurological complications was 0.2%[35]. Complications can be classified as neurological and non-neurological. Rare reported neurological complications are pontocerebellar junction infarct[36], brainstem vascular damage (vessel perforation) with venous subarachnoid hemorrhage[37], and cranial nerve palsies[38]. Cerebrovascular accidents are thought to be venous in origin and have been attributed to placement of a catheter in small intracranial vessels, which occurs during bilateral inferior petrosal sinus sampling but is less likely during jugular venous sampling. Variant venous anatomy or specific catheter use may lead to neurological complications. The adverse sequelae may be reduced or averted if immediate measures are taken upon development of new neurological signs or symptoms. Headache is a common neurological manifestation that may be provoked secondary to the contrast injection or the insertion of the catheter into a small inferior petrosal sinus. Ipsilateral ear pain may also occur if the catheter is inserted into a small inferior petrosal sinus. The patient may also hear strange noises in the ear on the side of the catheter insertion. Intravenous narcotics can be used to help relieve the discomfort during the procedure. Reassurance about the transient nature of these symptoms is valuable for the patient.

The most common complication, however, is non-neurological: a groin hematoma, estimated to have a frequency of around 3–4%[30]. One of the reasons may be that Cushing's syndrome patients are quite prone to developing ecchymoses, even with peripheral venipuncture. Interestingly, one of the most serious non-neurological complications is deep venous thrombosis, with or without pulmonary thromboembolism, which has been reported in different series[39,40]. It is believed that Cushing's disease patients are hypercoagulable, hence the importance of good heparinization during the test.

References

1. Baxendale S. The Wada test. *Current Opinions in Neurology* 2009;22:185–9.

2. Wada J. An experimental study on the neural mechanism of the spread of epileptic impulse. *Folia Psychiatrica Neurologica Japonica* 1951;4:289–301.

3. Kemp S, Wilkinson K, Caswell H, Reynders H, Baker G. The base rate of Wada test failure. *Epilepsy and Behavior* 2008;13:630–3.

4. Brassel F, Weissenborn K, Ruckert N, Hussein S, Becker H. Superselective intra-arterial amytal (Wada test) in temporal lobe epilepsy: basics for neuroradiological investigations. *Neuroradiology* 1996;38:417–21.

5. Vulliemoz S, Pegna AJ, Annoni JM, *et al.* The selective amobarbital test in the anterior choroidal artery: perfusion pattern assessed by intraarterial SPECT and prediction of postoperative verbal memory. *Epilepsy and Behavior* 2008;12:445–55.

6. Fitzsimmons BF, Marshall RS, Pile-Spellman J, Lazar RM. Neurobehavioral differences in superselective Wada testing with amobarbital versus lidocaine. *AJNR American Journal of Neuroradiology* 2003;24:1456–60.

7. Niimi Y, Berenstein A, Setton A, Pryor J. Symptoms, vascular anatomy and

endovascular treatment of spinal cord arteriovenous malformations. *Interventional Neuroradiology: Journal of Peritherapeutic Neuroradiology, Surgical Procedures and Related Neurosciences* 2000;6 Suppl 1:199–202.

8. Niimi Y, Sala F, Deletis V, Berenstein A. Provocative testing for embolization of spinal cord AVMs. *Interventional Neuroradiology: Journal of Peritherapeutic Neuroradiology, Surgical Procedures and Related Neurosciences* 2000;6 Suppl 1:191–4.

9. Niimi Y, Sala F, Deletis V, *et al.* Neurophysiologic monitoring and pharmacologic provocative testing for embolization of spinal cord arteriovenous malformations. *AJNR American Journal of Neuroradiology* 2004;25:1131–8.

10. Deveikis JP. Sequential injections of amobarbital sodium and lidocaine for provocative neurologic testing in the external carotid circulation. *AJNR American Journal of Neuroradiology* 1996;17:1143–7.

11. Loddenkemper T, Morris HH, Moddel G. Complications during the Wada test. *Epilepsy and Behavior* 2008;13:551–3.

12. Loddenkemper T, Morris HH 3rd, Perl J 2nd. Carotid artery dissection after the intracarotid amobarbital test. *Neurology* 2002;59:1797–8.

13. Loddenkemper T, Moddel G, Schuele SU, Wyllie E, Morris HH 3rd. Seizures during intracarotid methohexital and amobarbital testing. *Epilepsy and Behavior* 2007;10:49–54.

14. McIvor NP, Willinsky RA, TerBrugge KG, Rutka JA, Freeman JL. Validity of test occlusion studies prior to internal carotid artery sacrifice. *Head and Neck* 1994;16:11–16.

15. Linskey ME, Jungreis CA, Yonas H, *et al.* Stroke risk after abrupt internal carotid artery sacrifice: accuracy of preoperative assessment with balloon test occlusion and stable xenon-enhanced CT. *AJNR American Journal of Neuroradiology* 1994;15:829–43.

16. Whisenant JT, Kadkhodayan Y, Cross DT 3rd, Moran CJ, Derdeyn CP. Incidence and mechanisms of stroke after permanent carotid artery occlusion following temporary occlusion testing. *Journal of Neurointerventional Surgery* 2014;7:395–401.

17. Witt JP, Yonas H, Jungreis C. Cerebral blood flow response pattern during balloon test occlusion of the internal carotid artery. *AJNR American Journal of Neuroradiology* 1994;15:847–56.

18. Standard SC, Ahuja A, Guterman LR, *et al.* Balloon test occlusion of the internal carotid artery with hypotensive challenge. *AJNR American Journal of Neuroradiology* 1995;16:1453–8.

19. Devagupthapu SR, Khatri R, Qureshi AI. Balloon test occlusion with hypotensive challenge using a novel agent Fenoldopam: a first experience. *Journal of Neurosurgery and Anesthesiology* 2011;23:270–1.

20. Sorteberg A, Bakke SJ, Boysen M, Sorteberg W. Angiographic balloon test occlusion and therapeutic sacrifice of major arteries to the brain. *Neurosurgery* 2008;63:651–60; dicussion 60–1.

21. Abud DG, Spelle L, Piotin M, *et al.* Venous phase timing during balloon test occlusion as a criterion for permanent internal carotid artery sacrifice. *AJNR American Journal of Neuroradiology* 2005;26:2602–9.

22. van Rooij WJ, Sluzewski M, Slob MJ, Rinkel GJ. Predictive value of angiographic testing for tolerance to therapeutic occlusion of the carotid artery. *AJNR American Journal of Neuroradiology* 2005;26:175–8.

23. Zoarski GH, Seth R. Safety of unilateral endovascular occlusion of the cervical segment of the vertebral artery without antecedent balloon test occlusion. *AJNR American Journal of Neuroradiology* 2014;35:856–61.

24. Tarr RW, Jungreis CA, Horton JA, *et al.* Complications of preoperative balloon test occlusion of the internal carotid arteries: experience in 300 cases. *Skull Base Surgery* 1991;1:240–4.

25. Mathis JM, Barr JD, Jungreis CA, *et al.* Temporary balloon test occlusion of the internal carotid artery: experience in 500 cases. *AJNR American Journal of Neuroradiology* 1995;16:749–54.

26. Deipolyi AR, Hirsch JA, Oklu R. Bilateral inferior petrosal sinus sampling. *Journal of Neurointerventional Surgery* 2012;4:215–8.

27. Utz A, Biller BM. The role of bilateral inferior petrosal sinus sampling in the diagnosis of Cushing's syndrome. *Arquivos brasileiros de endocrinologia e metabologia* 2007;51:1329–38.

28. Testa RM, Albiger N, Occhi G, *et al.* The usefulness of combined biochemical tests in the diagnosis of Cushing's disease with negative pituitary magnetic resonance imaging. *European Journal of Endocrinology* 2007;156:241–8.

29. Findling J. Differential diagnosis of Cushing's syndrome. *Endocrinologist* 1996;7:17S–23S.

30. Miller DL, Doppman JL. Petrosal sinus sampling: technique and rationale. *Radiology* 1991;178:37–47.

31. Doppman JL, Oldfield EH, Nieman LK. Bilateral sampling of the internal jugular vein to distinguish between mechanisms of adrenocorticotropic hormone-dependent Cushing syndrome. *Annals of Internal Medicine* 1998;128:33–6.

32. Ilias I, Chang R, Pacak K, *et al.* Jugular venous sampling: an alternative to petrosal sinus sampling for the diagnostic evaluation of adrenocorticotropic hormone-dependent Cushing's syndrome. *The Journal of Clinical Endocrinology and Metabolism* 2004;89:3795–800.

33. Scott LV, Medbak S, Dinan TG. ACTH and cortisol release following intravenous desmopressin: a dose-response study. *Clinical Endocrinology* 1999;51:653–8.

34. Tsagarakis S, Vassiliadi D, Kaskarelis IS, *et al.* The application of the combined corticotropin-releasing hormone plus desmopressin stimulation during petrosal sinus sampling is both sensitive and specific in differentiating patients with Cushing's disease from patients with the occult ectopic adrenocorticotropin syndrome. *The Journal of Clinical Endocrinology and Metabolism* 2007;92:2080–6.

35. Brismar G, Brismar J, Cronqvist S. Complications of orbital and skull base phlebography. *Acta Radiologica: Diagnosis* 1976;17:274–80.

36. Gandhi CD, Meyer SA, Patel AB, Johnson DM, Post KD. Neurologic complications of inferior petrosal sinus sampling. *AJNR American Journal of Neuroradiology* 2008;29:760–5.

37. Bonelli FS, Huston J 3rd, Meyer FB, Carpenter PC. Venous subarachnoid hemorrhage after inferior petrosal sinus sampling for adrenocorticotropic hormone. *AJNR American Journal of Neuroradiology* 1999;20:306–7.

38. Lefournier V, Martinie M, Vasdev A, *et al.* Accuracy of bilateral inferior petrosal or cavernous sinuses sampling in predicting the lateralization of Cushing's disease pituitary microadenoma: influence of catheter position and anatomy of venous drainage. *The Journal of Clinical Endocrinology and Metabolism* 2003;88:196–203.

39. Blevins LS Jr., Clark RV, Owens DS. Thromboembolic complications after inferior petrosal sinus sampling in patients with Cushing's syndrome. *Endocrine Practice: Official Journal of the American College of Endocrinology and the American Association of Clinical Endocrinologists* 1998;4:365–7.

40. Obuobie K, Davies JS, Ogunko A, Scanlon MF. Venous thrombo-embolism following inferior petrosal sinus sampling in Cushing's disease. *Journal of Endocrinological Investigation* 2000;23:542–4.

41. Shiu PC, Hanafee WN, Wilson GH, Rand RW. Cavernous sinus venography. *American Journal of Roentgenology, Radium Therapy, and Nuclear Medicine* 1968;104:57–62.

42. Qureshi AI *Textbook of Interventional Neurology*. New York: Cambridge University Press, 2011.

43. Landolt AM, Schubiger O, Maurer R, Girard J. The value of inferior petrosal sinus sampling in diagnosis and treatment of Cushing's disease. *Clinical Endocrinology (Oxf)*. 1994;40:485–92.

Chapter 10

Role of neurocritical care in prevention and treatment of acute respiratory, cardiovascular, and neurological complications in the angiographic suite

Tenbit Emiru, Jose I. Suarez, and Adnan I. Qureshi

Most complications of neuroendovascular procedures occur during or within a few hours of the procedure. The patients often have a history of prior cerebrovascular and cardiovascular diseases predisposing them to adverse events during the procedure. The adverse events can be categorized as respiratory, cardiovascular, or neurological in nature and may be related to the inciting event, the procedure, or medications administered during the procedure. Complications can be minimized with appropriate patient selection, adequate intensity of patient monitoring, thorough understanding of the pharmacology of the medications used, anticipation of commonly encountered adverse events, and timely response to such complications.

Preprocedure assessment of patients

It is important to review the patient's medical history including previous catheterization, complications with anesthesia, time since last meal, list of current medications and allergies, history of cigarette smoking, alcohol intake, and any history of illicit drug use prior to endovascular procedure. This information has implications for the choice of anesthetic agents, procedural technique and timing, and medications prescribed during and after the procedure. It is particularly important to ask about history of any cardiac diseases, problems with chest pain or palpitations, respiratory issues such as asthma, chronic obstructive pulmonary disease, cough or recent upper respiratory infection, history of acid reflux, diabetes mellitus, kidney disease, liver disease, coagulation abnormalities, and transmittable blood-borne infections. This allows an opportunity to understand and monitor the current health status of the patient, and respond to any adverse events.

Complete physical examination including respiratory, cardiovascular, and neurological systems should be performed and clearly documented so that any changes can be identified after the procedure. A complete set of laboratory values including basic metabolic panel, complete blood count, and coagulation markers are helpful. Recent echocardiograms, if available, need to be reviewed especially in the elderly and those with prior cardiac disease. Depending on the elective or emergent nature of the procedure, the patient's medical status can be optimized to minimize the risks of the procedure and improve outcome. For example, a patient

Complications of Neuroendovascular Procedures and Bailout Techniques, ed. Rakesh Khatri, Gustavo J. Rodriguez, Jean Raymond and Adnan I. Qureshi. Published by Cambridge University Press.
© Cambridge University Press 2016.

with severe coronary artery disease needs to be evaluated thoroughly and treated with beta-blockers; those who are at risk for bronchospasm require bronchodilators; those with coagulation abnormalities may require transfusions of blood products if necessary; and those who are at risk for aspiration will require gastric emptying by fasting or increasing gastric motility.

Monitoring during endovascular procedures

Clinical observation and, when possible, interaction with the patient is the mainstay of monitoring during endovascular procedures but is often augmented by the use of monitoring devices. The most frequently monitored parameters are vital signs including blood pressure (BP), heart rate (HR), respiratory rate (RR), oxygen saturation (SPO$_2$), and cardiac rhythm. In addition to these basic modalities monitored during most procedures, neuroendovascular procedures also require the following to be monitored: frequent levels of activated clotting time (ACT), blood glucose levels, neurological exam and findings, and, depending on the nature and the length of the procedure, intracranial pressures (ICP) may be monitored.

Blood pressure can be monitored using either invasive or non-invasive methods. With good patient selection, and correct cuff size and positioning, non-invasive BP monitoring using automated cuff measurement is adequate for short neurointerventional procedures. Scenarios such as active bleeding secondary to trauma in patients undergoing therapeutic embolization, hypotensive challenge, or pre-existing BP lability may require invasive BP monitoring via intra-arterial catheter. This is preferred, and should be placed prior to the start of the procedure.

Cardiac rhythm and rate are often monitored with electrocardiography (ECG). A limited number of electrodes are placed on the chest to record rate and rhythm of patients during the endovascular procedure.

A **pulse oximeter** is one of the most commonly used monitoring devices used in patient care, and is placed on the patient's fingers, toes, earlobe, or forehead. It non-invasively measures the oxygen saturation of blood in the capillary, that is, oxygen content of blood per gram of hemoglobin and oxygen supply to the tissues. It uses differential absorption of light by oxyhemoglobin and deoxyhemoglobin.

Other monitoring parameters such as temperature and blood glucose level are often instituted on a case by case basis. For example, temperature is often monitored if general anesthesia is used since both hypothermia and hyperthermia can be complications of anesthesia. On the other hand, intermittent monitoring of blood glucose levels is indicated especially for patients with diabetes mellitus, those with labile blood glucose levels, and those with liver failure.

Patients are frequently examined during endovascular procedures to assess their neurological functioning because thromboembolic phenomena can lead to new neurological deficits. The National Institute of Health Stroke Scale (NIHSS) is impractical to carry out during endovascular procedures owing to the relative immobility of the patient, limited visibility due to sterile drapes covering the patient, image intensifiers in proximity to the head, introducer sheath in the common femoral artery, and catheters in position within the neck and brain. A shorter scale termed the endovascular procedure-specific neurological examination scheme (NES) evaluates six aspects of neurological function (see Figure 10.1), including language tested by comprehension and expression aspects of speech; gaze deviation; visual field assessed in a neutral position and then by confrontational testing; cranial nerve testing limited to detecting asymmetry in eye closure and naso-labial fold elevation; and the upper and lower extremity function tested by three motor activities, all of which can be executed and assessed within the confines of the intraprocedural position (upper extremity: extension of the wrist, finger grip, and flexion of the elbow; lower extremity: straight flexion

Component	Task	Performance: Score	Image
Language	Ask patient to give full name, repeat a sentence, and follow 1 command, e.g., to open and close the eyes	No task: 2 1 or 2 tasks: 1 All tasks: 0	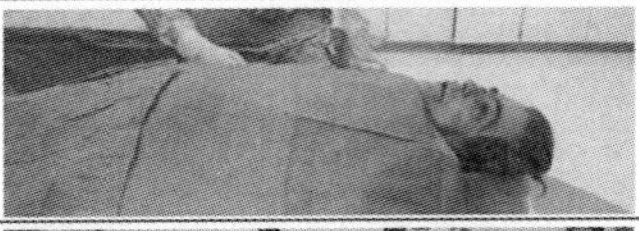
Gaze deviation	Ask patient to follow finger from one visual field (left) into the other visual field (right) and back	Gaze deviation or preference: 1 Voluntarily moves eyes in both directions without restriction/preference: 0	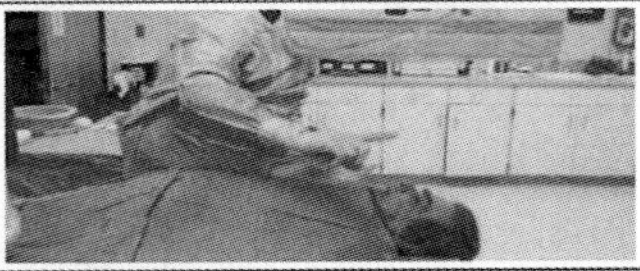
Visual fields	Ask patient to look at 1 or 2 fingers simultaneously in each visual field and to count the fingers and subsequently look toward the moving finger	No task: 1 Both tasks: 0	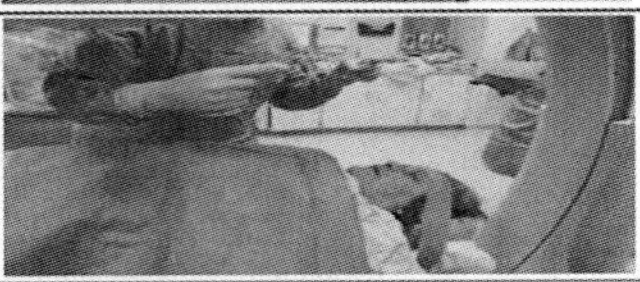
Cranial nerve	Ask patient to show teeth and close eyes in separate requests	No task: 1 Both tasks: 0	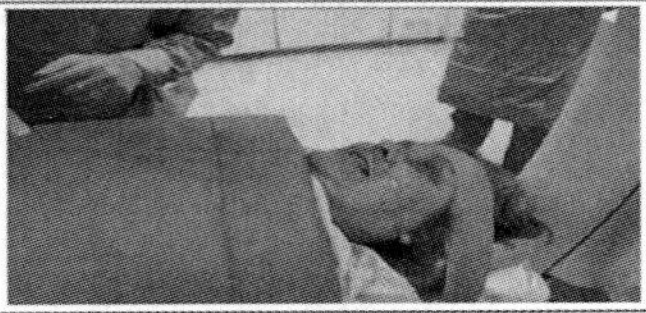

Begin with suspected normal extremity

Component	Task	Performance: Score	Image
Upper extremity (left)	Assess extension of wrist	Grade for each of 3 tasks: No movement: 2	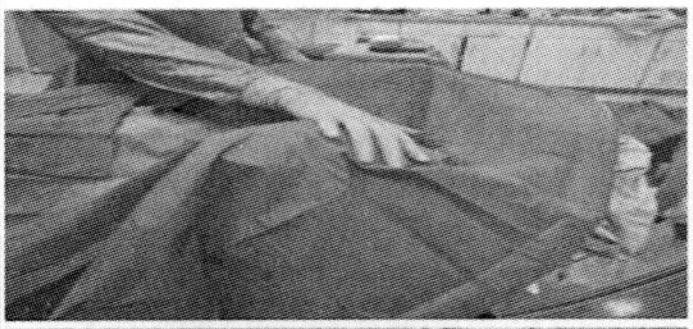 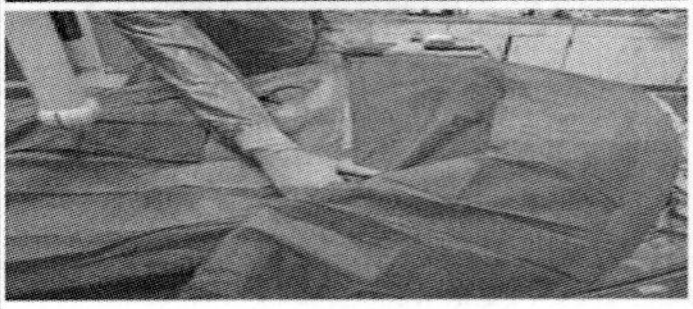
	Assess finger grip	Some effort against resistance but clear asymmetry between upper extremities (asymmetrical movement): 1	
	Assess flexion of elbow	Good effort against resistance without a clear asymmetry between upper extremities (symmetrical movements): 0	
Upper extremity (right)	Assess extension of wrist	Grade for each of 3 tasks: No movement: 2	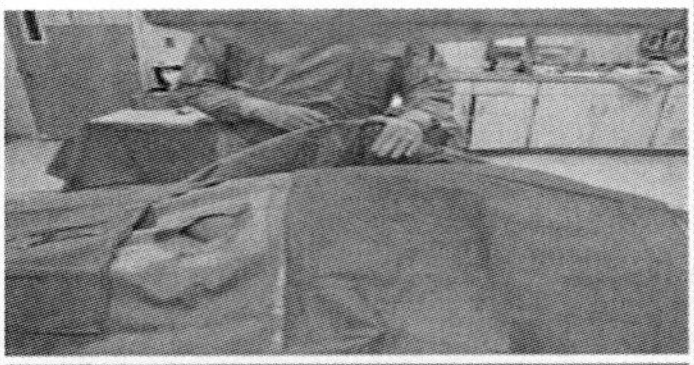 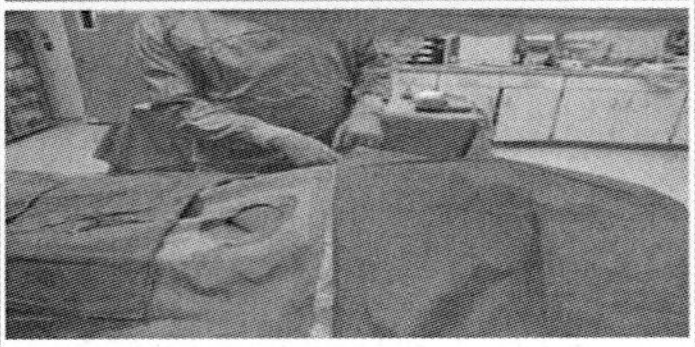
	Assess finger grip	Some effort against resistance but clear asymmetry between upper extremities (asymmetrical movement): 1	
	Assess flexion of elbow	Good effort against resistance without a clear asymmetry between upper extremities (symmetrical movements): 0	

Figure 10.1 The endovascular procedure-specific neurological examination scheme (NES). Reprinted with permission from ref. [1].

Begin with suspected normal extremity

Component	Task	Performance: Score	Image
Lower extremity (left)	Assess straight flexion at hip joint	Grade for each of 3 tasks: No movement: 2	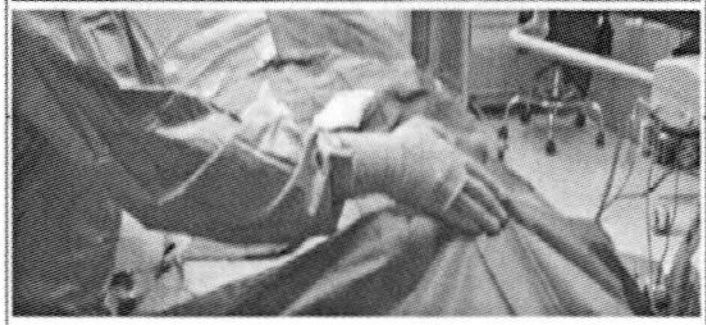 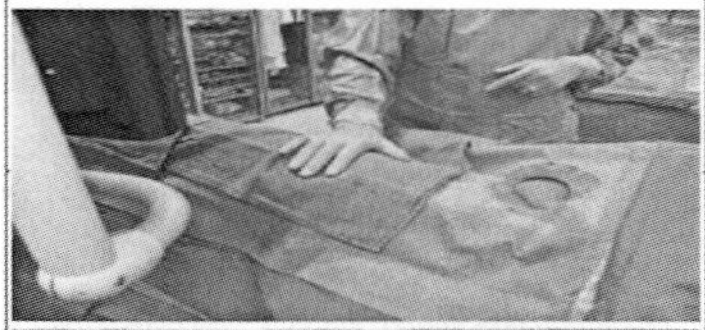
	Assess plantar flexion	Some effort against resistance but clear asymmetry between lower extremities (asymmetrical movement): 1	
	Assess plantar dorsiflexion	Good effort against resistance without a clear asymmetry between lower extremities (symmetrical movements): 0	
Lower extremity (right)	Assess straight flexion at hip joint	Grade for each of 3 tasks: No movement: 2	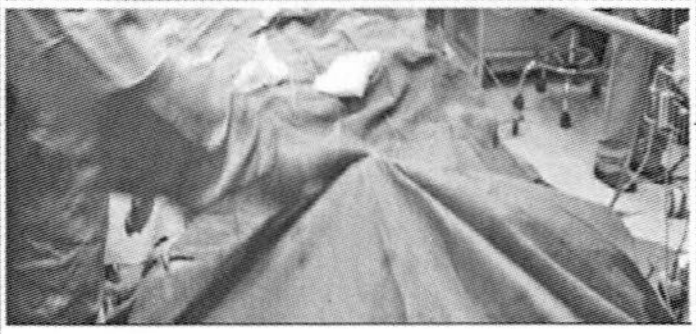 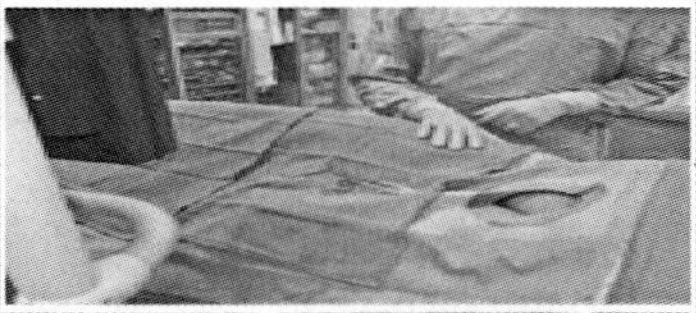
	Assess plantar flexion	Some effort against resistance but clear asymmetry between lower extremities (asymmetrical movement): 1	
	Assess plantar dorsiflexion	Good effort against resistance without a clear asymmetry between lower extremities (symmetrical movements): 0	

Figure 10.1 (cont.)

at the hip joint, plantar flexion, and dorsiflexion)[1]. There was a high level of agreement between the endovascular procedure-specific NES and the NIHSS assessment (the Spearman rank correlation coefficient was 0.96 ($p = 0.001$). The positive predictive value of the endovascular procedure-specific NES compared with the NIHSS score was 100%.

Respiratory complications

The most frequent reasons for hypoxemic or hypercarbic respiratory failure in the endovascular suite is central nervous system (CNS) depression of respiration secondary to medications or new intracranial event such as intracranial hemorrhage or ischemic event, upper airway collapse and obstruction from inability to protect airway, lower airway obstruction from prior respiratory problem, and ineffective air exchange from pneumonia, edema, or shunting. Respiratory complications are often first detected by reduction in SPO_2 by the pulse oximeter. The unique aspect of respiratory insufficiency is the low tolerance during endovascular procedures because of the patient's supine position and immobility, and need for additional sedation required to continue the procedure. Dyspnea and agitation pose additional limitations on successful continuation of the procedure. Awaiting response to diuresis, bronchodilators and frequent tracheal suctioning delays the procedure at a critical stage. Therefore, early intubation and mechanical ventilation should be considered in such scenarios.

Inadequate oxygenation: Hypoxemia results when the systemic oxygen demand is greater than the supply provided by pulmonary oxygen exchange. Such a balance is dependent on the adequacy of pulmonary gas exchange, amount of hemoglobin in blood, competence of the cardiovascular system, and demand of tissues for oxygen. If hypoxemia is detected (SPO_2 measurements <90% or a difference of more than 5% from baseline values), the following measure should be taken.

(1) Confirm the placement of the pulse oximeter probe and the tracings if available on the monitoring device. It may give inaccurate readings if not placed in opposition to the skin; if the patient is hypothermic; if there is poor peripheral circulation; or if there is significant motion artifact. The patient should be monitored closely as artifact is being excluded.

(2) Supplemental oxygen can be provided by using nasal cannula or non-rebreathing mask depending upon the severity of the hypoxemia, patient preference. and the amount of fraction of inspired oxygen (FiO_2) needed to improve oxygenation to an acceptable range. Nasal cannula can provide low flow rate (up to 5–6 l/min) of oxygen and FiO_2 of 40–50%, while different face masks can provide higher flow rates and FiO_2 up to 80% depending on the mask. Continued hypoxemia can lead to cardiac arrhythmias, hypotension, myocardial injury, and cardiac arrest.

Inadequate ventilation: Hypoventilation and apnea are indications for intubation and mechanical ventilation. An early response to patient's inadequate level of consciousness and any deterioration is mandatory. Arterial blood gas analysis demonstrating presence of low pH and high partial pressure of CO_2 ($PaCO_2$) also confirms the presence of inadequate ventilation. Depression of the CNS respiratory center by medications or because of intracranial pathology, failure to maintain airway patency resulting in airway obstruction, weakness or paralysis of respiratory muscles, and altered lung mechanics lead to failure to ventilate. Assessment of level of consciousness prior to the procedure helps in determining whether the patient will protect his or her airway and be able to tolerate the procedure without assisted ventilation. For example, a Glasgow Coma Scale (GCS) score of <8 has been used as a cutoff for intubation and mechanical ventilation. Although a cutoff system has not been developed for stroke, patients with very high NIHSS scores are often intubated prior to undergoing endovascular treatments. If large doses of sedatives are anticipated, if the patient is unable to follow simple commands, is agitated, or has severe dysarthria and dysphagia with inability to control oral secretions, respiratory compromise during the endovascular treatment should be anticipated.

Aspiration of gastric contents into the tracheobronchial system can occur during the procedure owing to altered level of consciousness because of sedation, oropharyngeal muscle weakness or paralysis, passive regurgitation secondary to gastro-esophageal reflex disease, anesthesia given to patients with full stomachs, large amount of air in the stomach secondary to difficult intubation or prolonged positive pressure mask ventilation, ineffective cricoid pressure during intubation, or active vomiting. The immediate signs of aspiration are oxygen desaturation, dyspnea, coughing, inability to control secretions, and visible gastric contents in the oral cavity. Aggressive but not prolonged deep suctioning should precede intubation. Temporary measures such as turning the head to the side and elevation of head may be required but interruption of ongoing neurological procedure is unavoidable. Placement of nasogastric tube and decompression of stomach may be necessary. High FiO_2 and positive end expiratory pressure (PEEP) may be required after intubation to maintain adequate oxygenation. Pneumonia, pneumonitis, sepsis, and infrequently acute respiratory distress syndrome (ARDS) are expected sequelae.

Failure of conscious sedation

Neuroendovascular procedures can be performed under local anesthesia in patients who are alert, have no language deficits, can follow direction, and are going to be discharged home after the procedure[2,3]. Conscious sedation keeps the patient immobile but comfortable, with adequate spontaneous ventilation, minimal supplemental oxygen and hemodynamic changes, and with a possibility of rapid return to consciousness when needed for neurological assessment. Table 10.1 lists dose, onset, peak, and duration of most commonly used narcotics, sedatives, and anesthetics, and their effect on cerebral metabolic rate, cerebral blood flow, and ICP[3,4]. Conversion to general endotracheal anesthesia is infrequently necessary in a small proportion of patients. Use of general endotracheal anesthesia reduces motion artifacts and improves the quality of images especially in children or uncooperative adults, and for complex procedures that are of long duration such as embolization of arteriovenous malformations (AVM), embolization of aneurysms, and imaging and treatment of spinal vascular pathology. However, preprocedural intubation has been associated with increasing rate of poor outcomes in endovascularly treated stroke patients[5-8]. Hassan et al. looked at the rate of poor outcome in 136 acute ischemic stroke patients who received endovascular treatment (83 of whom received local sedation without intubation and 53 of whom were intubated) and found that after adjusting for age, gender, and NIHSS score, poor outcome at discharge (defined as modified Rankin Score (mRS) score ≥3) and in-hospital mortality were significantly higher among intubated patients[5]. In addition, after adjusting for pneumonia, the effect of intubation on poor outcome at discharge and in-hospital mortality remained significant, leading to the conclusion that this increased rate is not explained by higher rates of subsequent aspiration pneumonia[5]. Therefore, there is increasing interest in performing endovascular procedures under awake condition and thus avoiding intubation and mechanical ventilation. Another study by Hassan et al. reported that from a total of 520 endovascular procedures initiated with the intent to perform under conscious sedation, 9 (1.7%) procedures required emergent conversion to general anesthesia; however, favorable clinical outcome or in-hospital mortality in patients requiring emergent conversion from conscious sedation to general anesthesia and those initiated with general anesthesia was not statistically different[9]. Therefore, practitioners must be aware of the risk of failure of conscious sedation in patients undergoing endovascular procedures and be prepared to respond accordingly. Table 10.2 shows the steps necessary for conversion to general anesthesia during the procedure.

Cardiovascular complications

Hypertension

Pre-existing hypertension (HTN) is common in patients with cerebrovascular disease. Common causes of HTN during endovascular procedures are pre-existing HTN, acute hypertensive response associated with stroke, hypoxemia or hypercarbia, increased ICP,

Table 10.1 Commonly used narcotics, sedatives and anesthetics and their effect on cerebral metabolic rate, cerebral blood flow, and intracranial pressure

Drug class	Dose	Onset	Duration	Effect on CMR, CBF, and ICP
Benzodiazepines				Mild decrease in all
Midazolam	1–5 mg	2–4 min	1–2 hours	
Lorazepam	2–4 mg	5–10 min	6–8 hours	
Diazepam	5–10 mg	3–6 min	4–8 hours	
Opioids				Mild decrease in all
Morphine	5–10 μg	3–10min	3–4 hours	
Hydromorphone	0.2–1 mg	15 min	4–5 hours	
Fentanyl	50–100 μg	2–4min	30–60 min	
Alfentanil	0.5–1.5 μg/kg	1–2min	10 min	
Remifentanil	0.5–1 μg/kg	1 min	3–10min	
Sufentanil	0.5–10 μg/kg	1–4 min	10 min–1 hour	
Others				
Ketamine	1–2 mg/ kg bolus 40 mg/kg/min infusion	1–2 min	5–10 min	Unchanged CMR, increased CBF and ICP
Propofol	1–3 mg/kg bolus 10–100 mg/hr infusion	2–5 min	10–20 min	Reduction in all
Dexmedetomidine	1 μg/kg/hr bolus 0.2–0.7 μg/kg/hr infusion	30 min	4 hours	Unknown
Antagonist				
Naloxone	0.1–0.4 mg	1–2 min	30 min–1 hour	
Flumazenil	0.1–0.5 mg	1–5 min	1–3 hours	

CMR=cerebral metabolic rate, CBF=cerebral blood flow, ICP=intracranial pressure, min=minutes, μg/kg/min=microgram per kilogram per minute

inadequate anesthesia, rebound HTN from withholding preprocedure antihypertensive mediations, and pain or discomfort associated with the procedure. First, the accuracy of BP recording needs to be verified. There are a number of different medications that can be given in boluses or as continuous infusions to treat HTN and to titrate BP into a desired range. Table 10.3 lists the dose, onset, peak, and duration of actions of the commonly used

Table 10.2 Special consideration for intubation during procedure

1. Discontinue procedure and remove intracranial catheters or guidewires within extracranial arteries that may injure arteries during head positioning and neck movements.

2. Secure femoral catheter.

3. Preserve sterile field.

4. Move cephalad part of angiographic table away from the image intensifiers to allow space for temporary ventilation via ambo-bag and subsequent intubation.

5. Remove head or neck collars placed for immobility during the procedure.

6. Anticipate post-intubation hypotension and have short-term vasopressor bolus infusions ready.

7. Assess the position of the endotracheal tube under immediately available fluoroscopy.

8. Intraventricular catheter can be placed after intubation and mechanical ventilation if necessary.

9. Do not delay administration of hypertonic saline or mannitol for intubation.

Table 10.3 Commonly used antihypertensive medications

Drug	Class	Dose	Onset	Duration
Labetolol	Strong beta-blocker; mild alpha-blocker	10–20 mg; q 10–20 min	2–5 min	2–6 hours
Nicardipine	Calcium channel blocker	5–30 mg/hr	5–15 min	4–6 hours
Enalaprilat	Angiotensin converting enzyme inhibitor	0.625–1.25 mg; q 6 hours	5–10 min	2–6 hours
Nitroprusside	Vasodilator	0.5–5 µg/kg/min	1 min	1–2 min
Nitroglycerin	Venodilator	5–400 µg/min	1–5 min	5–10 min
Hydralazine	Vasodilator	10–20 mg; q 10 min	5–10 min	2–6 hours

min=minutes, µg/kg/min=microgram/kilogram/minute

antihypertensive medications. If repeated bolus administration or infusion of such medications is anticipated, an arterial line placement for close monitoring and titration of BP is indicated. Cheung and Hobson recommend that systolic blood pressure be maintained below 140 mmHg in the first 48 hours after carotid endarterectomy or carotid stent placement for most patients, and below 120 mmHg for those patients at high risk for reperfusion syndrome, keeping in mind that there is an increased propensity for hypotension and bradycardia in the postprocedure period[10]. There are no guidelines on the recommended range of BP after intracranial angioplasty and stenting; however, generally BP is kept in the range of 120–140 mmHg to prevent hyperperfusion injury.

Hypotension

Hypotension is a fall in systolic BP to a value less than 90 mmHg. It is usually seen because of high dose of intravenous (IV) sedation and hypnotics, baroreceptor stimulation during carotid angioplasty and stent placement, and retroperitoneal or access site hemorrhage. If hypotension is sudden and is encountered during the procedure, verify that the BP recording is accurate and obtain repeated measurements. IV fluid boluses and infusions of either crystalloids or colloids using a large bore or a central IV catheter should be initiated and given as fast as possible, using a pressure bag if available, to expand intravascular volume. IV vasopressor or inotropic agents should be used early because volume depletion alone is less likely to be the cause of hypotension, since continuous infusion of fluids is often a part of endovascular procedures. Table 10.4 lists the most commonly used vasopressors and inotropic agents. In the event of protracted hypotension, IV vasopressors such as dopamine (2–20 micrograms/kg/min particularly in patients with bradycardia) or norepinephrine (5–20 micrograms/min) may be initiated and titrated to response during the procedure. If femoral access site hemorrhage is suspected, a careful evaluation of the site is warranted. If bleeding is continued, sufficient pressure, injection of vasoconstricting agent, reversal of anticoagulation and closure of site may be necessary. If access site is secured and further hemorrhage is suspected, imaging with computed tomography (CT) may be required to rule out retroperitoneal hematoma. If retroperitoneal hemorrhage is identified, peripheral vascular surgery consultation may be required to surgically secure the site of bleeding in the femoral or iliac artery. Hemoglobin and hematocrit levels as well as type and cross should be obtained, as blood transfusion may be necessary.

Arrhythmias

Bradycardia is commonly seen post-carotid artery angioplasty and stent placement, owing to mechanical compression and manipulation of baroreceptors leading to impaired baroreflex mechanism. Baroreceptors are stretch receptors located at the carotid bifurcation; they detect the pressure change and adjust sympathetic and parasympathetic activity through vagal modulation of the heart rate. During carotid angioplasty and stent placement, the atherosclerotic plaque is compressed into the vessel wall, stimulating the baroreflex mechanism and leading to increased parasympathetic output, thus leading to decreased HR and BP. This phenomenon has been recognized to subside in a few days[11]. If there is

Table 10.4 Commonly used vasopressors and inotropic agents

Drug	Main action	Dose
Norepinephrine	Strong alpha-agonist, mild beta-agonist	1–2 µg/min bolus; 5–20 µg/min infusion
Phenylephrine	Pure alpha-agonist	0.1–0.5 mg bolus; 2 µg/kg/min infusion
Vasopressin	Alpha-agonist*	0.01–0.04 U/min; no titration
Ephedrine	Alpha-agonist	10–50 mg
Dopamine	Alpha- and beta-agonist	2–20 µg/kg/min
Dobutamine	Beta-agonist	2–15 µg/kg/min

*Also causes contraction of the smooth muscle of the gastrointestinal tract and is antidiuretic.

protracted hypotension or clinical symptoms, bradycardia should be treated. Common medications used to treat significant bradycardia are atropine 0.4–0.8 mg IV and glyco-pyrrolate 0.2–0.4 mg IV. If bradycardia is persistent and refractory to medications, trans-cutaneous pacing should be initiated. Myocardial ischemia or infarction can occur in patients with pre-existing coronary artery disease, peripheral vascular disease, or unstable angina, owing to tachycardia introduced by baroreceptor manipulation and/or hypoten-sion. Increased myocardial oxygen demand or decreased oxygen delivery may lead to ST changes due to myocardial ischemia or infarction visible on the continuous electrocardi-ography monitor. An awake patient may complain of chest pain, dyspnea, or shortness of breath. If the BP is stable, it is reasonable to reduce the heart rate using IV beta-blockers or calcium channel blockers. In most instances, the ST elevation or depression may resolve with reduction in heart rate and subsequent reduction in myocardial oxygen consumption. Severe hypotension and cardiac arrest are medical emergencies that require interruption of endovascular procedures and following advanced cardiac life support (ACLS) and hospital guidelines for further triage and treatment of the patient.

Neurological complications

Neurological complications are the most anticipated complications during neuroendovas-cular procedures. The three most common scenarios for neurocritical care in the endovas-cular suite are new neurological deficits, increase in ICP, and seizures.

New neurological deficits

New neurological deficits can result from cerebral ischemic events or new intracranial hemorrhage (described in the later section on ICP elevation). Careful attention to the patient's vital signs is important, in addition to possible new neurological deficits such as pupillary dilation, gaze abnormalities, hemiparesis or hemiplegia, and increased tone, which are indicators of transtentorial herniation from a rapidly expanding supratentorial lesion such as edema or hemorrhage, leading to increased ICP. Cerebral angiographic images of the arterial distribution associated with neurological deficits may identify an arterial occlusion which differentiates the ischemic nature of deficits from intracranial hemorrhage. A less specific finding may be delayed flow of contrast in affected arterial distribution. Such delay is secondary to multiple emboli that occlude the microvessels and cause ischemic deficits. In patients with high ICP, there may be global decrease in contrast flow within the hemisphere. In presence of very high ICP, the angiographic findings may mimic the flow arrest that can be seen in patients with brain death. Contrast extravasation on angiographic images may also support the diagnosis of new intracranial hemorrhage. In the presence of new neurological deficits, the patient's level of cooperativeness may change to an unacceptable level for continuation of endovascular procedure. Therefore, decisions regarding continuation of procedure and steps required to ensure patient safety may require careful evaluation.

Elevation in ICP

Increased ICP is an important cause of secondary brain injury, and its severity and duration is associated with patient outcome and should be treated emergently. A change in the neurological examination, sudden increase in BP, changes in HR and RR, and possibly agitation and restlessness can be the manifestation of sudden increase in ICP. In patients with an existing ICP monitor, the ICP values can provide a higher degree of information

Table 10.5 The "brain code" protocol

Suggested steps for reversing transtentorial herniation
- Follow general guidelines of resuscitation with airway, breathing, and circulation
- Hyperventilation (keeping the PaCO$_2$ between 25 and 30 mmHg)
- Elevation of the head of the bed and removing any restrictive objects around the neck
- Osmotic therapy consisting of either mannitol or hypertonic saline
  - Mannitol given in boluses of 0.5–1.5 gram/kg and
  - Hypertonic saline in the form of 23.4% sodium chloride given in boluses of 30 ml to keep the ICP to a normal range.
  - Hypertonic saline can also be continued in the form of 2% or 3% sodium chloride infusion to increase and maintain serum sodium between 140–155 mmol/l.
- Brain imaging
- Emergency ventricular CSF drainage

regarding severity and response to treatment. Brain tissue is essentially incompressible, so any increase in ICP due to brain swelling initially results in extrusion of cerebrospinal fluid (CSF) and (mainly venous) blood from the intracranial cavity. Once this compensatory capacity is exhausted, any further increases in intracranial volume may lead to a precipitous increase in ICP and displacement of brain tissue (herniation syndrome). The general guidelines of resuscitation with airway, breathing, and circulation are addressed first. If there is significant alteration of consciousness, endotracheal intubation and mechanical ventilator support are required. Arterial carbon dioxide (CO$_2$) reactivity is a vigorous mechanism that alters vascular tone thus ICP. Therefore, hyperventilation (keeping the PaCO$_2$ between 25–30 mmHg) may reduce ICP on a short-term basis. Elevation of the head of the bed and removing any restrictive objects around the neck to facilitate venous drainage are simple measures to decrease ICP. Osmotic therapy consisting of either mannitol or hypertonic saline has been used to increase serum osmolarity and increase osmotic gradient from the interstitial tissue to intravascular compartment therefore reducing brain water content. Mannitol is given in boluses of 0.5–1.5 gram/kg and hypertonic saline in the form of 23.4% sodium chloride given in boluses of 30 ml to keep the ICP to a normal range. Hypertonic saline can also be continued in the form of 2% or 3% sodium chloride infusion to increase and maintain serum sodium between 140 and 155 mmol/l. Any patient with a change in neurological examination should then undergo brain imaging. Emergency ventricular CSF drainage may be necessary. While there are no standardized protocols for management of patients with increased ICPs and mortality after transtentorial herniation is high, some have recommended adaptation of "brain code", a timely medical intervention for reversing transtentorial herniation that can result in a potential preservation of neurologic function[12]. The "brain code" protocol is presented in Table 10.5. In the neuroendovascular suite, the most common reason for elevation in ICP is intracranial hemorrhage either due to rupture of intracranial aneurysm or AVM or primary artery rupture. Emergent identification and correction of medication induced coagulopathy is crucial and described in later sections.

Brain death

At times the neurointerventionalist is called to perform an ancillary test to confirm brain death. The diagnosis of brain death is mainly clinical and entails the absence of cerebral or brainstem function and an apnea not explained otherwise that is irreversible. Occasionally, through various circumstances, there is a need to perform an ancillary test: one of the ancillary tests is cerebral angiography[13]. A selective four-vessel cerebral angiography or an aortic arch run using a pigtail at high pressure focused on the head will demonstrate the absence of filling of the carotid and vertebral arteries above the dura mater with presence of filling of the external carotid branches. Opacification of the superior longitudinal sinus can be seen, owing to filling by meningeal or emissary veins[14]. False-negative cerebral angiograms where some intracranial blood vessels are visualized have been reported in cases where ICP is lowered by surgery, trauma, and ventricular shunts, or in infants with pliable skulls. Rarely, angiography may demonstrate contrast stasis or delayed filling in intracranial arteries, perhaps as an evolutionary stage preceding absent filling. In a more recent approach in the angiographic interpretation, it appears that the absence of a capillary phase or a venous phase would be more reliable (Figure 10.2)[15,16].

Seizures

Seizures during neuroendovascular procedure are rare but could occur in patients with large ischemic stroke, subarachnoid hemorrhages, and intra-procedural hemorrhages. In a large prospective hospital-based stroke registry in Germany of 58,874 patients with transient ischemic attacks (TIA), acute ischemic strokes, or intracerebral hemorrhages, acute post-stroke seizures were more frequent in younger patients, those with a higher stroke severity, acute non-neurologic infection, or a history of diabetes mellitus or preceding TIA[17]. Practitioners must be aware of the higher risk in such patients who are undergoing endovascular procedures. Patients who have a prior history or who had a seizure prior to arrival in the endovascular suite are at higher risk for developing more seizures. If a patient has a seizure during the endovascular procedure, the operator must ensure that catheters and microwires are removed from the intracranial arteries to avoid inadvertent displacement and arterial injury. The access site may also be vulnerable to compromise owing to movement of lower extremities. Benzodiazepines are the first line of treatment for seizure because of their fast onset of action and ease of availability. Lorazepam in 2 mg doses up to 8 mg is generally recommended. Emergent intubation and mechanical ventilation may be necessary if seizure activity continues, if the patient fails to return to the baseline neurological status, if the patient's neurological status can no longer be reliably assessed, and/or if the patient's respiratory status is compromised. Sedation with infusion of short-acting benzodiazepine such as midazolam or other anesthetic agents can prevent further seizure activity. In addition, IV bolus of anti-epileptic drug such as phenytoin, levetiracetam, or valproic acid is instituted. Complete laboratory studies including electrolyte levels should be investigated. Further brain imaging should be considered to rule out new lesions such as hemorrhages associated with the procedure or hemorrhagic transformation of ischemic stroke. All patients should also undergo EEG to look for continuous subclinical seizure activity in the event of lack of adequate response to initial doses of benzodiazepines.

Complications related to coagulopathy

Intra-arterial thrombosis is a major concern during endovascular procedures and may lead to ischemic events. Patients are typically treated for a variable number of days before the procedure with a single or a combination of antiplatelet agents in varying doses. In addition, unfractionated heparin is administered by intermittent boluses or continuous infusion

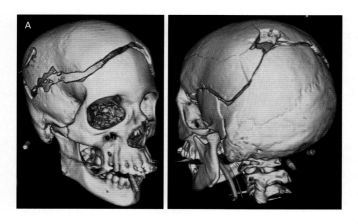

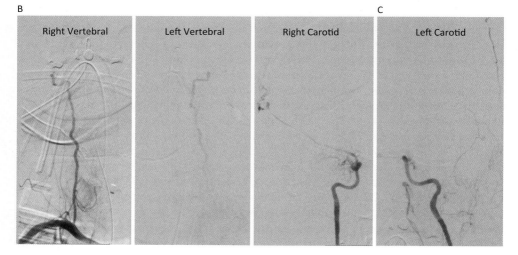

Figure 10.2 A 50-year-old female who suffered a gunshot wound to the head (A). She did not have brainstem reflexes. Apnea test could not be performed owing to the hemodynamic instability. The patient was brought to the angiography suite for diagnostic cerebral angiography as a confirmatory test. Four-vessel cerebral angiography (B) demonstrated absent intracranial flow except in the injection of right internal carotid artery where flow was noted in middle cerebral artery with fistulous connection and flow in extracranial space. There is no capillary or venous filling noted, suggesting absent cerebral perfusion. (C) Four-vessel cerebral angiography demonstrated absent intracranial flow except in the injection of right internal carotid artery where flow is noted in the middle cerebral artery with fistulous connection and flow in extracranial space. There is no capillary or venous filling noted, suggesting absent cerebral perfusion.

throughout the procedure. Some patients also receive continuous platelet glycoprotein IIb/IIIa inhibitors which may add to the anticoagulant activity of heparin. Anticoagulation is monitored by measuring ACT during the procedure with target ranges between 200 to 350 seconds depending upon the operator and the nature of the procedure. Anticoagulation is mostly discontinued after the procedure although infrequently it may be continued for up to 24 hours after the procedure. Heparin is not reversed and ACT elevation is allowed to resolve spontaneously[18]. In cases of hemorrhagic complications (access site complications or intracranial hemorrhage) during or after endovascular procedures, operators must be aware of the intraprocedural use of heparin and potentially the need to reverse anticoagulation activity induced by heparin using protamine sulfate (1 mg per 100 U of heparin).

Rare complications

Anaphylactic reaction: Most medications including hypnotics, opioids, local anesthetics, antiplatelet agents, heparin, iodinated contrast media (ICM), antiseptics, disinfectants, latex, and colloids that are used during endovascular procedures can cause an allergic reaction. Allergic reactions range from mild itching, hives, and rash to swelling, cardiovascular collapse or airway obstruction. Anaphylaxis is a clinical diagnosis. Epinephrine is the first and most important drug that must be administered emergently in 0.1–0.5 mg (1:1000 concentration) every 15 minutes as needed. If signs and symptoms of respiratory compromise are detected, anesthesiology team must be notified for possible difficult intubation owing to the possibility of airway and oropharyngeal edema. Inhaled beta-2 agonist should be given for bronchodilation in the event of bronchospasm. Histamine antagonists such as diphenylhydramine (25–50 mg every 2–4 hours as needed for a maximum dose of 100 mg in 4 hours) are valuable in mild anaphylactic reactions manifesting in itching, hives, and rash. IV glucocorticosteroids (variable doses) are often given for prolonged courses of anaphylaxis to reduce anti-inflammatory reaction and reduce airway edema. Aggressive replacement of volume with crystalloids and vasopressor infusions are crucial in severe anaphylactic shock. Patients suffering from anaphylactic shock should be observed in an intensive care unit. The cause of the reaction has to be investigated, and the patient should be evaluated by an allergist and immunologist.

References

1. Qureshi, A.I., An endovascular procedure-specific neurological examination scheme for intraprocedural monitoring in awake patients. *J Endovasc Ther*, 2011. 18(4): p. 531–7.

2. Hashimoto, T., Gupta, D.K., Young, W.L., Interventional neuroradiology –anesthetic considerations. *Anesthesiol Clin North America*, 2002. 20(2): p. 347–59, vi.

3. Young, W.L., Anesthesia for endovascular neurosurgery and interventional neuroradiology. *Anesthesiol Clin*, 2007. 25(3): p. 391–412, vii.

4. Jones, M., Leslie, K., Mitchell, P., Anaesthesia for endovascular treatment of cerebral aneurysms. *J Clin Neurosci*, 2004. 11(5): p. 468–70.

5. Hassan, A.E., Chaudhry, S.A., Zacharatos, H. *et al.*, Increased rate of aspiration pneumonia and poor discharge outcome among acute ischemic stroke patients following intubation for endovascular treatment. *Neurocrit Care*, 2012. 16(2): p. 246–50.

6. Jumaa, M.A., Zhang F., Ruiz-Ares, G., *et al.*, Comparison of safety and clinical and radiographic outcomes in endovascular acute stroke therapy for proximal middle cerebral artery occlusion with intubation and general anesthesia versus the nonintubated state. *Stroke*, 2010. 41(6): p. 1180–4.

7. Nichols, C., Carrozzella, J., Yeatts, S. *et al.*, Is periprocedural sedation during acute stroke therapy associated with poorer functional outcomes? *J Neurointerv Surg*, 2010. 2(1): p. 67–70.

8. Schumacher, H.C., Meyers, P.M., Higashida, R.T., *et al.*, Reporting standards for angioplasty and stent-assisted angioplasty for intracranial atherosclerosis. *J Vasc Interv Radiol*, 2009. 20(7 Suppl): p. S451–73.

9. de Bruijn, N.P., Hlatky, M.A., Jacobs, J.R., *et al.*, General anesthesia during percutaneous transluminary coronary

angioplasty for acute myocardial infarction: results of a randomized controlled clinical trial. *Anesth Analg*, 1989. 68(3): p. 201–7.

10. Cheung, A.T., Hobson, R.W. 2nd, Hypertension in vascular surgery: aortic dissection and carotid revascularization. *Ann Emerg Med*, 2008. 51(3 Suppl): p. S28–33.

11. Demirci, M., Saribaş, O., Uluç, K., *et al.*, Carotid artery stenting and endarterectomy have different effects on heart rate variability. *J Neurol Sci*, 2006. 241(1–2): p. 45–51.

12. Qureshi, A.I., Geocadin, R.G., Suarez, J.I., Ulatowski, J.A., Long-term outcome after medical reversal of transtentorial herniation in patients with supratentorial mass lesions. *Crit Care Med*, 2000. 28(5): p. 1556–64.

13. Combes, J.C., Chomel, A., Ricolfi, F., d'Athis, P., Freysz, M., Reliability of computed tomographic angiography in the diagnosis of brain death. *Transplant Proc*, 2007. 39(1): p. 16–20.

14. Wijdicks, E.F., Varelas, P.N., Gronseth, G.S., Greer, D.M. Evidence-based guideline update: determining brain death in adults: report of the Quality Standards Subcommittee of the American Academy of Neurology. *Neurology*, 2010. 74(23): p. 1911–8.

15. Savard, M., Turgeon, A.F., Gariépy, J.L., Trottier, F., Langevin, S., Selective 4 vessels angiography in brain death: a retrospective study. *Can J Neurol Sci*, 2010. 37(4): p. 492–7.

16. Ergun, O., Birgi, E., Tatar, I.G., Oztekin, M.F., Hekimoglu, B., Can arteriovenous malformation prevent the diagnosis of brain death? *Emerg Radiol*, 2015. 22(2): p. 199–201.

17. Krakow, K., Sitzer, M., Rosenow, F., *et al.*, Predictors of acute poststroke seizures. *Cerebrovasc Dis*, 2010. 30(6): p. 584–9.

18. Schumacher, H.C., Meyers, P.M., Higashida, R.T., *et al.*, Reporting standards for angioplasty and stent-assisted angioplasty for intracranial atherosclerosis. *Stroke*, 2009. 40(5): p. e348–65.

Periprocedural planning for neuroendovascular procedures

Alluru S. Reddi, Wondwossen G. Tekle, and Neil Kothari

Introduction

A significant proportion of periprocedural complications related to endovascular procedures can be mitigated with appropriate preprocedural planning and preparations. Meticulous patient selection through thorough knowledge of each patient's medical history, including medication use, allergies, and metabolic profile, is of paramount importance prior to bringing them into the neuroangiography suite. In this chapter, we focus on practical "screening tools" that could be used by the neurointerventionalist as a preprocedural checklist. We have covered cardiovascular and pulmonary diseases in Chapter 10. We will focus on pertinent points in this chapter that were not covered in Chapter 10 including allergy to contrast and heparin, peripheral vascular disease, and detailed discussion about contrast-induced nephropathy.

Allergy
Contrast medium allergy

- Both acute and delayed contrast-medium-related adverse reactions are known to occur after exposure to intravenous (IV) contrast medium.
- Methods to avoid contrast allergy:
  i.   Pretreatment with steroids and antihistamine as given below in Table 11.1. (Adapted from *American College of Radiology Manual* 2013; http://aegysgroup.com)
  ii. Oral administration of steroids is preferable to IV administration, and prednisone and methylprednisolone are equally effective. It is preferred that steroids be given beginning at least 6 hours prior to the injection of contrast media, regardless of the route of steroid administration, whenever possible.
  iii. Severity of contrast allergy can be dose-dependent – use the minimum amount needed to complete procedure[1].
  iv. Use of non-ionic contrast is associated with lower risk of allergy/intolerance.

- The most serious acute contrast allergy is anaphylactic reaction. Call the emergency response team while taking steps to stabilize the patient.
- Management of acute contrast reaction is discussed briefly in Table 11.2. (Adapted from *American College of Radiology Manual* 2013; http://aegysgroup.com)

Complications of Neuroendovascular Procedures and Bailout Techniques, ed. Rakesh Khatri, Gustavo J. Rodriguez, Jean Raymond and Adnan I. Qureshi. Published by Cambridge University Press. © Cambridge University Press 2016.

Table 11.1 Specific recommended premedication regimens

Elective premedication: Two frequently used regimens
1. Prednisone – 50 mg by mouth at 13 hours, 7 hours, and 1 hour before contrast media injection, plus diphenhydramine (Benadryl®)* – 50 mg intravenously, intramuscularly, or by mouth 1 hour before contrast medium.
2. Methylprednisolone (Medrol®) – 32 mg by mouth 12 hours and 2 hours before contrast media injection. An antihistamine (as in option 1) can also be added to this injection regimen.
If the patient is unable to take oral medication, 200 mg of hydrocortisone intravenously may be substituted for oral.

Emergency premedication (in decreasing order of desirability)
1. Methylprednisolone sodium succinate (Solu-Medrol®) 40 mg or hydrocortisone sodium succinate (Solu-Cortef®) 200 mg intravenously every 4 hours (q4h) until contrast study required plus diphenhydramine 50 mg IV 1 hour prior to contrast injection.
2. Dexamethasone sodium sulfate (Decadron®) 7.5 mg or betamethasone 6.0 mg intravenously q4h until contrast study must be done in patient with known allergy to methylprednisolone, aspirin, or non-steroidal anti-inflammatory drugs, especially if asthmatic. Also diphenhydramine 50 mg IV 1 hour prior to contrast injection.
3. Omit steroids entirely and give diphenhydramine 50 mg IV.

Note: IV steroids have not been shown to be effective when administered less than 4 to 6 hours prior to contrast injection.
 * Note: all forms can cause drowsiness; intramuscular (IM)/IV form may cause or worsen hypotension.

- Delayed reaction (symptoms that occurred 1 hour or more after the study) usually includes minor skin lesions, nausea/vomiting, headache, and fever.

Heparin allergy
- Heparin is routinely used as anticoagulant during neuroendovascular procedures to prevent thromboembolic complications.
- Heparin allergy can represent both acute severe allergy[2] and delayed-type hypersensitivity reactions (e.g. eczematous skin lesion).
- Alternative therapy should be planned if allergy/intolerance known.
  i.   Bivalirudin (Angiomax) is a direct thrombin inhibitor and has been shown to be safe for both cardiovascular and neurovascular procedures[3].
  ii. Argatroban is another synthetic thrombin inhibitor which can be used as alternative anticoagulation for patients with heparin intolerance[4].
  iii. Other thrombin inhibitors such as lepirudin have been used as alternative anticoagulation to heparin in cardiac patients.

Peripheral arterial disease
Peripheral arterial disease (PAD) poses significant challenges related to access in neuroendovascular procedures:
- Difficult/unsuccessful access via transfemoral route.
- Higher risk of complications including femoral artery or branch artery occlusion, dissection, distal embolization, retroperitoneal hematoma, external iliac/common iliac perforation, and shock.

Table 11.2 Reactions with contrast medium and their management

Hives

Mild	Moderate	Severe
No treatment often needed; however, if symptomatic, can consider diphenhydramine (Benadryl®)* 25–50 mg PO or fexofenadine (Allegra®)** 180 mg PO	Monitor vitals Preserve IV access Consider diphenhydramine (Benadryl®)* 25–50 mg PO or fexofenadine (Allegra®)** 180 mg PO or Consider diphenhydramine (Benadryl®)* 25–50 mg IM or IV (administer IV dose slowly over 1–2 min)	Monitor vitals Preserve IV access Consider diphenhydramine (Benadryl®)* 25–50 mg IM or IV (administer IV dose slowly over 1–2 min) May also consider: epinephrine (IM) IM 0.3 mg (0.3 ml of 1:1,000 dilution) or IM EpiPen® or equivalent (0.3 ml of 1:1000 dilution, fixed) or epinephrine (IV) IV 1–3 ml of 1:10,000 dilution; administer slowly into a running IV infusion of saline

Diffuse erythema

Preserve IV access, monitor vitals, pulse oximeter, O_2 by mask 6–10 l/min

Normotensive	Hypotensive	Refractory hypotension
No other treatment usually needed	IV fluids 0.9% normal saline 1000 ml rapidly or lactated Ringer's 1,000 ml rapidly	Epinephrine (IV)*** IV 1–3 ml of 1:10,000 dilution; administer slowly into a running IV infusion of saline; can repeat every 5–10 minutes up to 10 ml total

Bronchospasm

Preserve IV access, monitor vitals, pulse oximeter O_2 by mask 6–10 l/min

Mild	Moderate	Severe
Beta-agonist inhaler (Albuterol®) 2 puffs (90 µg/puff) for a total of 180 µg; can repeat	Epinephrine (IV)*** IV 1–3 ml of 1:10,000 dilution; administer slowly into a running IV infusion of saline; can repeat up to 1 mg total	Epinephrine (IV)*** IV 1–3 ml of 1:10,000 dilution; administer slowly into a running IV infusion of saline; can repeat up to 1 mg total

Laryngeal edema

Preserve IV access, monitor vitals, pulse oximeter, O_2 by mask 6–10 l/min
Epinephrine (IV)*** IV 1–3 ml of 1:10,000 dilution; administer slowly into a running IV infusion of saline; can repeat up to 1 mg total
Call emergency response team

 * Note: all forms can cause drowsiness; IM/IV form may cause or worsen hypotension.
** Note: second-generation antihistamines cause less drowsiness; may be beneficial in patients who need to drive themselves home.
***Note: in hypotensive patients, the preferred route of epinephrine delivery is IV, as the extremities may not be perfused sufficiently to allow for adequate absorption of IM administered drug.

Prevention strategies:

- Knowledge of the severity and location (which side) of PAD and past treatments (e.g. stents) is helpful before the procedure.
- In emergency situations, a quick look at the patient's medical records or any relevant previous radiographic studies/reports may reveal such information.
- An alternative approach such as the transradial option should be considered.
- Ultrasound-guided access using micropuncture needle is recommended.
- Be vigilant in picking up postprocedure complications such as retroperitoneal/groin hematoma, limb ischemia (dissection or distal thromboembolism).

  - Retroperitoneal hematoma

    - Back pain is a very sensitive symptom of retroperitoneal hematoma. Hypotension and drop in hematocrit are usually late signs of continued bleeding.
    - Emergent computed tomography (CT) of the abdomen and pelvis aids in diagnosis.
    - Emergent surgical consultation should be done.
    - May need to reverse heparin, platelet transfusion, or packed red blood cell infusion. This should be decided on a case by case basis.
    - Vascular surgeon consultation should be done on emergent basis

  - Limb ischemia

    - Signs of ischemia: decreased/absent pedal pulses (use manual and Doppler ultrasound), decreased temperature, pain, and ankle-brachial index (ABI) <0.90.
    - Consider anticoagulation with IV heparin.
    - Consider consulting interventional radiology or vascular surgery.

Contrast-induced nephropathy

Intravascular administration of iodinated contrast media for imaging studies is routinely performed both in hospitalized and ambulatory patients for diagnostic and therapeutic considerations. While these procedures are extremely helpful, they are not without complications. One of the most important complications of iodinated contrast media is the development of acute kidney injury (AKI), and is frequently called contrast-induced nephropathy (CIN). Although minor increases in serum creatinine levels occur following the contrast study, CIN is an established entity that causes prolonged hospital stay and higher short-term and long-term morbidity and mortality, as well as higher cost. In this chapter, we will define CIN, and review briefly the incidence, risk factors and risk assessment, pathophysiology, clinical evaluation, and strategies for prevention of CIN. A brief discussion of the physicochemical properties of the contrast media is helpful in choosing the appropriate medium for the procedure. In addition, a brief discussion of the use and complications of non-iodinated contrast media (gadolinium chelates) is presented.

Iodinated contrast media

Definition of CIN: CIN was variously defined as an increase in serum creatinine levels of 0.3 to 2.0 mg/dl from baseline, 1 to 5 days following exposure to contrast media.

This definition has created confusion regarding the rate of incidence and management of CIN. Recently, several reports and consensus panels have redefined CIN as an increase in serum creatinine levels of 0.5 mg/dl (>44 µmol/l) above baseline, or 25% increase in serum creatinine levels, or a decrease in estimated glomerular filtration rate (eGFR) by >25% within 48 h following an IV or intra-arterial administration of contrast material. As stated above, CIN is associated with prolonged hospital stay and short-term as well as long-term morbidity. Some patients may require renal replacement therapy. Early and late cardiovascular complications are rather common following CIN. Oral contrast does not cause AKI because it is not absorbed by the gastrointestinal tract.

Incidence of CIN: AKI occurs not only with iodinated contrast media, but with non-iodinated gadolinium-containing contrast media as well. The incidence of AKI is increasing as the number of imaging studies with contrast media is increasing. CIN is the third most common cause of AKI in hospitalized patients after renal ischemia and nephrotoxins[5]. The incidence of CIN varies among studies. The incidence is 1–2% in patients with normal renal function even in the presence of diabetes; however, the incidence is as high as 25–40% in patients with risk factors such as pre-existing renal disease, coexisting chronic kidney disease (CKD) and diabetes, elderly subjects, patients with congestive heart failure, or patients receiving antibiotics or any other nephrotoxins. The reason for increased incidence of nephrotoxicity in renal impairment is mostly related to delayed excretion by the kidneys and prolonged exposure of the kidneys to contrast media.

Properties of contrast media: In addition to the patient-related risk factors, contrast media have also been identified as risk factors for CIN because of their intrinsic chemical properties such as osmolality, ionic or non-ionic status, viscosity, degree of polymerization, and the volume injected. Table 11.3 shows the properties of various contrast media. As evident, iodine is the only element that can be used as contrast medium to provide radiopacity. Iodine is not suitable for magnetic resonance imaging (MRI) studies because it is not a paramagnetic atom. Generally, contrast media are divided into high-osmolality, low-osmolality, and iso-osmolality agents[6]. Currently, low- and iso-osmolality agents are used for contrast studies. The monomers shown in Table 11.3 contain one benzene (hexagonal) ring with three iodine atoms at the C2,4,6 positions, and the dimers contain two benzene rings with six iodine atoms. High-osmolality contrast media (HOCM) consist of a negatively charged anion (e.g. iothalamate) and a positively charged cation (e.g. Na^+ or meglumine or both), whereas low-osmolality contrast media (LOCM) are non-ionic agents with only uncharged triiodinated benzene ring compounds. Thus, all non-ionic monomer contrast media dissociate in water into non-radiopaque cations (Na^+ and meglumine) and a radiopaque anion (iodine), giving an iodine:molecule ratio of 3:2. Because of the presence of two cations, the media is hyperosmolar. Ionic dimers yield an iodine:molecule ratio of 6:2. On the other hand, non-ionic chemicals do not dissociate, and a non-ionic dimer dissociates into an iodine:molecule ratio of 6:1.

For simplicity, viscosity is viewed as thickness of the media. For example, honey is thicker than water. The flow of less viscous fluids is much faster than that of highly viscous fluids. Experimental evidence suggests that contrast media with high viscosity and low osmolality are associated with decreased renal medullary blood flow, pO_2 content, and erythrocyte concentration. Osmolality alone does not cause such changes. Therefore, viscosity and osmolality act differently.

The incidence of CIN is much higher with HOCM than LOCM. Patients with CKD are at more risk than patients with normal renal function. Although some studies found

Table 11.3 Properties of some contrast media

Generic name	Trade name	Ionic nature	Polymeri-zation	Osmolality (mOsm/kg H_2O	Iodine content (mg/ml)	Viscosity (cP@ 37 °C)
HOCM						
Diatrozate	Renograffin-76	Ionic	Monomer	1940	370	9.1
Iothalamate	Conray	Ionic	Monomer	1400	282	4.3
LOCM						
Ioxalate	Hexabrix 320	Ionic	Dimer	580	320	7.5
Iohexol	Omnipaque 300	Non-ionic	Monomer	640	300	6.1
Iobitridol	Xenetix 300	Non-ionic	Monomer	695	300	6.0
Iomeprol	Iomeron	Non-ionic	Monomer	618	350	7.0
Iopamidol	Isovue	Non-ionic	Monomer	300–340	150	1.5
Iopromide	Ultravist 300	Non-ionic	Monomer	620	300	4.6
Ioversol	Optiray 300	Non-ionic	Monomer	645	300	5.5
IOCM						
Iodixanol	Visipaque 320	Non-ionic	Dimer	290	320	11.4
Iotrolan*	Isovist 300	Non-ionic	Dimer	320	300	8.1

HOCM, high-osmolality contrast media; LOCM, low-osmolality contrast media; IOCM, iso-osmolality contrast media; cP, centipoise
*Withdrawn because of delayed adverse reactions, particularly in Japanese studies.

iso-osmolality agents to be less nephrotoxic than LOCM, other studies did not find any clinical significance between these two types of contrast media [7].

There is a relationship between the volume of contrast agent injected and the extent of nephropathy. The general consensus is that small doses of contrast media (<70 ml) cause less nephropathy than large doses of any osmolality. One study[8] reported that none of the patients required dialysis following the administration of <100 ml of contrast media for coronary studies. However, another study[9] reported that diabetic patients with serum creatinine >5 mg/dl are at risk of nephropathy even with 20–30 ml of contrast media. In diabetic patients, a correlation between the volume and the degree of nephropathy has been established[10]. For example, each 100 ml increment in the amount of contrast medium caused a 30% increase in the odds of CIN. Thus, there is a relationship between the volume of contrast media administered and the incidence of nephropathy, particularly in patients with CKD and diabetes.

Route of contrast administration seems to have some impact on the incidence of CIN. It has been suggested that the intra-arterial route causes higher incidence of CIN than the IV route, because the former route delivers more contrast to the kidneys. However, it was subsequently shown that the volume of contrast through the intra-arterial route is larger, because of diagnostic and interventional procedures, than for the IV route which requires a fixed dose of contrast (CT angiography), and this may account for different incidences in CIN.

Table 11.4 Risk factors for contrast-induced nephropathy[11]

Non-modifiable factors	Modifiable factors
Chronic kidney disease (eGFR <60 ml)	Contrast media volume
Diabetes mellitus (type 1 and type 2)	Volume depletion
Age >70 yr	Hypotension
Emergent situations (benefit outweighs risk)	Anemia (hematocrit <35 g/l)
Left ventricular ejection fraction <40%	Intra-aortic balloon pump
Acute myocardial infarction	Hypoalbuminemia (<3.5 g/dl)
Severe hypertension	Drugs (diuretics, non-steroidal anti-inflammatory drugs (NSAIDs), antibiotics, or anti-infectives)
Conditions with decreased effective arterial blood volume (congestive heart failure, cirrhosis, nephrotic syndrome)	<72 h between first and second study
Renal transplant	

Risk factors for CIN: Table 11.4 identifies a number of modifiable and non-modifiable risk factors for CIN. In general, coexistence of chronic kidney disease (eGFR <60 ml/min) and diabetes carries more risk than either condition alone. Also, volume depletion and conditions of decreased arterial blood volume such as congestive heart failure predispose to CIN. Elderly subjects with age >70 years are also at risk for CIN. Repeat exposure to contrast media within 72 hours is an unnecessary added risk. A common clinical situation is diagnostic angiography in one hospital, and transfer of the same patient to another hospital the following day for intervention.

Risk assessment of CIN: Several risk factors for CIN are known. However, their cumulative effect on the prediction and the incidence of CIN has only been recently addressed. Two predictive models have been proposed: one preprocedure[12] and the other postprocedure[13]. Brown et al.[12] developed a risk score system with the preprocedural characteristics of patients who underwent a percutaneous coronary intervention. This scoring system predicts those patients who are at risk for developing severe renal dysfunction. Based on the number of points, as shown in Table 11.5, the risk for CIN can be stratified into low (0–7 points), medium (8–14 points), and high-risk (≥15 points) groups. This stratification would help the clinician to identify high-risk patients and manage them aggressively to prevent CIN.

Mehran et al.[13] have analyzed several risk factors (postprocedure) by assigning weighted integer scores in a study of patients who underwent percutaneous coronary intervention. Based on the calculation of scores, these investigators derived the incidence of CIN risk as well as the risk for dialysis. As shown in Table 11.6, a score of 5 was given to each of hypotension (systolic blood pressure <80 mmHg for at least 1 hour requiring inotropic support), intra-aortic balloon pump within 24 hours postprocedurally, and congestive heart failure (class III–IV by the New York Heart Association classification and/or history of pulmonary edema). Age >75 years was assigned 4 points. Anemia (baseline hematocrit <39% for men and <36% for women) and diabetes were each given 3 points. If serum creatinine was >1.5 mg/dl, 4 points were assigned. Patients also received different scores based on their eGFRs (2 for 40–60; 4 for 20–40; and 6 for <20 ml/min/1.73 m^2). Excess use of contrast medium also received points.

Table 11.5 Preprocedure scoring system[12]

Variable	Points
Age >80 yr	2
Female	1.5
Diabetes	3
Urgent intervention	2.5
Emergent intervention	3.5
Congestive heart failure	4.5
Preprocedure use of intra-aortic balloon pump	13
Serum creatinine 1.3–1.9 mg/dl	5
Serum creatinine >2.0 mg/dl	10

Table 11.6 Mehran scoring system[13]

Risk factor	Integer score	Risk calculation		
		Cumulative score	CIN risk (%)	Dialysis risk (%)
Hypotension	5	0–5	7.5	0.04
IABP	5	6–10	14	0.12
CHF	5	11–16	26.1	1.09
Age >75 yr	4	>16	57.3	12.6
Anemia	3			
Diabetes	3			
Volume of contrast	1 (for each 100 ml)			
eGFR (ml/min/1.73 m^2)				
40–60	2			
20–40	4			
<20	6			

IABP, intra-aortic balloon pump; CHF, congestive heart failure

Pathogenesis of CIN: The pathogenesis of CIN is not completely understood. However, several possible mechanisms have been proposed, including decreased renal blood flow (RBF), direct tubular injury, medullary hypoxia with impaired microcirculation, and tubular obstruction[14,15].

Contrast agents have a biphasic effect on RBF. Initially, vasodilation of the afferent arterioles causes a transient increase in RBF, followed by prolonged vasoconstriction and a decrease in RBF. Vasoconstriction is due to the release of endothelin and adenosine, and a decrease in nitric oxide and PGE_1 and PGE_2 production. Adenosine, for example, causes afferent arteriolar vasoconstriction and efferent arteriolar vasodilation, resulting in compromised GFR and AKI. This is the basis for the use of theophylline, which antagonizes the effects of adenosine.

It has long been known that iodine has a cytotoxic effect on bacteria. Iodine causes direct damage to membrane proteins, leading to the loss of cell membrane integrity. Thus, a direct injury to the renal tubules has been proposed. Direct tubular injury by contrast media is mediated by the generation of reactive oxygen species (ROS). Apoptosis with loss of cellular membrane proteins and loss of cytochrome C from mitochondria have been observed in renal tubular epithelial cells. Also, pathologically, vacuolization in the proximal tubular cells has been observed. In animal studies, antioxidants prevented nephrotoxicity induced by contrast media. These studies formed the basis for the use of antioxidants such as N-acetylcysteine and ascorbic acid in humans to prevent CIN. Also, it was shown that $NaHCO_3$ can act as an antioxidant, and prevent nephrotoxicity.

Renal medullary hypoxia is an important mechanism for CIN. Normally, renal medulla functions at low O_2 tension (30 mmHg), as compared with the cortex where O_2 tension is very high. Contrast media reduce outer medullary O_2 tension substantially to as low as 10 mmHg. This medullary portion (thick ascending limb of Henle's loop) of the nephron segment requires high O_2 tension because of active transport mechanisms. Also, contrast media increase the viscosity in both the tubular fluid and vasa recta with subsequent red blood cell aggregation. These changes cause low blood supply and O_2 to the medulla, resulting in medullary hypoxia. ROS generation is stimulated with subsequent membrane injury and DNA damage. Mitochondrial enzyme activity is also impaired, leading to depletion of intracellular energy. The net result is cell necrosis and apoptosis.

High-osmolality contrast media induce osmotic diuresis via the release of atrial natriuretic peptide. Excess delivery of NaCl to the macula densa activates the tubuloglomerular feedback mechanism via adenosine, resulting in afferent arteriolar constriction and a decrease in GFR.

Finally, contrast media promote the excretion of uric acid and oxalate. If not adequately hydrated postprocedurally, the patient may develop precipitation of urate and oxalate crystals in the tubular lumen, causing obstruction and a decrease in GFR. Figure 11.1 summarizes various mechanisms in the pathogenesis of CIN.

Clinical evaluation of patients with CIN: History and physical examination are important components of clinical evaluation.

(1) Past medical history such as kidney disease, diabetes, hypertension, hyperlipidemia, heart failure, and nephrotoxic drugs can identify patients at high risk for CIN.

(2) Assessment of volume status is essential in both hospitalized and ambulatory patients.

(3) eGFR is a better marker than serum creatinine of renal function. Determination of baseline serum creatinine or eGFR[16] is necessary to assess renal function prior to the study and more frequent estimations are required following the study for comparison.

(4) Serum cystatin C levels, if available, can also be used in association with serum creatinine levels. Increase of >10% in serum cystatin levels is indicative of AKI. In the future, markers such as NGAL (neutrophil gelatinase-associated lipocalin) may play a role in early detection (hours) of AKI following contrast study. Urinalysis is variable, but usually not helpful. Also, fractional excretion of Na^+, which is <1% in CIN, is misleading because it indicates pre-renal azotemia rather than CIN.

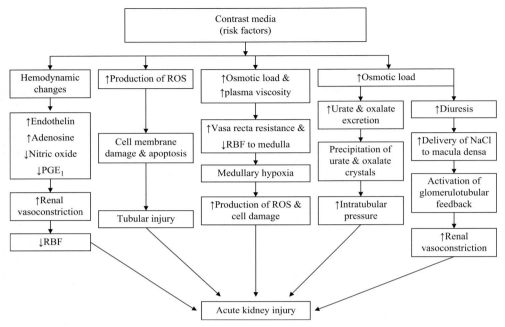

Figure 11.1 Pathogenesis of contrast-induced nephropathy.

In the emergency situation where the benefit of contrast study outweighs the risk of waiting, the procedure can be done even in the absence of serum creatinine or eGFR and the risk for development of AKI is high.

Although the fractional excretion of Na^+ (FE_{Na}) in acute tubular necrosis (ATN) due to antibiotics is >2%, it is <1% in contrast-induced ATN. This suggests that patients with CIN have low intravascular volume. Renal biopsy is not indicated.

Clinical course of CIN: The clinical course of CIN in patients with no risk factors is simple. Many individuals may have a transient increase (<0.5 mg/dl) in serum creatinine levels. Such minor increases improve following good oral or IV intake of fluids. In patients with risk factors, oliguric AKI develops with serum creatinine increase by >0.5 mg/dl. Typically, serum creatinine starts increasing in 24 hours and reaches peak concentrations in 3–4 days with improvement in 7–13 days. A few patients require short-term dialysis; however, some patients with both diabetes and serum creatinine levels >4.0 mg/dl may require chronic dialysis. CIN risk increases with an increase in baseline creatinine and addition of risk factors. Estimating eGFR from serum creatinine is only valid if the patient is in steady state. However, Table 11.7 gives an approximation of GFR loss with an increase of serum creatinine by 0.5 mg/dl after contrast study from baseline creatinine levels of 1 to 2.0 mg/dl.

Preventive strategies of CIN

Several non-pharmacologic and pharmacologic therapeutic modalities have been applied to prevent and reduce the incidence and severity of nephropathy, as shown in Table 11.8. Of all these modalities, adequate hydration with appropriate fluids has been reported to be the most accepted non-pharmacologic therapeutic measure for prevention of CIN. In addition

Table 11.7 Approximate loss of GFR in patients with CIN

Baseline creatinine (mg/dl)	Creatinine after increase by 0.5 mg/dl	Change in GFR (ml/min)	% loss of GFR
1.0	1.5	100 – 67	33
1.5	2.0	67 – 50	25
2.0	2.5	50 – 40	20

Table 11.8 Prevention of CIN[17–19]

Preprocedure management
Determine baseline serum creatinine and eGFR
Identify high-risk patient
Estimate preprocedure risk score
Avoid intravascular volume depletion (or dehydration)
Start IV hydration with either isotonic (0.9%) saline or isotonic $NaHCO_3$ or 0.45% saline plus 75 mEq of $NaHCO_3$
Start either oral or IV N-acetylcysteine (NAC)
Withdraw all nephrotoxins
Hold metformin 24–48 h before procedure if possible and avoid its use for at least 48 h postexposure, as it may cause lactic acidosis (rare)
Avoid diuretics, mannitol, fenoldapam, endothelin, and adenosine receptor blockers
Avoid prophylactic renal replacement therapy (hemodialysis)
Renal consult for CKD patients

Management during procedure
Continue hydration
Maintain systolic blood pressure >120 mmHg
Minimize the dose of contrast media
Use either iso-osmolality or low-osmolality contrast medium

Postprocedure management
Continue hydration and NAC
Monitor hemodynamic status, if indicated
Maintain urine output >100 ml/h
Maintain urine pH >6.5, if isotonic $NaHCO_3$ is used
Calculate postprocedure risk score
Obtain serum creatinine and eGFR daily for 4 days (in-hospital patients), and then as needed
Start renal replacement therapy (hemodialysis or hemofiltration) early, as needed
Avoid repeat contrast procedure until serum creatinine returns to baseline

to hydration, pharmacologic agents such as N-acetylcysteine, ascorbic acid, theophylline, endothelin receptor blockers, statins, fenoldopam, and other agents have been used. However, only N-acetylcysteine is accepted as a prophylactic antioxidant because of its low adverse effects and cost. Therefore, discussion pertinent only to hydration and N-acetylcysteine is presented below.

Hydration: Following the identification of a high-risk patient, the most important preventive measure is hydration. IV hydration is superior to oral hydration in preventing

CIN. Volume expansion improves RBF and blood pressure, dilutes contrast material in renal tubules, removes contrast from renal parenchyma, prevents tubular obstruction, and reduces the actions of renin–angiotensin–aldosterone as well as antidiuretic hormone. Also, adequate volume expansion improves endogenous production of nitric oxide and vasodilatory prostaglandins. Three types of IV solutions have been used in clinical studies: (1) 0.45% saline (half-normal saline), (2) 0.9% saline (normal saline); and (3) isotonic $NaHCO_3$. Initial studies have used 0.45% saline, whereas subsequent studies found that use of normal saline is superior to half-normal saline in reducing the incidence of CIN. Most of the CIN Consensus Working Panels recommend normal saline as the fluid of choice.

Oral hydration is usually recommended for outpatients, as IV administration is not feasible. Generally, patients are advised to drink 1–2 liters of water, or water with salt-containing liquids such as soup. Infusion of normal saline a few hours before and few hours after the procedure has also been recommended.

Recently, $NaHCO_3$ has gained popularity over saline because of the hypothesis that alkalinization of tubular fluid with bicarbonate may reduce generation of ROS in medulla. Because of this antioxidant property, some studies[20] favored the use of $NaHCO_3$ and found less nephropathy, as compared with 0.9% saline for CIN prophylaxis. Also, it has been proposed that the Cl^- in NaCl may cause renal vasoconstriction. Despite these advantages, other studies[21] did not show $NaHCO_3$ superiority. $NaHCO_3$ is available as 8.4% (1 ml = 1 mEq) solution or can be prepared in 1 liter of 5% dextrose in water (D5W) with 154 mEq of $NaHCO_3$. This solution can be used in non-diabetics. Despite the availability of $NaHCO_3$ solutions, many practicing physicians take advantage of the beneficial effects of both saline and $NaHCO_3$, and use the combination of 0.45% saline and 75 mEq of $NaHCO_3$ as an isotonic solution.

Although routine use of isotonic $NaHCO_3$ is not recommended, its administration is supported in certain patients: (1) those who require an emergent percutaneous intervention where infusion is performed in an hour prior to procedure; (2) during an acute intervention with renal impairment; or (3) high-risk CKD patients. CKD patients with low serum bicarbonate may benefit more than patients with near-normal serum bicarbonate from administration of $NaHCO_3$, as metabolic acidosis promotes ROS generation.

N-acetylcysteine (NAC): NAC scavenges free radicals. It also improves RBF by stimulating vasodilators such as nitric acid and prostaglandins. Because of these beneficial properties, particularly in patients with renal impairment, NAC has gained popularity for CIN prevention. Although several studies failed to prove a prophylactic effect, NAC is routinely used because of its low adverse reactions and cost[22]. Adverse reactions are more common with IV than oral use.

Protocols for fluid and NAC administration: Several protocols for fluid and NAC administration have been followed in clinical trials, with variable results. Postprocedure hydration is extremely important to improve RBF and urine output. The following preventive and therapeutic measures seem to satisfy most of the protocols for CIN management.

Hemodialysis (HD) and hemofiltration (HF): Nephrologists are often called for HD or HF or continuous renal replacement therapies after contrast study to prevent CIN. These procedures remove contrast agents because of their small size, small volume of distribution, low protein binding, and water solubility. In addition, HD removes excess fluid and, therefore, improves congestive heart failure in those with low ejection fraction. Contrast

Table 11.9 Suggested preventive and therapeutic measures of CIN

Low- to moderate-risk patient

Inpatient (ejection fraction (EF) > 45%): 0.9% saline at 1–1.5 ml/kg/min (up to 100 ml/h) 12 h before and 6–24 h after procedure.

Inpatient (EF < 40%): 0.9% saline at 0.5 ml/kg/h (or 50 ml/h) as above

Outpatient: 0.9% saline at 1–1.5 ml/kg/min (up to 100 ml/h) 3 h before and 12 h after procedure (depending on timing of the discharge)

NAC: 600 mg orally b.i.d. before the day and continue 600 mg orally b.i.d (total of four doses) for a day after procedure for both inpatients and outpatients.

High-risk patient

Inpatient (EF > 45%): Isotonic $NaHCO_3$ (preferred to isotonic saline) at 3 ml/kg/h for 1 h before and 1 ml/kg/h for 6–12 h after procedure. Follow for signs of pulmonary edema in CHF and CKD 4–5 patients and adjust the dose as needed.

NAC: 1200 mg orally b.i.d. before the day and continue 600 mg orally b.i.d. (total of four doses) for a day after procedure

Emergent procedure

Low-risk patient (serum creatinine <1.5 mg/dl or eGFR >60 ml/min)

0.9% saline bolus of 300–500 ml 1 h before, and NAC 600 mg oral or IV, as indicated. Continue 0.9% saline at 1 m/kg/h for 12–24 h after procedure. NAC 600 mg b.i.d. for 24h oral or IV, as indicated

High-risk patient (serum creatinine >1.5 mg/dl or eGFR <60 ml/min)

Isotonic $NaHCO_3$ (preferred to isotonic saline) at 3 ml/kg/h for 1 h before and 1 ml/kg/h for 6–12 h after procedure. Follow for signs of pulmonary edema in CHF and CKD 4–5 patients and adjust the dose, as needed.

NAC: 1200 mg oral or IV, as indicated, prior to procedure with two more doses after procedure (total doses three)

Note: NAC and isotonic $NaHCO_3$ use is preferred by some operators. Their use is still controversial. Hydration is the mainstay of treatment.

agents cause hyperkalemia by solvent drag. Thus, HD removes contrast and fluid, and corrects hyperkalemia. Peritoneal dialysis is also effective in removing contrast media, but it takes longer than HD.

Because of the removal of contrast agents by HD and HF, some investigators have used these procedures before, during, and after the study. The results are mixed, and prophylactic use of HD is not suggested. The only study that showed positive results with HF for CIN prophylaxis is in CKD patients with creatinine >2 mg/dl who underwent coronary intervention. A recent systematic review showed no benefit of renal replacement therapy in CIN prophylaxis. In fact, the review suggested that HD increased the risk for CIN. However, HD is indicated in the following patients: (1) those whose serum creatinine does not improve despite adequate standard preventive therapy, (2) those at risk for fluid overload, and (3) those with CKD stage 5 who have some residual renal function.

Gadolinium-based contrast agents

There are several case reports in the literature about the use of gadolinium (Gd)-based contrast in situations where iodine-based contrast cannot be used due to severe contrast allergy. However, there are several limitations to the use of Gd as an X-ray contrast agent.

It is inferior to iodinated agents for image contrast, although digital subtraction postprocessing can resolve that problem to some extent. The total dosage of Gd is limited to 0.4 mmol/kg per examination, and the safety dose is ≤40–70 ml of Gd at one examination per patient. Operators need to be cautious about the volume when performing cerebral angiography in these patients.

Properties: Currently, there are nine Gd^{3+}-based contrast agents (GBCAs) approved for use in the United States and the European Union (Table 11.10). The GBCAs can be classified on the basis of their structure (linear vs. macrocyclic), their ionicity (ionic vs. non-ionic), or whether they are albumin-binding. Macrocyclic molecule binds Gd^{3+} tightly than linear chelate with lower dissociation. Negligible or low albumin-binding drugs have a good tolerability profile, whereas drugs that are albumin-bound may have poor tolerability and induce nausea and vomiting. Following injection, GBCAs are distributed in the extracellular space except for gadobenate disodium, which can be taken up by the liver. GBCAs are not metabolized, and are excreted unchanged by the kidneys. The half-life of GBCAs is about 1.5 hours and >90% of the drug is excreted in 24 hours. The molecular weight ranges from 559 to 1058 daltons. Release of Gd^{3+} from the chelate is an important property of GBCAs, because free Gd^{3+}, as stated above, is toxic. Endogenous cations such as Cu^{2+}, Ca^{2+}, and Zn^{2+} can displace Gd^{3+} and promote toxicity. Macrocyclic chelates such as gadoterate (Doterem), gadoteridol (ProHance), and gadobutrol (Gadovist) are more stable and release less free GD^{3+} than non-ionic linear chelates. Other properties of GBCAs are shown in Table 11.10.

Nephropathy: GBCAs are more nephrotoxic than iodinated contrast agents in equimolar concentrations. Because of the use of low volume for MRI and other studies, the incidence of nephrotoxicity with MRI agents is much lower than for iodinated contrast agents. However, in diabetics, non-dialysis patients with CKD stages 4–5, and dialysis patients, GBCAs induce nephrotoxicity called nephrogenic systemic fibrosis[18] even at standard doses,

Nephrogenic systemic fibrosis (NSF): NSF was first observed in 1997, and subsequently reported in 2000. It was originally identified as a cutaneous lesion with indurated plaques and papules on the extremities and trunk in patients on HD and in failed renal transplant patients. Thickening of the skin, resembling scleroderma, is a common feature. In 2006, a relationship between NSF and GBCAs was suggested.

Prevalence: NSF is not limited to skin only, but it also involves muscles, diaphragm, heart, lungs, and liver. Thus, it is a systemic disorder. The prevalence of NSF varies between 1.5 and 5% in biopsy-proven HD patients. It is even higher when clinical criteria are used. NSF develops anywhere from days to months (2 days to 18 months). Not only HD patients but also patients with CKD stages 4–5 and patients with AKI are prone to develop NSF when exposed to GBCAs. The risk of NSF is related to dose and the type of GBCAs. So far, 631 cases of NSF have been reported to the Food and Drug Administration (FDA). Of these, 382 cases were reported with the use of Omniscan, 155 with Magnevist, 35 with Optimark, 10 with MultiHance, and 9 with ProHance[23].

Risk factors: Any patient with eGFR <30 ml/min, whether on dialysis or not, is at risk for NSF. AKI is another risk factor. Many other risk factors have been postulated to explain why some patients develop NSF following exposure to GBCAs and others do not. These include metabolic acidosis, higher serum levels of iron, Ca^{2+}, phosphate, inflammation, and high doses of erythropoietin. However, the role of these factors has not been firmly established.

Table 11.10 Properties of GBCAs

Generic name (year introduced)	Trade name	Ionic nature	Structure	Osmolality (mOsm/kg H_2O)	Viscosity (mPa 37 °C)	Albumin-binding	Availability in USA
Gadopentate dimeglumine (1988)	Magnevist	Linear	Ionic	1960	2.0	No	Yes
Gadoterate meglumine (1989)	Dotarem	Cyclic	Ionic	1350	1.4	No	No
Gadodiamide (1993)	Omniscan	Linear	Non-ionic	790	1.4	No	Yes
Gadoteridol (1994)	ProHance	Cyclic	Non-ionic	630	1.3	No	Yes
Gadobenate disodium (1998)	MultiHance	Linear	Ionic	1970	5.3	Weak	Yes
Gadobutrol (1998)	Gadovist	Cyclic	Non-ionic	1600	4.96	No	No
Gadoversetamide (2000)	Optimark	Linear	Non-ionic	1110	2.0	No	Yes
Gadoextetate disodium (2004)	Eovist/Primivist	Linear	Ionic	688	1.19	No	Yes
Gadofosvest trisodium (2005)	Ablavar/Vasovist	Linear	Ionic	825	1.8	Strong	Yes

Clinical manifestations: Gd^{3+} is extremely toxic because of its deposition in skin, lungs, lymph nodes, bone, and other organs. It may stimulate many cytokines that promote fibrosis. Joint contractures and limitations in mobility are common. Deep vein thrombosis, pulmonary embolism, atrial thrombus, and clotting of arterio-venous fistulas have been reported in patients with NSF. These patients seem to have antiphospholipid antibody syndrome. Fibrosis of several organs, including lungs, muscle, and diaphragm, may lead to morbidity and mortality. Sudden death from respiratory failure has been reported.

Treatment: There is no proven treatment for NSF. Plasma exchange, ultraviolet light therapy, sodium thiosulfate, high-dose immunoglobulin, and angiotensin converting enzyme (ACE)-inhibitors have been tried with variable successes. Physical therapy improves joint mobility.

Prevention: The following measures are suggested for patients with AKI and different renal function.

CKD stage 1 (eGFR 90 ml/min): No NSF has been reported.

CKD stage 2 (eGFR 60–89 ml/min): The risk is low, and the lowest dose is recommended.

CKD stage 3a (eGFR 45–59 ml/ min) and CKD stage 3b (eGFR 30–44 ml/min): The risk is low, and the lowest dose is recommended.

CKD stage 4 (eGFR 15–29 ml/min) and stage 5 (eGFR <15 ml/min): Patients who are not on HD are at high-risk for NSF.

HD patients as well as patients with AKI:

(1) Identify the indication and risk:benefit ratio
(2) Consider alternative study
(3) If benefit outweighs the risk, explain to the patient the risks and advantages of the procedure
(4) Obtain consent
(5) Use lowest possible dose of contrast agent
(6) Use preferably macrocyclic low-molecular-weight agent
(7) DO NOT use Omiscan, Magnevist, or Optimark (contraindicated)
(8) Avoid multiple exposure, as cumulative dose is a risk factor
(9) Provide HD two to three times after study, if possible, or perform the study just before dialysis and HD later.

References

1. McCullough PA, Soman SS. Contrast-induced nephropathy. *Crit Care Clin* 2005;21:261–80.

2. Alban S. Adverse effects of heparin. *Handb Exp Pharmacol* 2012;207:211–63.

3. Harrigan, MR. *et al.* Bivalirudin for endovascular intervention in acute ischemic stroke: case report. *Neurosurgery* 2004;54:218–23.

4. Lewis, BE, *et al.* "Argatroban anticoagulant therapy in patients with heparin-induced thrombocytopenia." *Circulation* 2001;103:1838–43.

5. Nash K, Hafeez A, Hou S. Hospital-acquired renal insufficiency. *Am J Kidney Dis* 2002;39:930–36.

6. Grainger RG, Thomsen HS, Marcos SK, *et al.* Intravascular contrast media for radiology, CT and MRI. In: Adam A, Dixon AK, eds. *Grainger & Allison's Diagnostic Radiology. A Textbook of Medical Imaging.* 5th edn, Edinburgh, Elsevier Churchill Livingstone, 2007; 31–53.

7. Solomon RJ, Natarajan MK, Doucet S, *et al.* Cardiac angiography in renally impaired patients (CARE) study. A randomized double-blind trial of contrast-induced

nephropathy in patients with chronic kidney disease. *Circulation* 2007;115: 3189–96.

8. McCullough PA, Wolyn R, Rocher LL, *et al.* Acute renal failure after coronary intervention: incidence, risk factors, and relationship to mortality. *Am J Med* 1997;103:368.

9. Newhouse JH, Kho D, Rao QA, Starren J. Frequency of serum creatinine changes in the absence of iodinated contrast material: implications for studies of contrast nephrotoxicity. *Am J Roentgenol* 2008;191:376.

10. Nikolsky E, Mehran R, Turcot D *et al.* Impact of chronic kidney disease on prognosis of patients with diabetes mellitus treated with percutaneous coronary intervention. *Am J Cardiol* 2004;94: 300–305.

11. Mehran R, Nikolsky E. Contrast-induced nephropathy: Definition, epidemiology, and patients at risk. *Kidney Int* 2006;69: S11-S15.

12. Brown JR, DeVries JT, Piper WD, *et al.* Serious renal dysfunction after percutaneous coronary intervention can be predicted. *Am Heart J* 2008;155:260–66.

13. Mehran R, Aymong ED, Nikolsky E, *et al.* A simple risk score for prediction of contrast-induced nephropathy after percutaneous coronary intervention: development and initial validation. *J Am Coll Cardiol* 2004;44:1393–99.

14. Persson PB, Hansell P, Liss P. Pathophysiology of contrast medium-induced nephropathy. *Kidney Int* 2005;68:14–22.

15. Heyman SN, Rosen S, Khamaisi M, *et al.* Reactive oxygen species and the pathogenesis of radiocontrast-induced nephropathy. *Invest Radiol* 2010; 45:188–95.

16. Levey AS, Coresh J, Greene T *et al.* Chronic Kidney Disease Epidemiology Collaboration. Using standardized serum creatinine values in the modification of diet in renal disease study equation for estimating glomerular filtration rate. *Ann Intern Med* 2006;145(4): 247–54.

17. Pannu N, Wiebe N, Tonelli M. Prophylaxis strategies for contrast-induced nephropathy. *JAMA* 2006;295: 2765–79.

18. Mohammed NMA, Mahfouz A, Achkar K, *et al.* Contrast-induced nephropathy. *Heart Views* 2013;14:106–116.

19. Golshahi J Nasri H, Gharipour M. Contrast-induced nephropathy; A literature review. *J Nephropathol* 2014;3: 51–56.

20. Merten GJ, Burgess WP, Gray LV, *et al.* Prevention of contrast-induced nephropathy with sodium bicarbonate: a randomized controlled trial. *JAMA* 2004;291:2328.

21. Rihal CS, Textor SC, Grill DE, *et al.* Incidence and prognostic importance of acute renal failure after percutaneous coronary intervention. *Circulation* 2002; 105:2259.

22. Zagler A, *et al.* N-acetylcysteine and contrast-induced nephropathy: A meta-analysis of 13 randomized trials. *Am Heart J* 2006;151:140–145.

23. Cohan R, Chovke P, Cohen M, *et al.* Nephrogenic systemic fibrosis. *American College of Radiology Manual on Contrast Media. Version 7.* 2010:49–55.

Relevant pharmacology for neurovascular procedures

James J. Roy, Megan Straub, and Bryan M. Statz

All medication doses provided in this text are adult doses, unless otherwise stated. Unapproved indications or doses of some medications are discussed throughout this text and will be designated by the term "off-label".

Abbreviations

D5W	dextrose 5% in water
IU	international units
IV	intravenous
IM	intramuscular
LR	lactated Ringer's
Max	maximum
NS	normal saline
PO	orally
SUBQ	subcutaneously

Analgesia[1]

See Table 12.1.

I. Fentanyl (procedural sedation; for analgesia)

    a. 0.5 to 1 µg/kg IV (up to 50 µg/dose); May repeat every 3 minutes to desired effect

    b. Onset: 1 to 2 minutes

    c. Duration of analgesia: In low doses, about 20 minutes

II. Morphine

    a. 2.5 to 5 mg IV. May repeat every 5 minutes to desired effect

    b. Onset: 6–15 minutes

    c. Duration of analgesia: 2–4 hours

    d. Consider dose reduction in obstructive sleep apnea, pulmonary disease, or elderly patients

Complications of Neuroendovascular Procedures and Bailout Techniques, ed. Rakesh Khatri, Gustavo J. Rodriguez, Jean Raymond and Adnan I. Qureshi. Published by Cambridge University Press. © Cambridge University Press 2016.

Table 12.1 Opioid drug classes

Phenylpiperidines	Meperidine, fentanyl, sufentanil, remifentanyl
Diphenylheptanes	Methadone, propoxyphene
Morphine group	Morphine, codeine, hydrocodone, oxycodone, oxymorphone, hydromorphone, nalbuphine, butorphanol, levorphanol, pentazocine

Table 12.2 Local anesthetics

Ester type	Amide type
Chloroprocaine (Nesacaine®)	Dibucaine (Nupercainal®)
Cocaine	Lidocaine (Xylocaine®)
Procaine	Mepivacaine (Carbocaine®, Polocaine®)
Proparacaine (Alcaine®)	Prilocaine (Citanest®)
Tetracaine	

III. Antidote

   a. Naloxone

      i. 0.1 to 2 mg IV at intervals of 2 to 3 minutes

      ii. Onset: 1 minute

      iii. Duration: 15 to 30 minutes

Anesthetics, local[2]

See Table 12.2.

I. Allergic reactions

   a. True anaphylaxis is rare

   b. Allergic reactions to metabolites of "ester" type local anesthetics may occur

      i. p-aminobutyric acid (PABA) or structurally similar compounds (metabolites of "ester" type local anesthetics)

      ii. PABA-like preservatives may be present in both amide and ester type local anesthetics and may cause allergic reaction

II. Systemic toxicity

   a. Seizures

      i. Benzodiazepines preferred

      ii. Avoid propofol if signs of cardiovascular instability

   b. Cardiotoxicity – arrhythmias

      i. Avoid vasopressin, calcium channel blockers, beta-blockers, or local anesthetic

      ii. Reduce individual epinephrine doses to less than 1 μg/kg

      iii. Lipid emulsion 20% therapy[3] (in addition to airway management and basic ACLS (advanced cardiovascular life support) for cardiovascular collapse; unlabeled use)

1. Bolus 1.5 ml/kg (lean body mass) IV over 1 minute
2. Continuous IV infusion at 0.25 ml/kg/min
3. Repeat bolus once or twice for persistent cardiovascular collapse
4. Double the infusion rate to 0.5 ml/kg/min if blood pressure remains low
5. Continue infusion for at least 10 minutes after attaining circulatory stability
6. Recommended upper limit: approximately 10 ml/kg lipid emulsion over the first 30 minutes
7. Discontinue within 1 hour if possible

Anticonvulsants for status epilepticus[4,5]

For overt, generalized, convulsive seizures:

Initial steps: Secure airway; obtain IV access; provide vasopressor support if needed; check finger-stick blood glucose; reverse thiamine deficiency and treat hypoglycemia if present.

Benzodiazepines are the preferred first-line medication therapy, followed by fosphenytoin in most cases.

I. Benzodiazepines

   a. Lorazepam (Ativan®)

      i. Usual recommended dose: 4 mg given IV slowly (2 mg/min). May repeat 4 mg dose in 5 to 15 minutes one time if seizures continue or recur

      ii. IV administration

         1. Must be diluted with equal volume of compatible diluent (sterile water for injection, NS, D5W)

         2. Do not inject IV faster than 2 mg/min

         3. Contains propylene glycol as diluent

      iii. Elimination half-life: 14 hours

      iv. Pregnancy category D

      v. Antidote: Flumazenil (see dosing information below)

   b. Midazolam (Versed®) – Intubation may be necessary

      i. Status epilepticus refractory to standard therapy (off-label)

         1. Midazolam 0.2 mg/kg IV bolus; repeat 0.2–0.4 mg/kg every 5 minutes until seizures stop (max dose of 2 mg/kg)

         2. IV infusion: Initial 0.1 mg/kg/hr; maintenance 0.05–2 mg/kg/hr

            a. Increase rate by 0.05–0.1 mg/kg/hr every 3–4 hours

      ii. IV administration

         1. Dilute to 0.5 mg/ml in D5W or NS for IV use

         2. Does not contain propylene glycol

      iii. Pharmacokinetics

         1. Amnestic onset within 1 to 5 minutes

         2. Duration of action: usually less than 2 hours

         3. Elimination half-life: 1.8 to 6.4 hours (mean approximately 3 hours)

         4. Clearance reduced in elderly patients, congestive heart failure, liver disease, or conditions that diminish cardiac output and hepatic outflow

      iv. Pregnancy: category D

      v. Antidote: Flumazenil (see dosing information below)

  c. Toxicology

      i. Flumazenil

        1. Rapidly reverses the benzodiazepine effect

        2. May cause withdrawal symptoms (including seizures)

        3. Starting dose: 0.1 to 0.2 mg IV over 15 to 30 seconds and repeated every 60 seconds as needed to a max of 1 mg

        4. In the event of re-sedation, repeated doses may be given at 20 minute intervals if needed. Maximum dose of 1 mg at any given time and no more than 3 mg in any one hour.

        5. Compatible with D5W, NS, and LR

        6. Onset: 1 minute

        7. Duration: 45 minutes

II. Fosphenytoin

  a. Loading dose: 15 to 20 mg/kg (maximum 1500 mg) IV at 50 to 150 mg/min, or IM (only if IV access is impossible)

  b. Dilute fosphenytoin in D5W or NS for injection to a concentration ranging from 1.5 to 25 mg/ml

  c. Because of the risk of hypotension, fosphenytoin should be administered no faster than 150 mg/min. Continuous monitoring of the electrocardiogram, blood pressure, and respiratory function is essential, and the patient should be observed throughout the period where maximal serum phenytoin concentrations occur, approximately 10 to 20 minutes after the end of fosphenytoin infusions

  d. Initial maintenance dose: 4–6 mg/kg/day orally or parenterally

  e. Contraindications

      i. Patients with sinus bradycardia, sino-atrial block, second and third degree A-V block, and Adams–Stokes syndrome

  f. Avoid fosphenytoin use in local-anesthetic-induced seizures

      i. May potentiate toxicity (sodium channel blockade)

III. Propofol

  a. Status epilepticus refractory to standard therapy (off-label)

      i. Propofol 1 to 2 mg/kg IV bolus loading dose

      ii. IV infusion: initial 33 µg/kg/min; maintenance 30–200 µg/kg/min

        1. Titrate to desired effect (burst suppression on electroencephalogram (EEG))

        2. May increase risk of hypotension and/or propofol infusion syndrome if infused at greater than 80 µg/kg/min, especially if for greater than 48 hour duration

      iii. Intubation may be necessary

  b. Administration

      i. Strict aseptic technique must always be maintained during handling

      ii. Prepared for single-patient use only

      iii. Shake product well before use

      iv. The tubing and any unused portions of propofol injectable emulsion should be discarded after 12 hours because propofol injectable emulsion contains no preservatives and is capable of supporting growth of microorganisms

  c. Contraindications

      i. Known hypersensitivity to propofol emulsion or any of its components

      ii. Patients with allergies to eggs, egg products, soybeans, or soy products

  d. Warnings

      i. Has been associated with both fatal and life-threatening anaphylactic and anaphylactoid reactions

      ii. Some products contain a "sulfite" that may cause allergic type reactions including anaphylactic symptoms and life-threatening or less severe asthmatic episodes in certain susceptible people

      iii. Undesirable side effects, such as cardiorespiratory depression, are likely to occur at higher blood concentrations which result from bolus dosing or rapid increases in infusion rates

      iv. Propofol infusion syndrome: Has been associated with a constellation of metabolic derangements and organ system failures that have resulted in death. The syndrome is characterized by severe metabolic acidosis, hyperkalemia, lipemia, rhabdomyolysis, hepatomegaly, cardiac and renal failure. In the setting of prolonged need for sedation, increasing propofol dose requirements to maintain a constant level of sedation, or onset of metabolic acidosis during administration of propofol infusion, consideration should be given to using alternative means of sedation

Antithrombotics

I. Anticoagulants – oral agents

Currently there are no antidotes available for the reversal of selected non-vitamin K mediated oral anticoagulants (apixaban, rivaroxaban, etc.). Non-specific reversal agents have been studied, but the data are limited and sometimes conflicting. General hemostatic measures and a "watch and wait" approach are often the best treatment strategies, but that may not always be appropriate. The following recommendations are potential reversal strategies, based on limited data, and may be considered for use in emergent, life-threatening situations

  a. Apixaban (Eliquis®)

      i. Factor Xa (FXa) inhibitor

      ii. Half-life: 12 hours

      iii. Discontinue 24 to 48 hours prior to a procedure

      iv. Acute management of life-threatening bleed/bleeding

        1. Hold apixaban

        2. Obtain coagulation screen (most useful monitoring lab is Anti-FXa assay)

3. Provide supportive care (fluids, red blood cells (RBCs), control of bleeding source, and hemodynamic support as needed)
4. Oral activated charcoal may be given if last dose taken within 6 hours
5. Very limited data on procoagulant reversal strategies
   a. For possible strategies see "Acute management of life-threatening bleed/ bleeding" under Rivaroxaban, below
6. Monitoring
   a. Anti-FXa assay: exhibits a direct linear relationship with apixaban plasma concentration

b. Dabigatran (Pradaxa®)

i. Direct thrombin inhibitor (DTI)
ii. Half-life: 12 to 17 hours
iii. Prior to procedures, discontinue dabigatran for 1 to 2 days if CrCl $\geq$ 50 ml/min, and for 3 to 5 days if CrCl < 50 ml/min
iv. Acute management of life-threatening bleed/bleeding
   1. Hold dabigatran
   2. Obtain coagulation screen (most useful monitoring labs include: activated partial thromboplastin time (aPTT), thrombin time (TT), ecarin clotting time (ECT), and diluted thrombin time test (dTT; e.g. Hemoclot®))[6]
      a. If aPTT and TT are normal, then dabigatran levels are low or absent
      b. If aPTT and TT are prolonged, anticoagulant effect may be present
      c. If ECT or dTT is normal, then anticoagulant effect is absent
   3. Provide supportive care (fluids, RBCs, control of bleeding source, and hemodynamic support as needed)
   4. Consider Idarucizumab (Praxbind®)
      a. Dose: 5 g (administered as two separate 2.5 g doses no more than 15 minutes apart). If coagulation parameters (e.g. aPTT) re-elevate and clinically relevant bleeding occurs or if a second emergency surgery/urgent procedure is required and patient has elevated coagulation parameters, may consider administration of an additional 5 g (limited data to support)
         i. Prior to administration, flush preexisting IV line with sodium chloride 0.9%. Administer dose undiluted as an IV bolus either via syringe or as an infusion by hanging the vials. Infusion of each vial should take no longer than 5–10 minutes. Begin administration within 1 hour of removing solution from the vial.
         ii. Onset: Within minutes
         iii. Duration: Usually at least 24 hours
   5. Oral activated charcoal may be useful if last dose taken within 2 hours
   6. Consider hemodialysis if feasible (especially if patient has renal impairment)
      a. Active dabigatran concentrations can be reduced by 50–60% after 4 hours of hemodialysis
   7. Monitoring:[7]
      a. TT: Measurements of "peak levels" will be very prolonged or unmeasurable. Only useful for monitoring "trough levels". Qualitative measurement

  b. aPTT: Normal aPTT usually suggests little anticoagulant activity, but even a mildly elevated level could be associated with clinically relevant levels of dabigatran

  c. ECT: Provides a direct measure of the activity of dabigatran. A normal level generally excludes anticoagulant activity.

  d. dTT: Gold standard. Hemoclot® is a dTT developed for dabigatran use. Displays a linear relationship with dabigatran concentration. A normal dTT indicates no clinically relevant anticoagulant effect of dabigatran. A trough dTT (measured $\geq$12 h after the previous dose) of >200 ng/ml dabigatran plasma concentration (i.e. dTT approximately 0.65 seconds) is associated with an increased risk of bleeding

c. Rivaroxaban (Xarelto®)

 i. FXa inhibitor

 ii. Half-life: 5 to 9 hours

 iii. Discontinue 24 hours prior to a procedure

 iv. Acute management of life-threatening bleed/bleeding

  1. Hold rivaroxaban

  2. Obtain coagulation screen (most useful monitoring lab is Anti-FXa assay)

  3. Provide supportive care (fluids, RBCs, control of bleeding source, and hemodynamic support as needed)

  4. Oral activated charcoal may be given to help reduce absorption if last dose taken within 8 hours

  5. Consider giving non-activated 4-factor prothrombin complex concentrate (PCC), such as Beriplex® P/N or Kcentra® (off-label)[7,8]

   a. Dose: 25–50 IU/kg IV once

   b. Max infusion rate and dose will depend on brand of PCC

   c. There are limited data regarding the re-dosing of PCC for anticoagulation reversal, so the risks/benefits must be weighed carefully

  6. Monitoring:

   a. PT: Can detect presence of drug but results differ for different reagents. A normal PT in patients on rivaroxaban suggest very low drug levels

   b. Anti-Xa assays: Correlate with the concentration of FXa inhibitors; however, they must be calibrated for each individual drug in order to be of use

d. Warfarin (Coumadin®)[12–15]

 i. Inhibits factors II, VII, IX, and X

 ii. Half-life: 20 to 60 hours

 iii. Warfarin should be discontinued 1 to 5 days prior to a procedure, depending on the type of procedure, the anticipated bleeding risk, and the current international normalization ratio (INR)

 iv. Acute management of life-threatening bleed/bleeding

  1. Hold warfarin

  2. Provide fluid replacement and hemodynamic support as needed

Table 12.3 Beriplex® P/N and Kcentra® recommended dosing

Initial INR	Approximate dose* (ml/kg body weight)	Approximate dose IU (Factor IX)/kg
2–3.9	1	25
4–6	1.4	35
>6	2	50

*The single dose should not exceed 5000 IU (200 ml)

Table 12.4 Octaplex® recommended dosing

Initial INR	Approximate dose* (ml/kg body weight)
2–2.5	0.9–1.3
2.5–3	1.3–1.6
3–3.5	1.6–1.9
>3.5	>1.9

*The single dose should not exceed 3000 IU (120 ml)

3. Give vitamin K 5–10 mg IV slowly over 30 minutes (maximum infusion rate of 1 mg/min)
   a. Onset: 1 to 2 hours
   b. Peak effect: 12 to 14 hours
4. Give 4-factor PCC if available
   a. Dose: 25–50 IU/kg IV, once
   b. Max single dose and infusion rate depends on product:
      i. Octaplex®: 2–3 ml/min
      ii. Beriplex® P/N and Kcentra®: Not more than 3 IU/kg/min; max ~8 ml/min
   c. Dosing also depends on product (see Tables 12.3 and 12.4)
5. If 4-factor PCC is not available, give 3-factor PCC with fresh frozen plasma (FFP)
   a. Dose: 3-factor PCC 25–50 IU/kg once
   b. FFP at least 2 units (and repeat as required)
6. Recheck INR 30 minutes after PCC administration and again every 4 to 6 hours until INR normalized
   a. Owing to the long half-life, subsequent dosing is usually unnecessary
   b. If INR is still elevated after 6 hours and patient rebleeds, consider giving a subsequent dose of PCC (e.g. 25 IU/kg)
   c. There are limited data regarding the re-dosing of PCC, so the risks/benefits must be weighed carefully

II. Anticoagulants – parenteral agents
   a. Argatroban[12]
      i. Direct thrombin inhibitor

    ii. First-line option for anticoagulation in the presence of heparin-induced thrombocytopenia (HIT)

    iii. Dosing

        1. No initial bolus

        2. Initial IV infusion rate: 2 µg/kg/min

        3. Decrease initial infusion rate to 0.5–1.2 µg/kg/min in the presence of heart failure, anasarca, or multiple organ system failure

        4. Target aPTT 1.5–3 times baseline

    iv. Half-life: 40 to 50 minutes

    v. No direct antidote available

  b. Bivalirudin (Angiomax®)[12,16,17]

    i.   Direct thrombin inhibitor

    ii. Safe alternative to heparin in neuroendovascular procedures

    iii. Second-line option for anticoagulation in the presence of HIT

    iv. Dosing

        1. Neuroendovascular procedures

            a. Bolus: 0.6 mg/kg

            b. Initial IV infusion rate: 1.25 mg/kg/hr

            c. Target ACT: 300 to 350 seconds

            d. Additional boluses of 0.15 mg/kg can be given to attain target activated clotting time (ACT)

        2. Anticoagulation in the presence of possible or confirmed HIT

            a. No initial bolus

            b. Initial IV infusion rate: 0.15–0.20 mg/kg/hr

            c. Target aPTT: 1.5 to 2.5 times baseline

    v. Half-life: 25 minutes

    vi. No direct antidote available

  c. Fondaparinux (Arixtra®)[12]

    i.   Causes an antithrombin III-mediated selective inhibition of factor Xa

    ii. No effect on thrombin

    iii. Possible option for anticoagulation in the presence of HIT (limited evidence)

    iv. Case reports of fondaparinux-induced HIT

    v. Dosing

        1. Deep venous thrombosis (DVT) prophylaxis following surgery

            a. Fondaparinux 2.5 mg SUBQ once daily

        2. DVT and pulmonary embolism (PE) treatment

            a. 5 mg SUBQ once daily (weight <50 kg)

            b. 7.5 mg SUBQ once daily (weight 50 to 100 kg)

            c. 10 mg SUBQ once daily (weight >00 kg)

    vi. Half-life: 17 to 21 hours

    vii. No direct antidote available

    viii. Hemodialysis may increase fondaparinux clearance by 20%

d. Heparin[12]

    i. Forms a complex with antithrombin III to inactivate FXa and inhibit the formation of thrombin

    ii. Small amount of activity on factors IX, XI, and XII

    iii. Dosing

        1. DVT prophylaxis: 5000 units SUBQ three times a day

        2. IV – stroke (off-label)

            a. No bolus dose

            b. Initial infusion rate: 10–12 units/kg/hr

            c. Adjust dose to target aPTT (differs between institutions)

            d. Note: Most institutions have dosing and monitoring protocols

        3. Intra-arterial – stroke (off-label)

            a. Use caution in patients already receiving systemic anticoagulation

            b. Small doses may be considered for local effects

    iv. Effects can be partially reversed using protamine

        1. Administer 1 mg of protamine for every 100 mg of heparin

        2. Maximum dose of protamine is 50 mg

        3. Administer by slow IV infusion over 10 minutes

    v. HIT can be characterized by:

        1. Decrease in platelets by 50% from baseline

        2. Platelet count $<150 \times 10^3$/microliter

    vi. To diagnose HIT, must consider the timing of platelet decrease as related to initiation of heparin and previous heparin exposure, as well as other possible causes of thrombocytopenia

    vii. If HIT is suspected or confirmed with a platelet factor 4 (PF4) and/or serotonin release assay (SRA), heparin should be discontinued and an alternative anticoagulant started

e. Low-molecular-weight heparins (LMWHs)

    i. Inhibits FXa with minimal direct effect on factor II

    ii. Enoxaparin (Lovenox®) and dalteparin (Fragmin®)

    iii. Used for DVT prophylaxis and treatment of acute thrombotic conditions

    iv. Prophylaxis dosing

        1. Enoxaparin 40 mg SUBQ once a day

        2. Enoxaparin 30 mg SUBQ twice a day (hip or knee replacement surgery)

        3. Dalteparin 2500 or 5000 IU SUBQ once a day

    v. Acute thrombosis dosing

        1. Enoxaparin 1 mg/kg SUBQ twice a day

        2. Enoxaparin 1.5 mg/kg SUBQ once a day can be used for inpatient treatment of acute DVT or PE

    vi. Doses may need adjustments for renal insufficiency

    vii. Effects of LMWHs can be partially reversed by protamine

        1. Enoxaparin

        a. If ≤8 hours since last dose, administer 1 mg protamine per 1 mg enoxaparin

        b. If >8 hours since last dose, administer 0.5 mg protamine per 1 mg enoxaparin

  2. Dalteparin

        a. Administer 1 mg of protamine per 100 units of dalteparin

  3. If aPTT remains prolonged 2–4 hours after initial protamine dose, a second dose of 0.5 mg protamine per 1 mg enoxaparin or per 100 units dalteparin may be given

  viii. If HIT is suspected or confirmed with a PF4 and/or SRA, LMWHs should be discontinued and an alternative anticoagulant started

III. Antiplatelet agents

a. ADP (adenosine diphosphate) inhibitors[18,19]

  i. Bind to $P2Y_{12}$ class of ADP receptors (thienopyridine inhibitor)

    1. Irreversibly inhibit platelet activation and aggregation for the life of the platelet (about 7 days)

    2. Platelet transfusion may restore some platelet function

  ii. Clopidogrel (Plavix®)

    1. Half-life: 6 hours

    2. Dosing

        a. Loading dose: 300 mg or 600 mg PO once

        b. Maintenance dose: 75 mg PO once a day

  iii. Ticagrelor (Brilinta®)

    1. Half-life: 7 hours

    2. Dosing

        a. Loading dose: 180 mg PO once

        b. Maintenance dose: 90 mg PO twice a day

  iv. Prasugrel (Effient®)

    1. Half-life: 7 hours

    2. Only approved for use in acute coronary syndrome

    3. Limited evidence suggests prasugrel may be an alternative agent for patients who are clopidogrel-non-responders

    4. Patients may be at higher risk for hemorrhagic complications

    5. Dosing

        a. Loading dose: 60 mg PO once

        b. Maintenance dose: 10 mg PO once a day

b. Aspirin (acetylsalicylic acid, ASA)[18]

  i. Blocks cyclooxygenase-1 (COX-1), leading to inhibition of thromboxane A_2 (TXA_2)

    1. Irreversibly inhibits platelet aggregation for the life of the platelet (about 7 days)

  ii. Platelet transfusion may restore some platelet function

  iii. Typical dose: 75–325 mg PO once a day

c. Glycoprotein (GP) IIb/IIIa inhibitors

   i. Block the binding site for fibrinogen and vonWillebrand factor on GP IIb/IIIa

   ii. Inhibit platelet aggregation

   iii. Only approved for cardiovascular indications, including acute coronary syndrome and percutaneous coronary intervention

   iv. Both eptifibatide and Abciximab have shown to be effective when used as adjunctive therapy for the management of thromboembolic complications in neuroendovascular procedures

   v. Eptifibatide (Integrilin®)[20]

     1. Half-life: 2.5 hours

     2. Dosing

       a. Loading dose: 180 µg/kg

       b. Continuous infusion: 2 µg/kg/min

       c. Reduce continuous infusion to 1 µg/kg/min if CrCl <50 ml/min

   vi. Abciximab (Reopro®)[21,22]

     1. Half-life: 10 to 30 minutes

     2. Dosing

       a. Loading dose: 0.25 mg/kg

       b. Continuous infusion: 0.125 µg/kg/min (max 10 µg/min) for 12 hours

     3. High rate of intracranial hemorrhage with Abciximab has been observed

     4. Platelet transfusion may partially restore platelet function

IV. Thrombolytic agents[23]

a. Alteplase (Activase®)

   i. Tissue plasminogen activator (tPA)

   ii. Binds to fibrin, enhances conversion of plasminogen to plasmin, and creates local fibrinolysis

   iii. Half-life <5 minutes

   iv. Dosing – stroke

     1. Intravenous

       a. Alteplase 0.9 mg/kg (not to exceed 90 mg total dose)

         i. Administer 10% of total dose as IV bolus over 1 minute

         ii. Administer the remaining dose as IV infusion over 60 minutes

       b. Approved for use within 3 hours of onset of stroke symptoms

       c. In some clinical conditions, may consider extending the time frame to 4.5 hours from the onset of stroke symptoms (off-label)

     2. Intra-arterial (off-label)

       a. Usually patients have received IV tPA prior to intervention

       b. Small doses (i.e. 1–5 mg) may be considered for local thrombolysis

   v. Reversal

     1. Reversal of tPA may result in thrombosis

     2. No reversal needed 2 hours post tPA infusion

     3. If fibrinogen <100 mg/dl administer cryoprecipitate 0.10 units/kg IV once

    4. Repeat fibrinogen in 1 hour; if <100 again, repeat cryoprecipitate dose IV once

    5. Administer aminocaproic acid (Amicar®) 1 g/10 kg IV in 250 cc NS over 1 hour

Calcium channel blockers[24]

I. Nicardipine (Cardene®)

  a. Cerebral vasospasm – intra-arterial (off-label)

    i. Wide range of doses used in clinical studies

    ii. Usual total doses of 5 to 40 mg

    iii. Onset of action: 1 minute

    iv. Duration of action

      1. Initial redistribution: 2 to 5 minute effective half-life after bolus of 0.25–2 mg

      2. Elimination half-life: 14.4 hours

  b. Warning: Use with caution in patients with coronary artery disease, heart failure, or aortic stenosis (contraindicated in advanced aortic stenosis)

II. Verapamil[25,26]

  a. Radial Artery Cocktail (off-label to prevent arterial vasospasm with radial artery access)

    i. Usual dose: 2.5 mg diluted in NS and administered slowly IV

    ii. Onset of action: 1 to 5 minutes

    iii. Duration of action: 10 to 20 minutes

    iv. Half-life after single dose: 3 to 7 hours

  b. Cerebral vasospasm – intra-arterial (off-label)

    i. Usual dose: 1 to 20 mg per arterial distribution

  c. Warning: Use with caution in patients with poor left ventricular function or conduction disturbances

III. Toxicology[27,28]

  a. Treatment for either nicardipine or verapamil poisoning

  b. Mild hypotension (treatment)

    i. IV fluids

  c. Hypotension and bradycardia (treatment)

    i. Standard ACLS treatment (O_2, IV line, and fluids)

    ii. Atropine 0.5–1 mg IV every 2 to 3 minutes (max 3 mg)

    iii. Calcium (off-label to improve hemodynamics in calcium channel blocker toxicity)

      1. 10 ml calcium chloride 10% IV or 30 ml calcium gluconate 10% IV over 10 minutes. May repeat dose every 15–20 minutes

        a. Monitor ionized calcium after three doses IV calcium

    iv. Vasopressors[29]: See "Vasopressors" section for standard dosing recommendations. Much higher doses than standard recommendations (i.e. standard references) may be required

    v. Glucagon (off-label for calcium channel blocker and beta-blocker toxicity)

      1. 50–150 µg/kg (3–10 mg) IV up to cumulative dose of 10 mg. Repeat every 3 to 5 minutes as necessary

      2. If there is a favorable result, place on IV continuous infusion at 5–10 mg/hr (diluted in D5W)

      3. Rapid onset of action (rarely longer than 15 minutes)

      4. A potent emetic which increases aspiration risk with bolus doses greater than 50 µg/kg

        a. Metoclopramide and serotonin antagonists are often used

        b. Hyperglycemia and hypokalemia can be expected

    vi. High-dose insulin and dextrose[30] (off-label for calcium channel blocker and beta-blocker toxicity)

      1. Insulin 1 unit/kg IV bolus followed by an IV infusion of 0.5 to 1 unit/kg/hr; titrate in 1 to 2 unit/kg/hr increments every 10 to 15 minutes up to10 units/kg/hr to achieve clinical response

      2. Administer 50 ml dextrose 50% IV bolus if initial blood glucose <200 mg/dl. In all patients, administer 10% dextrose infusion IV starting at 100–250 ml/hr. Maintain blood glucose greater than 100 mg/dl

        a. If central line available, may use 50% dextrose infusion IV to avoid fluid overload

        b. Monitor blood glucose every 10 minutes initially, then every 30 to 60 minutes once glucose is stable

      3. Onset: 5 to 45 minutes

      4. Maintain serum potassium >3 mmol/l and <4.5 mmol/l

      5. Monitor magnesium and phosphorus concentrations

      6. Dextrose supplementation may be needed for up to 24 hours after insulin therapy stopped due to elevated insulin levels

      7. An attempt to wean off vasopressors should be considered while on high-dose insulin therapy

    vii. Lipid emulsion[3] (off-label for local anesthetic, calcium channel blocker, and beta-blocker toxicity)

      1. See dosing and administration information in "Anesthetics, local" section above, under lipid emulsion

    viii. Extracorporeal life support

Contrast media (IV)[31]

Management of acute reactions to contrast media

I. All reactions

    a. Maintain IV access

    b. Monitor vital signs

    c. Provide supplemental oxygen as needed

II. Bronchospasm

    a. Albuterol

        i. Two puffs via metered-dose inhaler (90 μg/inhalation)

        ii. 2.5 mg via nebulizer (2.5 mg/0.5 ml)

        iii. May repeat every 15 minutes for three doses

    b. Epinephrine (1:1,000 dilution) 0.3 mg IM (moderate)

    c. Epinephrine (1:10,000 dilution) 0.3 mg IV (severe)

        i. Administer slowly into a running saline infusion

        ii. May repeat every 5 to 15 minutes up to a total dose of 1 mg

III. Erythema (diffuse)

    a. Normotensive

        i. No additional treatment usually required

    b. Hypotensive

        i. NS or LR IV bolus 500–1000 ml

        ii. Epinephrine (1:10,000 dilution) 0.3 mg IV

            1. Administer slowly into a running saline infusion

            2. May repeat every 5 to 15 minutes up to a total dose of 1 mg

        iii. Epinephrine (1:1000 dilution) 0.3 mg IM (if no IV access)

IV. Hives

    a. Diphenhydramine 50 mg PO, IV (over 1 to 2 minutes), or IM

    b. Epinephrine (1:1000 dilution) 0.3 mg IM

V. Hypoglycemia

    a. If patient can safely swallow, administer 15 g oral glucose

    b. If patient cannot safely swallow

        i. 50% dextrose 25 g IV over 2 minutes

        ii. Glucagon 1 mg IM or SUBQ

VI. Hypotension

    a. Elevate legs at least 60 degrees

    b. NS or LR IV bolus 500–1000 ml

    c. Bradycardia with continued hypotension

        i. Consider atropine 1 mg IV

    d. Tachycardia with continued hypotension

        i. Consider epinephrine (1:10,000 dilution) 0.3 mg IV

            1. Administer slowly into a running saline infusion

            2. May repeat every 5 to 15 minutes up to a total dose of 1 mg

        ii. IM administration is not preferred in patients with hypotension as absorption may be inadequate due to decreased perfusion in the extremities

VII. Laryngeal edema

    a. Epinephrine (1:10,000 dilution) 0.3 mg IV

        i.   Administer slowly into a running saline infusion

        ii. May repeat every 5 to 15 minutes up to a total dose of 1 mg

    b. Epinephrine (1:1000 dilution) 0.3 mg IM

VIII. Pulmonary edema

    a. Elevate head of bed

    b. Furosemide 40 mg IV over 2 minutes

IX. Pulseless and unresponsive

    a. Follow standard ACLS protocols

X. Reaction rebound prevention

    a. IV corticosteroids are not useful for the acute treatment of allergic reactions, but may help to prevent short-term recurrence

    b. Hydrocortisone 5 mg/kg (max 200 mg) IV over 1 to 2 minutes

    c. Methylprednisolone 1 mg/kg (max 40 mg) IV over 1 to 2 minutes

Magnesium sulfate[32]

Intra-arterial in combination with nicardipine for cerebral vasospasm (off-label)

I.   Dilute magnesium sulfate 1 g (2 ml) in 28 ml of NS (final concentration 33.3 mg/ml)

II. Inject 0.25 to 1 g intra-arterially through microcatheter per vessel

    a. Usual recommended max infusion rate: 150 mg/min

III. Monitoring parameters: magnesium serum levels and respiratory rate

IV. Use with caution in patients with renal impairment, myasthenia gravis, or other neuromuscular diseases

V. Treat magnesium-induced hypotension with IV fluids, and dopamine or norepinephrine if unresponsive to fluids

Osmotic agents

For intracranial hypertension or cerebral edema

I.   Mannitol 20% or 25%

    a. Administer 0.25–1 g/kg dose IV over 20 to 30 minutes

    b. May repeat every 6 hours

    c. Maintain serum osmolality <300–320 mOsm/kg

    d. Monitor renal function

II. Sodium chloride 23.4%[33] (off-label)

    a. Administer 30 ml IV through a central line over 20 minutes

    b. May cause hypotension if injected too rapidly

Sedation

I. Benzodiazepines

    a. Lorazepam (Ativan®)

        i. Usual initial IV dose: 2 mg, or 0.044 mg/kg, whichever is smaller

            1. Administer 15 minutes prior to procedure for optimal effect, measured as lack of recall

            2. Larger doses of up to 0.05 mg/kg, up to a total of 4 mg, IV may be administered in those patients in whom a greater likelihood of lack of recall would be beneficial

            3. Doses of other injectable central nervous system (CNS) depressant drugs ordinarily should be reduced

        ii. IV administration

            1. Must be diluted with equal volume of compatible diluent (sterile water for injection, NS, D5W)

            2. Do not inject IV faster than 2 mg/min

        iii. Elimination half-life: 14 hours

        iv. Pregnancy Category D

    b. Midazolam (Versed®)

        i. Preprocedural sedation in healthy adults below 60 years of age

            1. Midazolam 1 to 2.5 mg IV over at least 2 minutes

                a. Reduce dose by 30% if narcotics or other CNS depressants are also used

        ii. Preprocedural sedation in patients age 60 or older, and debilitated or chronically ill patients

            1. Midazolam 1 to 1.5 mg IV over at least 2 minutes

                a. Reduce dose by 50% if narcotics or other CNS depressants are also used

        iii. Administration: Dilute to 0.5 mg/ml in D5W or NS for IV use

        iv. Pharmacokinetics

            1. Amnestic onset within 1 to 5 minutes

            2. Duration of action: usually less than 2 hours

            3. Elimination half-life: 1.8 to 6.4 hours (mean approximately 3 hours)

            4. Clearance reduced in elderly, congestive heart failure, liver disease, or conditions which diminish cardiac output and hepatic outflow

        v. Pregnancy Category D

    c. Paradoxical reactions to benzodiazepines[34]

        i. Agitation, emotional release, excitement, excessive movement

        ii. Occurs in less than 1% of patients

        iii. Predisposing factors include young and advanced age, alcoholism, and psychiatric disorders

        iv. Flumazenil can reverse this effect

    d. Antidote: Flumazenil rapidly reverses the sedation effect (See dosing information in "Anticonvulsants for status epilepticus" section under Benzodiazepines, Toxicology)

II. Propofol[35–38]

    a. Procedural sedation

        i. Recommended initial dose: 1 mg/kg IV followed by 0.5 mg/kg every 3 to 5 minutes as needed for sedation

        ii. Intubation may be necessary

    b. See contraindications, warnings, and administration instructions in "Anticonvulsants for status epilepticus" section under Propofol

Vasopressors[39,40]

I. Dobutamine (direct-acting positive inotrope, mild chronotrope)

    a. Cardiac decompensation: 0.5 to 20 µg/kg/min IV (max 40 µg/kg/min)

    b. Post cardiac arrest (American Heart Association [AHA] ACLS Guidelines, off-label) 5–10 µg/kg/min; titrate as needed

    c. Onset of action: 1 to 2 minutes

    d. Plasma half-life: 2 minutes

    e. May increase heart rate

    f. May exacerbate ventricular ectopy

    g. Ineffective therapeutically in the presence of severe aortic stenosis

II. Dopamine (positive inotrope and chronotrope; vasopressor)

    a. Hypotension, low cardiac output, poor perfusion of vital organs, or shock: Initiate at 2 to 5 µg/kg/min; titrate up to 20–50 µg/kg/min as needed

    b. Symptomatic bradycardia (AHA ACLS Guidelines, off-label): 2–10 µg/kg/min; titrate to response

    c. Inotropic and chronotropic effects predominate at 2–10 µg/kg/min IV infusion rates

    d. Vasopressor effects predominate at 10–20 µg/kg/min IV infusion rates

    e. Onset of action: within 5 minutes

    f. Plasma half-life: 2 minutes

    g. May exacerbate ventricular ectopy

    h. Initiate with 1/10 the usual dopamine dose in patients taking monoamine oxidase inhibitors within 2–3 weeks prior to dopamine initiation

    i. Hypotension may occur at lower IV infusion rates

    j. Infuse into a central line or large vein whenever possible to prevent extravasation into adjacent tissue

        i. If tissue ischemia occurs, mix 5–10 mg phentolamine (adrenergic blocking agent) in 10–15 ml NS and infiltrate ischemic area with phentolamine solution as soon as possible. Use a fine hypodermic needle. Do not exceed 0.1 to 0.2 mg/kg (5 mg total). If dose is effective, normal skin color should return to the blanched area within 1 hour

III. Epinephrine (positive inotrope, vasopressor; when given by slow IV injection, vasodilation of the skeletal muscle vasculature occurs)

    a. Asystole, pulseless arrest, pulseless VT/VF (AHA ACLS Guidelines, off-label): Epinephrine 1 mg IV every 3 to 5 minutes until return of spontaneous circulation

b. Via endotracheal tube (off-label): 2 to 2.5 mg diluted in 5 to 10 ml sterile water or NS
c. Usual IV infusion dose: 2 to 10 µg/min
d. Anaphylaxis:

   i. 0.3 to 0.5 mg IM or SUBQ (1 mg/ml concentration), repeated every 5 to 10 minutes as needed
   ii. AHA ACLS Guidelines (off-label): 0.2 to 0.5 mg IM every 5 to 15 minutes as needed
   iii. For anaphylactic shock where patient is not in cardiac arrest: 0.05 to 0.1 mg IV has been used. An IV infusion of 5 to 15 µg/min may also be considered

e. Asthma (AHA ACLS dosing, off-label): 0.01 mg/kg divided into three doses of approximately 0.3 mg SUBQ at 20 minute intervals (1 mg/ml concentration)
f. Symptomatic bradycardia as a second line treatment (AHA off-label dosing): Initial dose 2–10 µg/min IV and titrate to response
g. Symptomatic hypotension (AHA ACLS Guidelines, off-label): 0.1 to 0.5 µg/kg/min IV for severe hypotension. Titrate to response
h. May exacerbate ventricular ectopy
i. Use caution in patients taking monoamine oxidase inhibitors
j. Infuse into a central line or large vein whenever possible to prevent extravasation into adjacent tissue

   i. See phentolamine dosing under dopamine section (section II above)

IV. Norepinephrine (positive inotrope, strong vasopressor)

a. Hypotension, acute

   i. Norepinephrine 8 to 12 µg/min IV
   ii. AHA ACLS Guidelines (off-label): Initial dose 0.1 to 0.5 µg/kg/min (as base) IV; titrate to desired effect

b. Post cardiac arrest (AHA ACLS Guidelines, off-label): 0.1 to 0.5 µg/kg/min (as base) IV; titrate to desired effect
c. Should be diluted in D5W or D5W-NS. Dextrose solutions reduce drug oxidation. Administration in NS alone is not recommended
d. Reduce infusions of norepinephrine gradually; avoid abrupt withdrawal
e. Use extreme caution if patient receiving monoamine oxidase inhibitors or antidepressants of the triptyline or imipramine types. Severe, prolonged hypertension may result
f. Infuse into a central line or large vein whenever possible to prevent extravasation into adjacent tissue

   i. See phentolamine dosing under dopamine section (section II above)

V. Phenylephrine (vasopressor)

a. Severe hypotension and shock

   i. Initiate IV infusion at 0.5 µg/kg/min. Titrate to desired response, up to 6 µg/kg/min IV
   ii. AHA ACLS Guidelines (off-label): phenylephrine 0.5 to 2 µg/kg/min IV

   b. Perioperative setting (surgical procedures with either neuraxial anesthesia or general anesthesia)

      i. Phenylephrine 0.5 to 1.4 µg/kg/min IV titrated to blood pressure goal

      ii. Intravenous bolus: 50–250 µg IV (usual dose 50–100 µg)

   c. Onset of effect IV: immediate

   d. Duration of effect IV: 15–20 minutes

   e. Produces vasoconstriction with reflex bradycardia (no beta-receptor effects)

   f. Reduce dose when used with monoamine oxidase inhibitors

   g. Tricyclic antidepressants and oxytocic drugs may potentiate phenylephrine effects

   h. Infuse into a central line or large vein whenever possible to prevent extravasation into adjacent tissue

      i. See phentolamine dosing under dopamine section (section II above)

VI. Vasopressin[41] (vasopressor – off-label)

   a. Vasodilatory shock/septic shock refractory to fluids and norepinephrine

      i. Initiate at 0.01 to 0.04 units/min IV infusion

   b. Onset of action: 1 to 3 minutes

   c. Duration of action: 20 to 30 minutes

   d. Produces vasoconstriction without inotropic or chronotropic effects

      i. Stimulates V_{1A} receptors on vascular smooth muscle

   e. Wean off catecholamine vasopressor(s) prior to weaning off IV vasopressin

   f. Wean off IV vasopressin slowly

   g. Doses greater than 0.04 units/min may induce cardiac ischemia and/or bradycardia

   h. Infuse through central line

   i. Monitor fluid and electrolyte status

   j. Infuse into a central line or large vein whenever possible to prevent extravasation into adjacent tissue

      i. See phentolamine dosing under dopamine section (section II above)

References

1. Patanwala AE, Keim SM, Erstad BL. Intravenous opioids for severe acute pain in the emergency department. *Ann Pharmacother*. 2010;44: 1800–09.

2. McDowell TS, Durieux ME. Pharmacology of local anesthetics. In: Hemmings HC, Hopkins PM, eds. *Foundations of anesthesia*. 2nd edn. Mosby: Elsevier; 2006. Available at http://sciencedirect.com. Accessed May 2013.

3. Weinberg GL. Lipid emulsion infusion: Resuscitation for local anesthetic and other drug overdose. *Anesthesiology*. 2012;117:180–7.

4. Hirsch LJ, Gaspard N. Status epilepticus. *Epilepsy*. 2013;19(3):767–94.

5. Brophy GM, Bell R, Claassen J, *et al.* Guidelines for the evaluation and management of status epilepticus. *Neuro Crit Care*. 2012;17(1):3–23.

6. Huisman MV, Lip GY, Diener HC, *et al.* Dabigatran etexilate for stroke prevention

in patients with atrial fibrillation: resolving uncertainties in routine practice. *Thromb Haemost.* 2012;107(5):838–47.

7. Marlu R, Hodaj E, Paris A *et al.* Effect of non-specific reversal agents on anticoagulant activity of dabigatran and rivaroxaban: a randomized crossover ex vivo study in health volunteers. *Thromb Haemost.* 2012;108(2):217–24.

8. Eerenberg ES, Kamphuisen PW, Sijpkens MK, *et al.* Reversal of rivaroxaban and dabigatran by prothrombin complex concentrate: a randomized, placebo-controlled, crossover study in healthy subjects. *Circulation.* 2011;124(14):1573–9.

9. Dager WE, Gosselin RC, Roberts AJ. Reversing dabigatran in life-threatening bleeding occurring during cardiac ablation with factor eight inhibitor bypassing activity. *Crit Care Med.* 2013;41(5):e42–e46.

10. Khoo TL, Weatherburn C, Kershaw G *et al.* The use of FEIBA® in the correction of coagulation abnormalities induced by dabigatran. *Int J Lab Hematol.* 2013;35(2):222–4.

11. Zhou W, Schwarting S, Illanes S, *et al.* Hemostatic therapy in experimental intracerebral hemorrhage associated with the direct thrombin inhibitor dabigatran. *Stroke.* 2011;42(12):3594–9.

12. American College of Chest Physicians. Antithrombotic therapy and prevention of thrombosis, 9th edn: American College of Chest Chysicians evidence-based clinical practice guidelines. *Chest.* 2012; 141(2 Suppl):1S–801S.

13. Makris M, Van Veen JJ, Tait CR, *et al.* Guideline on the management of bleeding in patients on antithrombotic agents. *Br J Haematol.* 2013;160(1):35–46.

14. Cabral KP, Fraser GL, Duprey J, *et al.* Prothrombin complex concentrates to reverse warfarin-induced coagulopathy in patients with intracranial bleeding. *Clin Neurol Neurosurg.* 2013;115 (6):770–4.

15. Woo CH, Patel N, Conell C, *et al.* Rapid warfarin reversal in the setting of intracranial hemorrhage: a comparison of plasma, recombinant activated factor vii,

and prothrombin complex concentrate. *World Neurosurg.* 2014;81(1):110–5.

16. Georgiadis A, Shah Q, Suri MF, Qureshi AI. Adjunct bivalirudin dosing protocol for neuro-endovascular procedures. *J Vasc Interv Neurol.* 2008;1(2):50–53.

17. Hassan AE, Memon MZ, Georgiadis AL, *et al.* Safety and tolerability of high-intensity anticoagulation with bivalirudin during neuroendovascular procedures. *Neurocrit Care.* 2011;15(1):96–100.

18. Fiorella D. Anti-thrombotic medications for the neurointerventionist: aspirin and clopidogrel. *J Neurointerv Surg.* 2010;2 (1):44–9.

19. Akbari SH, Reynolds MR, Kadkhodayan Y, Cross DT III, Moran CJ. Hemorrhagic complications after prasugrel (Effient) therapy for vascular neurointerventional procedures. *J Neurointerv Surg.* 2012;5(4):337–43.

20. Dumont TM, Kan P, Snyder KV, *et al.* Adjunctive use of eptifibatide for complication management during elective neuroendovascular procedures. *J Neurointerv Surg.* 2013;5(3):226–30.

21. Velat GJ, Burry MV, Eskioglu E, *et al.* The use of Abciximab in the treatment of acute cerebral thromboembolic events during neuroendovascular procedures. *Surg Neurol.* 2006;65(4):352–8.

22. Walsh RD, Barrett KM, Aguilar MI, *et al.* Intracranial hemorrhage following neuroendovascular procedures with Abciximab is associated with high mortality: a multicenter series. *Neurocrit Care.* 2011;15(1):85–95.

23. Abdihalim MM, Hassan AE, Qureshi AI. Off-label use of drugs and devices in the neuroendovascular suite. *Am J Neuroradiol.* 2013;34(11):2054–63.

24. Weant KA, Ramsey CN, Cook, AM. Role of intrarterial therapy for cerebral vasospasm secondary to aneurysmal subarachnoid hemorrhage. *Pharmacotherapy.* 2010; 30(4):405–17.

25. Ruiz-Salmeron RJ, Mora R, Masotti M, Betriu A. Assessment of the efficacy of phentolamine to prevent radial artery

spasm during cardiac catheterization procedures: a randomized study comparing phentolamine vs. verapamil. *Catheter Cardiovasc Interv.* 2005;66(2):192–8.

26. Sehy JV, Holloway WE, Lin SP, *et al.* Improvement in angiographic cerebral vasospasm after intra-arterial verapamil administration. *Am J Neuroradiol.* 2013;31:1923–8.

27. Marraffa JM, Cohen V, Howland MA. Antidotes for toxicological emergencies: A practical review. *Am J Hosp Phar.* 2012;69(3):199–212.

28. Kerns W II. Management of β-adrenergic blocker and calcium channel antagonist toxicity. *Emerg Med Clin North Am.* 2007;25:309–31.

29. Levine M, Curry SC, Padilla-Jones A, Ruha AM. Critical care management of verapamil and diltiazem overdose with a focus on vasopressors: A 25 year experience at a single center. *Ann Emerg Med.* 2013;62 (3):252–8.

30. Holger JS, Stellpflug SJ, Cole JB, Harris CR, Engebretsen KM. High-dose insulin: A consecutive case series in toxin-induced cardiogenic shock. *Clin Tox.* 2011;49: 653–658.

31. American College of Radiology. *Manual on Contrast Media* 9th edn. Reston, VA: ACR; 2013.

32. Shah QA, Memon MZ, Suri MFK, *et al.* Super-selective intra-arterial magnesium sulfate in combination with nicardipine for the treatment of cerebral vasospasm in patients with subarachnoid hemorrhage. *Neurocrit Care.* 2009;11:190–8.

33. Lazaridis C, Neyens R, Bodle J, DeSantis SM. High-osmolarity saline in neurocritical care: Systematic review and meta-analysis. *Crit Care Med.* 2013;41(5):1353–40.

34. Mancuso CE, Tanzi MG, Gabay M. Paradoxical reactions to benzodiazepines: Literature review and treatment options. *Pharmacotherapy* 2004;24(9): 1177–85.

35. Miner JR, Danahy M, Moch A, Biros M. Randomized clinical trial of etomidate versus propofol for procedural sedation in the emergency department. *Ann Emerg Med* 2005;49(1):15–22.

36. Burton JH, Miner JR, Shipley ER, *et al.* Propofol for emergency department procedural sedation and analgesia: a tale of three centers. *Acad Emerg Med* 2006;13(1): 24–30.

37. Miner JR, Bachman A, Kosman L, *et al.* Assessment of the onset and persistence of amnesia during procedural sedation with propofol. *Acad Emerg Med* 2005;12(6): 491–6.

38. Miner JR, Biros M, Krieg S, *et al.* Randomized clinical trial of propofol versus methohexital for procedural sedation during fracture and dislocation reduction in the emergency department. *Acad Emerg Med* 2003; 10:931–7.

39. 2010 American Heart Association Guidelines for Cardiopulmonary Resuscitation and Emergency Cardiovascular Care. *Circulation.* 2010; 122(18)(suppl 3):S640–S933.

40. ECC Committee, Subcommittee and Task Forces of the American Heart Association. 2005 American Heart Association guidelines for cardiopulmonary resuscitation and emergency cardiovascular care. *Circulation.* 2005; 112(24)(suppl): IV1–IV203.

41. Bauer SR, Lam SW. Arginine vasopressin for the treatment of septic shock in adults. *Pharmacotherapy.* 2010;30(10): 1057–71.

Chapter 13

Radiation-related complications of neuroendovascular procedures

Venkata K. Lanka and Gustavo J. Rodriguez

In the early 1900s, medical radiologists alerted their colleagues to the risks of radiation and the possibility of some cancers and cataracts being caused by fluoroscopy use. They recognized the need for safe practices to prevent such health hazards. In recent years, fluoroscopically guided interventional procedures have increased greatly in Europe and the United States because of their tremendous advantage over invasive surgical procedures[1]. Interventional fluoroscopically guided procedures are minimally invasive, but are associated with radiation exposure for both patients and caregivers[2]. Neuroendovascular practitioners use the fluoroscopic unit, which produces ionizing radiation, to help to guide the manipulation of catheters and devices to the target lesion. To avoid undesirable radiation effects – including both acute skin injuries and latent effects such as cataracts and cancer – there is a need for a detailed understanding of radiation physics, biological effects, radiation-related complications, and ways of controlling exposures to patients and healthcare providers.

Ionizing versus non-ionizing radiation

High-energy electromagnetic radiation – that is, radiation beyond the ultraviolet region of the spectrum, such as X-rays and gamma-rays – possesses sufficient energy to eject an electron from its orbit, producing ionized atoms and molecules. It is thus known as ionizing radiation[3] (Figure 13.1). Radiation at frequencies less than the ultraviolet region of the electromagnetic spectrum does not possess enough energy to eject an electron from the

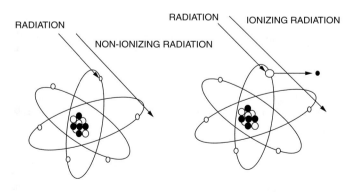

RADIATION

RADIATION   IONIZING RADIATION

NON-IONIZING RADIATION

Figure 13.1 Non-ionizing and ionizing radiation

Complications of Neuroendovascular Procedures and Bailout Techniques, ed. Rakesh Khatri, Gustavo J. Rodriguez, Jean Raymond and Adnan I. Qureshi. Published by Cambridge University Press. © Cambridge University Press 2016.

orbit of an atom and is called non-ionizing radiation (e.g. visible light, infrared light, TV and radio broadcast waves, and cell phone radiation).

X-ray production, voltage (kVp) and current (mA)

X-rays are produced when high-speed electrons from a filament hit a metal target in a vacuum tube. X-rays are a short-wavelength, high-energy part of the electromagnetic spectrum (Figure 13.2).

When X-rays are used in interventional procedures, some of the radiation is absorbed within the body while some emerges on the other side of the body, where a film is exposed to the radiation (or the radiation is absorbed by a digital detector) to create an image. The strength of the X-rays is described in two terms: voltage and current.

The voltage, which is related to the energy of the X-rays, affects the image contrast, while the current affects the density. Voltage is expressed as kilovoltage peak (kVp) and ranges from 60 to 125 kVp in fluoroscopy equipment. For higher kVp, the electrons are attracted more strongly to the target and have higher kinetic energy. This produces an X-ray emission spectrum with higher peak energy, reducing the differentiation between tissues (contrast).

The current in an X-ray tube is expressed in mA (milliamperes), which is the flow of electrons through the tube. The current controls the rate at which X-rays are produced. Fluoroscopic procedures are performed at tube currents of up to 5 mA. Higher mA values indicate that more electrons are striking the tungsten target, therefore producing more X-rays.

The higher the tube current or mA, the higher is the radiation dose to the patient. A change in the X-ray tube current does not affect the ultimate X-ray image contrast, but a change in the tube voltage (kVp) does.

Image contrast is dependent on the number of photons that are absorbed by the different densities inside the patient. The image quality, however, is dependent on how many X-rays reach the film. The total number of X-ray photons produced at a set kVp depends directly on the product of mA and exposure time, also known as mA-s. The goal in imaging is to keep the mA as low as possible and the kVp as high as possible, thereby negotiating between image quality (contrast) and radiation dose to the patient.

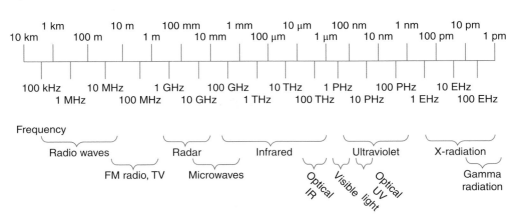

Figure 13.2 Electromagnetic spectrum

Radiation quantities and units

The radiation absorbed by the body contributes to the "radiation dose" to the patient. One joule of energy deposited in a kilogram of matter or tissue is termed a gray (Gy), and a milligray (mGy) is 1/1000 of a Gy. Another unit used to quantify radiation exposures is the sievert (Sv) or millisievert (mSv). A sievert is the dose equivalent which predicts biological effectiveness; it is the product of the absorbed dose (Gy) and the radiation quality factor, which is approximately equivalent to one (1) in the case of diagnostic X-rays[4]. Since the sensitivity of different organs of the body varies, the effective dose for each organ is measured by multiplying the dose equivalent and the organ weighting factor, as indicated in International Commission on Radiation Protection (ICRP) reports, in units of Sv or mSv.

Peak skin dose (PSD) is the highest radiation dose received at any area of the patient's skin, and it is very difficult to measure[5]. As an alternative methodology similar to the PSD, dose area product (DAP) was developed to measure the dose to the area of the skin. DAP is the product of the dose in air (air KERMA; see below), in Gy, and the exposed area of the skin in square centimeters (cm^2). DAP is used to measure radiation output from fluoroscopy, in units of Gy-cm^2 or mGy-cm^2, and may be used to estimate total energy delivered to the patient during a procedure. Kinetic energy released in matter (KERMA) is the amount of energy transferred from an X-ray beam to the charged particles per unit mass in the medium of interest. Air KERMA, measured in the units of Gy, is essentially the energy deposited in air at the position of interest. If we know the air KERMA measured at a point surface of the skin (entrance skin exposure), the absorbed dose in the tissue will be just about equal to the air KERMA. For diagnostic radiographs, air KERMA is the dose delivered to that volume of air. The KERMA–area product (KAP) is also known as DAP[6].

Interpreting DAP measurements is very difficult. DAP may not be used to evaluate skin injury but provides cumulative skin dose at the interventional reference point (IRP).

As shown in Figure 13.3, the relationship between the cumulative skin dose (DAP) and the PSD is highly variable. However, for estimating the PSD, the Joint Commission, a hospital accreditation agency in the United States, recommends calculating skin dose based on a fraction, say 75%, of the cumulative dose (DAP) measurements. In the RAD-IR study, the relationship between the PSD and DAP is stated as follows:

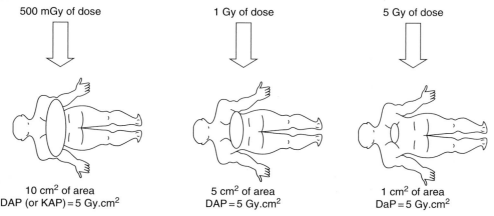

500 mGy of dose	1 Gy of dose	5 Gy of dose
10 cm^2 of area	5 cm^2 of area	1 cm^2 of area
DAP (or KAP) = 5 Gy.cm^2	DAP = 5 Gy.cm^2	DaP = 5 Gy.cm^2

Figure 13.3 Same DAP values for different skin areas

$$PSD(mGy) = 249 + 5.2\,DAP(Gy.cm^2) \tag{13.1}$$

This conversion formula is approximate and includes both computed tomography (CT) scan and fluoroscopy radiation exposures.

Biological effects of radiation

Radiation deposited in tissue results in ionization inside the living cells. Ionization is the removal of electrons from atoms, resulting in charged species known as ions. The ions formed can go on to react with other atoms or molecules in the cell, causing damage. An example of this would be an X-ray passing through a cell and causing the water molecules near the DNA to be ionized. The ions might react with and disrupt the DNA strands.

The biological effects are classified into two categories: stochastic, and deterministic or non-stochastic effects. Stochastic effects are those that occur by chance and consist primarily of cancer and genetic effects. They are associated with long-term, low-level (chronic) radiation exposures at any dose. At lower levels of exposure, damage can occur at the cellular level and may disrupt the control processes of the cell, giving rise to altered DNA and resulting in mutations and cancer.

Non-stochastic effects (acute effects) are those in which the severity of effects varies with the dose, for which a threshold dose exists (Table 13.1). Manifestation of the early effects of radiation exposure to skin, such as erythema or epilation, can occur with short-term, high-level exposure (referred to as acute dose), but only when certain threshold dose levels are exceeded[4]. At lower dose levels, the effects may not be induced because only a minimal number of cells are damaged. The threshold dose at which such effects will be seen varies with the patient and depends on individual patient conditions, previous exposure to radiation, and/or exposure to chemicals. The index of deterministic effective dose is the entrance skin dose (ESD), whereas the effective dose (a calculated value taking into account absorbed dose to all organs, radiation quality, and sensitivity of each organ to radiation) is the index of stochastic effects.

Fluoroscopy system

The purpose of fluoroscopy is to observe real-time motion of internal anatomical structures, and of catheters and devices. While performing procedures, the operator should

Table 13.1 Deterministic effects of ionizing radiation in neuroendovascular procedures

Tissue	Effect	Acute threshold dose (Gy)	Time to effect
Skin	Early transient erythema	2	Hours
	Temporary epilation	3	3–6 weeks
	Main erythema	6–8	3–6 weeks
	Permanent epilation	7	3–6 weeks
	Moist desquamation	10	4–6 weeks
	Dermal necrosis	18	>10 weeks
Eye	Lens opacity	2	Variable
	Cataract	5	>1 year
Parotid glands	Reduced function	3	Hours

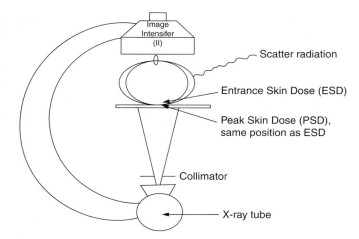

Figure 13.4 X-ray system

understand the machine parameters and be aware of the parameters that affect radiation exposure to the patient. A brief description of fluoroscopy is as follows:

A diverging uniform X-ray beam, produced from an X-ray tube (Figure 13.4), enters the patient's body and interacts with various tissues within the body. The X-rays that do not interact will exit from the patient as a non-uniform beam representing the image. The absorbed dose is greater where the X-rays enter the patient's body (i.e. ESD) and lower where the X-rays exit the body. For an average patient, the absorbed dose at the exit point is approximately 1% of the entrance absorbed dose. When the X-rays exit the patient, they are captured by an image intensifier. The image intensifier converts the X-ray into a "live" image that can be displayed on a monitor.

In conventional fluoroscopy, each image on the monitor represents 1/30 of a second, and the image may be blurred since the X-rays are produced continuously. In pulsed fluoroscopy, images are acquired using short pulses of X-rays with no X-ray production during the interval between pulses, enhancing the image quality; if 30 frames per second are utilized in a procedure, the average tube current and dose rate to the patient do not change, but the net result will be an increase in image quality. To reduce the dose, one may reduce the number of pulses per second.

Modern fluoroscopy systems are equipped with digital angiography (DA), digital subtraction angiography (DSA), or cine fluoroscopy modes (termed fluorography), in order to acquire and digitally record higher-quality static images. In complex neuroendovascular procedures, the use of fluoroscopy could be as high as 30% and cine fluorography use may range up to 70%. In fluorography, a high radiation dose rate is used to obtain high-resolution images with reduced image noise. The radiation dose per frame is approximately 15 times greater than for fluoroscopy[7].

To help to reduce the dose to the patient, several enhancements are available on modern fluoroscopy units. Automatic brightness control (ABC) features provide consistent image quality during dynamic imaging. When using ABC, the image intensifier output is monitored by the system and then adjusts automatically to maintain constant brightness. The ABC compensates brightness loss caused by the decreased image intensifier X-ray reception by generating more X-rays (increasing mA and/or kVp). If the image is too bright, the ABC adjusts the brightness level by reducing mA and/or kVp. "Last frame hold" is also a useful tool. When the fluoroscopist takes his/her foot off the fluoroscopy pedal, the "last frame hold" feature enables the last "live" image to be shown continuously on the monitor until the fluoroscopy pedal is depressed. This convenient feature holds the frame as long as necessary with no additional radiation to the patient.

Road mapping software is another very useful tool in modern fluoroscopy systems for neuroendovascular procedures. This system employs two side-by-side monitors and allows the operator to capture an image, usually using a catheter. The image will be displayed on one monitor while the "live" fluoroscopy image is shown on the other.

The neuroendovascular surgeon can also utilize image magnification for better viewing purposes. The first method is geometric magnification, which is accomplished by moving the image intensifier farther from the patient, moving the X-ray tube closer to the patient, or both. The second method is electron magnification, in which the size of the beam is restricted to only one portion of the image intensifier. The resulting image will be magnified to fill the entire display area. In both cases, the patient dose will be increased; however, geometric magnification should not be used because this mode increases radiation exposure without sharpening the image. Although the patient dose will be slightly higher with electronic magnification than with the geometric magnification, it is recommended to employ electron magnification during clinical procedures[8].

Radiation dose to operators and patients

Evaluating the severity of deterministic effects such as skin injury requires knowledge of the locally delivered dose (entrance skin exposure, ESE) and fluoroscopy time used in each procedure[7]. The more complex the procedure, the longer the fluoroscopy time. Several studies have examined patient doses in endovascular procedures and found that in cerebral embolization procedures, 4% of the patients received a peak skin dose of greater than 5 Gy; 17% received greater than 3 Gy; and the remaining patients received a peak skin dose from 1 Gy to 3 Gy. It is evident that many interventional fluoroscopy procedures have the potential to produce a high radiation dose and may cause some type of injury to the skin as shown in Table 13.2. Serious injuries are uncommon. Fluoroscopy time in the above procedures ranges up to 275 minutes. Lengthy fluoroscopy time and high entrance X-ray exposure to a patient creates high scatter radiation from the patient and will expose the operator to high doses of radiation[9]. The scatter radiation exposure may cause some stochastic effects, such as cataracts or cancer, in the operator.

Occupational exposure limits: Based on the latest biological and physical information, the ICRP and the US National Council on Radiation Protection and Measurements (NCRP) have recommended radiation exposure limits for both occupational workers and the public. Many of these recommendations have been included as requirements in countries around the world[2,10].

Radiation dose management

The US Food and Drug Administration (FDA) has recommended that physicians performing interventional procedures be aware of the potential for serious, radiation-induced skin injury caused by long periods of fluoroscopy during these procedures.

Prior to performing the procedure, the previous radiation exposure history or the area of the skin that was irradiated prior to the present exposure must be considered. If it is the same area, the risk of the deterministic effect will increase. The pregnancy status of the

Table 13.2 Recommended dose limits for occupational exposure and public exposure

Type of limit	NCRP	ICRP
Occupational exposure: stochastic effects		
Effective dose	50 mSv/yr	20 mSv/yr, averaged over 5 years with no more than 50 mSv in any 1 year
Deterministic effects		
Equivalent dose to lens of the eye	150 mSv/yr	20 mSv/yr
Equivalent dose to skin	500 mSv/yr	500 mSv/yr
Equivalent dose to hands and feet	500 mSv/yr	500 mSv/yr
Embryo or fetus exposure	5.0 mSv/yr for gestation period of 0.5 mSv/month	1 mSv (total)
Public exposure: stochastic effects		
Effective dose	1 mSv/yr	1 mSv/yr
Deteministic effects		
Equivalent dose to lens of the eye	50 mSv/yr	15 mSv/yr
Equivalent dose to skin	50 mSv/yr	50 mSv/yr
Equivalent dose to hands and feet	50 mSv/yr	

proposed patient must be considered, as it requires special considerations owing to the risk of radiation-induced cancer to the unborn child. In this case, the dose to the embryo or fetus can be minimized by using low-dose fluoroscopy, which will reduce any deterministic effects. Physicians performing interventional fluoroscopic procedures should estimate absorbed skin doses for the different procedures in order to avoid skin injuries. Patients should also be advised to report signs and symptoms of radiation-induced injury to their attending physician.

All controls of fluoroscopy have to be optimized to reduce exposure. Fluoroscopy time and peak skin dose have a direct relationship in determining the deterministic effects. **Recording fluoroscopy time for each patient procedure is required for risk estimates.** The use of many features of the fluoroscopy unit, such as proper use of collimation, low dose mode, and limiting the use of magnification modes, optimizes the patient dose[11]. Always use the lowest possible electronic magnification to reduce radiation exposures. Utilizing the last image hold feature and tapping the foot pedal only while viewing the video monitor decreases the patient dose. Employ dose-saving pulsed fluoroscopy, if available. Increasing the source-to-skin distance and minimizing the air-gap between the patient and the image intensifier reduce the dose to the patient and reduce scatter radiation to the operator. Care must be taken to ensure that other unintended body parts of the patient's body, such as arms, are kept outside the radiation field to avoid skin injuries. Spreading the skin dose over a large area reduces the skin injury. Peak skin dose can be reduced by utilizing gantry angulation, couch movement, and collimation. This will help to reduce the maximum dose to any location of the skin. In addition, while performing cerebral embolization procedures, special consideration should be given to the dose to the lens of the eye.

The equipment used for any interventional procedure must be able to estimate and display cumulative dose in mGy and DAP measurements. Monitoring radiation measurements throughout the procedure helps in reducing exposure to the patient. The radiation dose level notification helps the interventionalist by allowing him or her to add the previous radiation dose levels already received by the patient.

If the patient is pregnant, the interventionalist and the medical physicist should evaluate the potential risk to the embryo or fetus prior to the start of the procedure. Limiting the dose to the embryo or fetus to no more than 50 mGy should be considered. Avoiding exposure to the embryo or fetus from the primary beam will greatly reduce exposure. The dose can be minimized by using a low dose mode, employing narrow beam collimation, and reducing the number of fluorography images.

The FDA recommends that the patient dose information be recorded in the patient's record at the conclusion of each procedure, as this permits estimation of the cumulative absorbed dose to the skin from all procedures. All patients with estimated skin doses of 3 Gy should be followed up 10–14 days post exposure. A system to identify repeat procedures should be set up for managing the dose to the patient.

Radiation protection program

All radiation exposures should be kept As Low As Reasonably Achievable (ALARA). At times, the interventionalist's hands are in the primary beam, resulting in high exposure to the hands. In addition, the operator and the staff in the fluoroscopy procedure room are exposed to leakage radiation from the X-ray tube, as well as scatter radiation from the patient. The leakage radiation from the X-ray tube ranges from 0.001 to 0.01 mGy/h at 1 meter. The staff assisting the interventionalist may receive about 0.1% of patient entrance radiation exposure at 1 meter from the patient. While planning an interventional suite, a radiation protection program must be established to shield an existing or new facility to limit the radiation exposure levels to no more than 0.1 mGy/yr, including the control room, to protect the employees and the public. Each individual present in the interventional procedure room should receive annual radiation safety training, including some dry runs of the clinical procedure with appropriate dose reduction techniques.

ICRP and NCRP recommend that the dose to the embryo or fetus of a pregnant radiation worker should be no more than 0.05 mGy per month. It is very difficult to estimate the dose to the embryo or fetus, but the ICRP and NCRP recommend approximating it by taking half of the measured dose on the dosimeter inside the lead apron to the estimate dose to the embryo or fetus.

Based on the recent data, the ICRP[2] recommended limiting the radiation exposure to the occupational radiation worker's lens of the eye to 20 mSv/yr averaged over 5 years and 50 mSv in any single year.

Use of dosimeters and personal protective equipment

For measuring occupational radiation exposure and compliance with regulatory agency requirements, the interventional fluoroscopy operators and staff in the procedure rooms must wear a collar badge and a whole body badge. A collar badge, worn outside the lead apron and at the collar level, is used to measure skin and thyroidal doses, whereas the whole body badge, worn inside the lead apron between the neck and the waist, is used to measure a whole body effective dose. During the procedure, the operator's hands may be exposed to a primary beam. A ring dosimeter may be used by the operator for measuring the dose to the fingers and hands.

Employers are responsible for providing radiation protective equipment, including mobile leaded shields for all employees who have potential to receive radiation exposures during interventional procedures. Evidence demonstrates that staff working within a one (1) meter distance from the X-ray tube or the patient interventional reference point receive higher radiation exposure. All personnel present in the endoscopy procedure room, except the staff behind the mobile leaded shield, must wear a radiation protective garment to shield them from scatter radiation. The thickness of the radiation protective garment (lead apron) should be sufficient to attenuate scatter radiation. The lead apron should be of an acceptable weight; to reduce the weight, a lightweight apron made up of non-lead materials (composite materials) that have the same attenuation or better may be used. A 0.5 mm lead or lead-equivalent material attenuates the incident radiation (scatter X-rays) by approximately 95%.

The thyroid gland is sensitive to radiation, and exposure may lead to radiation-induced cancer. To protect the thyroid from such stochastic effects, a thyroid collar with 0.5 mm lead or lead-equivalent material must be worn at all times during the fluoroscopy procedure.

It is known that high radiation exposure may occur to the eye lens of a physician performing endovascular procedures. To keep the exposures ALARA, leaded eye glasses, corrected to prescription, sized, and fitted to the individual's face, should be worn to protect the lens of the eye. Where practical, it is advisable to use ceiling-mounted, clear leaded glass while performing any fluoroscopy procedures. Ceiling-mounted leaded glass provides protection to the whole head, including the eyes.

Reduction of hand exposure can be achieved using flexible, sterile, radiation-attenuating surgical gloves during the procedure. Transparent mobile leaded shields are beneficial in protecting the required ancillary staff present during fluoroscopy procedures. Leaded flaps, which are mounted at the side of the table, are designed to protect the lower extremities of the operator and should not be removed from the table.

Techniques to minimize radiation exposure to patient and staff

Increasing the distance between the X-ray tube and the patient skin entrance area greatly reduces the exposure to the patient and reduces the potential injury to the skin. In addition, it reduces scatter radiation to the staff. The law that relates to distance is the "inverse square law," which states that the radiation exposure decreases inversely proportional to the square of distance. If the distance is doubled between the operator and the source of radiation, the radiation exposure decreases to a quarter of the original exposure. **Since increasing the distance reduces exposure to staff, the NCRP recommends that personnel stand at least 2 meters away from the X-ray tube, whenever possible.** As per the FDA regulations, most of the fluoroscopy units come with a spacer device which is placed on the X-ray port area to maintain minimum separation from the skin to the X-ray port area. Radiation exposure intensity is decreased with spacer use owing to the increase in distance from the patient's skin, thereby reducing potential injury to the skin.

A typical fluoroscopic system is equipped with an X-ray "beam-on" foot pedal. Most units also have a beam-on button or a switch that the user can operate by hand. This is called a "dead man" switch. When pressure is applied on the "dead man" switch, X-rays are produced. When the operator is not observing the monitor during the procedure, the pressure on the switch should be released to turn off continuous X-ray production. Using short taps of the fluoroscopy beam-on control reduces the exposure to the patient. Keeping the image receptor as close to the patient as possible not only reduces scatter radiation to the operator and the staff, but also minimizes the concentration of X-rays at the patient's skin surface. Also, if the collimator is tightly confined to the area of interest, this reduces the patient's total skin entrance exposure, improves the contrast, and decreases the scatter radiation exposure to the staff. Utilizing the lowest magnification modes consistent with clinical procedure optimizes the radiation exposure to the patient. Scatter radiation distorts the image quality. A flat plate called a grid, which is placed in front of the image intensifier, improves the image contrast by stopping the scatter radiation. Using low dose mode or a lower pulse rate when possible minimizes exposure to the patient. Positioning the X-ray tube underneath the patient table reduces scatter radiation to the operator. For lateral and oblique projections, position the C-arm so that the X-ray tube is on the opposite side of the patient from where you are working. This will reduce the scatter radiation reaching the operator[12].

Sometimes a physician's height complicates the procedure and increases the radiation exposure to the patient. Tall operators can maintain good geometry; however, for the vertically challenged operator, the table height needs to be lowered. This brings the patient nearer to the X-ray source and causes a higher radiation dose to the patient. Using long extension tubing from the manifold to the catheter reduces a physician's hand exposure. Inadvertent use of the biplane system (by activating both lateral and frontal X-ray tubes) with exposure to the same skin area, as shown in Figure 13.5, may cause serious skin injury.

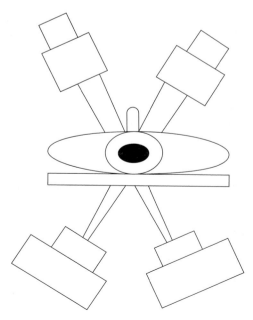

Figure 13.5 Biplane system – cause of injury.

Summary

An operator's body and lens of the eye receive high radiation exposures from scatter radiation. Hands in the primary beam also receive a large radiation dose. In addition, the patient receives higher radiation exposure at the X-ray beam entrance site. These procedures require the operator to wear and use protective devices. Careful manipulation of the equipment is required to reduce exposure to the patient and the staff. At each institution, a committee that includes physicians, technologists, medical physicists, and administrators should be formed to discuss problems that complicate procedures and corrective actions to prevent such complications. Neurointerventionalists should adhere to basic radiation protection ALARA principles to achieve the desired safety parameters.

References

1. Miller DL. Overview of contemporary interventional fluoroscopy procedures. *Health Phys* 2008;95:638–44.

2. The 2007 Recommendations of the International Commission on Radiological Protection. *ICRP publication 103. Ann ICRP* 2007;37:1–332.

3. Walsh SR, Cousins C, Tang TY, Gaunt ME, Boyle JR. Ionizing radiation in endovascular interventions. *J Endovasc Ther* 2008;15:680–7.

4. Mooney RB, McKinstry CS, Kamel HA. Absorbed dose and deterministic effects to patients from interventional neuroradiology. *Br J Radiol* 2000;73:745–51.

5. Miller DL, Balter S, Cole PE, *et al.* Radiation doses in interventional radiology procedures: the RAD-IR study. Part II: skin dose. *J Vasc Interv Radiol* 2003;14:977–90.

6. Miller DL, Balter S, Cole PE, *et al.* Radiation doses in interventional radiology procedures: the RAD-IR study. Part I: overall measures of dose. *J Vasc Interv Radiol* 2003;14:711–27.

7. Panuccio G, Greenberg RK, Wunderle K, *et al.* Comparison of indirect radiation dose estimates with directly measured radiation dose for patients and operators during complex endovascular procedures. *J Vasc Surg* 2011;53:885–94 e1; discussion 94.

8. Stecker MS, Balter S, Towbin RB, *et al.* Guidelines for patient radiation dose management. *J Vasc Interv Radiol* 2009;20: S263–73.

9. McParland BJ. A study of patient radiation doses in interventional radiological procedures. *Br J Radiol* 1998;71:175–85.

10. Linton OW. The National Council on Radiation Protection and Measurements: a growing structure. *Radiology* 2014;271:1–4.

11. Balter S, Schueler BA, Miller DL, *et al.* Radiation doses in interventional radiology procedures: the RAD-IR Study. Part III: Dosimetric performance of the interventional fluoroscopy units. *J Vasc Interv Radiol* 2004;15:919–26.

12. Haqqani OP, Agarwal PK, Halin NM, Iafrati MD. Minimizing radiation exposure to the vascular surgeon. *J Vasc Surg* 2012;55:799–805.

Index